Bill Wells.

Phonological Development
and Disorders in Children

Child Language and Child Development: Multilingual–Multicultural Perspectives
Series Editor: Professor Li Wei, *University of Newcastle-upon-Tyne, UK*
Editorial Advisors:
Professor Gina Conti-Ramsden, *University of Manchester, UK*
Professor Kevin Durkin, *The University of Western Australia*
Professor Susan Ervin-Tripp, *University of California, Berkeley, USA*
Professor Jean Berko Gleason, *Boston University, USA*
Professor Brian MacWhinney, *Carnegie Mellon University, USA*

Children are brought up in diverse yet specific cultural environments; they are engaged from birth in socially meaningful and appropriate activities; their development is affected by an array of social forces. This book series is a response to the need for a comprehensive and interdisciplinary documentation of up-to-date research on child language and child development from a multilingual and multicultural perspective. Publications from the series will cover language development of bilingual and multilingual children, acquisition of languages other than English, cultural variations in child rearing practices, cognitive development of children in multicultural environments, speech and language disorders in bilingual children and children speaking languages other than English, and education and healthcare for children speaking non-standard or non-native varieties of English. The series will be of particular interest to linguists, psychologists, speech and language therapists, and teachers, as well as to other practitioners and professionals working with children of multilingual and multicultural backgrounds.

Recent Books in the Series
Culture-Specific Language Styles: The Development of Oral Narrative and Literacy
    Masahiko Minami
Language and Literacy in Bilingual Children
    D. Kimbrough Oller and Rebecca E. Eilers (eds)
Phonological Development in Specific Contexts: Studies of Chinese-Speaking Children
    Zhu Hua
Bilingual Children's Language and Literacy Development
    Roger Barnard and Ted Glynn (eds)
Developing in Two Languages: Korean Children in America
    Sarah J. Shin
Three is a Crowd? Acquiring Portuguese in a Trilingual Environment
    Madalena Cruz-Ferreira
Childhood Bilingualism: Research on Infancy through School Age
    Peggy McCardle and Erika Hoff (eds)

Other Books of Interest
Foundations of Bilingual Education and Bilingualism
    Colin Baker
Learning to Request in a Second Language: A Study of Child Interlanguage Pragmatics
    Machiko Achiba
Language Acquisition: The Age Factor (2nd edition)
    David Singleton and Lisa Ryan

For more details of these or any other of our publications, please contact:
Multilingual Matters, Frankfurt Lodge, Clevedon Hall,
Victoria Road, Clevedon, BS21 7HH, England
http://www.multilingual-matters.com

CHILD LANGUAGE AND CHILD DEVELOPMENT 8
Series Editor: Li Wei, University of Newcastle

Phonological Development and Disorders in Children
A Multilingual Perspective

Edited by
Zhu Hua and Barbara Dodd

MULTILINGUAL MATTERS LTD
Clevedon • Buffalo • Toronto

Library of Congress Cataloging in Publication Data
Phonological Development and Disorders in Children: A Multilingual
Perspective/Edited by Zhu Hua and Barbara Dodd.
Child Language and Child Development: 8
Includes bibliographical references and index.
1. Language acquisition. 2. Language disorders in children. 3. Grammar, Comparative
and general–Phonology. 4. Bilingualism in children. I. Hua, Zhu. II. Dodd, Barbara.
III. Series.
P118.P475 2006
401'.93–dc22   2006001482

British Library Cataloguing in Publication Data
A catalogue entry for this book is available from the British Library.

ISBN 1-85359-889-5 / EAN 978-1-85359-889-0 (hbk)

Multilingual Matters Ltd
UK: Frankfurt Lodge, Clevedon Hall, Victoria Road, Clevedon BS21 7HH.
USA: UTP, 2250 Military Road, Tonawanda, NY 14150, USA.
Canada: UTP, 5201 Dufferin Street, North York, Ontario M3H 5T8, Canada.

Copyright © 2006 Zhu Hua, Barbara Dodd and the authors of individual chapters.

All rights reserved. No part of this work may be reproduced in any form or by any
means without permission in writing from the publisher.

Typeset by Techset Composition Ltd.
Printed and bound in Great Britain by the Cromwell Press Ltd.

Contents

Acknowledgements vii
Contributors. viii

Part 1: Introduction

1 A Multilingual Perspective on Phonological Development
  and Disorders
  Zhu Hua and B. Dodd 3
2 The Need for Comparable Criteria in Multilingual Studies
  Zhu Hua. 15

Part 2: Monolingual Context

3 English Phonology: Acquisition and Disorder
  B. Dodd, A. Holm, Zhu Hua, S. Crosbie and J. Broomfield 25
4 Evidence from German-Speaking Children
  A.V. Fox 56
5 The Normal and Disordered Phonology of Putonghua
  (Modern Standard Chinese)-Speaking Children
  Zhu Hua. 81
6 Cantonese Phonological Development: Normal
  and Disordered
  L.K.H. So 109
7 Phonological Development of Maltese-Speaking Children
  H. Grech. 135
8 Syllabic Constraints in the Phonological Errors of
  Children with Pre-lingual Hearing Loss: A Perspective
  from Telugu
  D. Vasanta 179
9 Phonological Development and Disorders: Colloquial
  Egyptian Arabic
  Wafaa Ammar and Ranya Morsi 204
10 Phonological Acquisition and Disorders in Turkish
   S. Topbaş and M. Yavaş 233

Part 3: Bilingual Context

11 Aspects of Bilingual Phonology: The Case of Spanish–English Bilingual Children
    M. Yavaş and B. Goldstein 265
12 Phonological Development and Disorder of Bilingual Children Acquiring Cantonese and English
    A. Holm and B. Dodd..................................... 286
13 Phonological Acquisition in Bilingual Pakistani Heritage Children in England
    C. Stow and S. Pert 326
14 Phonological Development and Disorder of Bilingual Children Acquiring Welsh and English
    M.J. Ball, N. Müller and S. Munro 346
15 Phonological Acquisition by Arabic–English Bilingual Children
    G. Khattab.. 383
16 Phonological Development of Cantonese–Putonghua Bilingual Children
    L.K.H. So and C.S.S. Leung.............................. 413

Part 4: Coda

17 Towards Developmental Universals
    Zhu Hua and B. Dodd 431

References 450
Appendix.. 474
Index 477

Acknowledgements

We are most grateful for the inspiring work of all the contributors whose dedication to and enthusiasm for the field make our editing effort worthwhile. We would like to acknowledge the support provided by our publishers, Multilingual Matters, who enabled the contributors to meet and discuss the project at a special workshop held in Newcastle-upon-Tyne in 2003. The editing process also benefited from an international research fellowship awarded to Zhu Hua by MARCS laboratory, University of West Sydney, Australia. We owe an immense debt to the series editor, Li Wei, who has given us support in various ways right through the project. A special thank you is due to Brigid O'Connor who proofread several of the chapters.

Contributors

Wafaa Ammar
Department of Phonetics, Faculty of Arts, University of Alexandria, Egypt

Martin Ball
Department of Communication Disorders, University of Louisiana at Lafayette, USA

Jan Broomfield
Middlesbrough Primary Care Trust, UK

Sharon Crosbie
Perinatal Research Centre, Royal Brisbane and Women's Hospital, University of Queensland, Australia

Barbara Dodd
Perinatal Research Centre, Royal Brisbane and Women's Hospital, University of Queensland, Australia

Annette Fox
Department of Health, Section Speech Therapy, University of Applied Sciences Europa Fachhochschule, Fresenius, Idstein, Germany

Brian Goldstein
Department of Communication Sciences, Temple University, USA

Helen Grech
Communication Therapy Division, Institute of Health Care, University of Malta, Malta

Alison Holm
Perinatal Research Centre, Royal Brisbane and Women's Hospital, University of Queensland, Australia

Ghada Khattab
School of Education, Communication and Language Sciences, University of Newcastle upon Tyne, UK

Cheung Shing Samuel Leung
Division of Speech & Hearing Sciences, Faculty of Education, University of Hong Kong, Hong Kong

Contributors

Ranya Morsi
School of Psychology and Clinical Language Studies, University of Reading, UK

Nicole Müller
Department of Communication Disorders, University of Louisiana at Lafayette, USA

Siân Munro
Speech Therapy Section, University of Wales Institute, Cardiff

Sean Pert
Rochdale Primary Care Trust, UK

Lydia K. H. So
Division of Speech & Hearing Sciences, Faculty of Education, University of Hong Kong, Hong Kong

Carol Stow
Rochdale Primary Care Trust, UK

Seyhun Topbaş
Centre for Speech and Language Disorders, Department of Speech and Language Pathology, Anadolu University, Eskişehir, Turkey

Duggirala Vasanta
Department of Linguistics, Osmania University, Hyderabad, India

Mehmet Yavaş
Linguistics Program, Florida International University, USA

Zhu Hua
School of Education, Communication and Language Sciences, University of Newcastle upon Tyne, UK

Part 1
Introduction

Chapter 1
A Multilingual Perspective on Phonological Development and Disorders

ZHU HUA and B. DODD

Why are Multilingual Studies Important?

Multilingual studies contribute to our understanding of language acquisition by evaluating and challenging theoretical claims about development. Their value lies not only in their capacity to appraise claims about universal patterns of language acquisition, but also in their potential to examine whether and how differences in specific target languages result in differences in acquisition patterns. Differences between monolingual children learning different languages and the characteristics of the language acquisition of bilingual and multilingual children, in comparison to monolingual peers, provide evidence about the role of specific linguistic exposure on patterns of language acquisition. Another crucial source of evidence examines the ways in which the acquisition process can go awry in different languages and in bilingual children. Multilingual studies can evaluate the boundaries of theories of typical and atypical language acquisition. The purpose of this volume is to integrate research on a range of languages to examine phonological acquisition and disorder.

While English remains the best researched language in the field of child language acquisition and disorder, multilingual studies have been expanding rapidly since the 1980s. Here, we use the term 'multilingual' to refer to studies of monolingual acquisition in different language contexts (usually referred to as cross-linguistic studies) as well as dual language and multilingual language acquisition. The languages examined in this book include: English, German, Putonghua, Cantonese, Maltese, Telugu, Colloquial Egyptian Arabic, Turkish, Spanish, Mirpuri/Punjabi/Urdu, Arabic, and Welsh. Both monolingual and bilingual contexts are studied, in both typical and atypical development.

The data are presented so that they can be used by speech and language pathologists in their professional work. In the following sections of this introduction, we emphasise four important issues in multilingual research: developmental universals, theoretical accounts of phonological acquisition, bilingualism, and clinical populations.

Developmental Universals

By definition, 'universals' should be features or tendencies shared by all. The first general claim of developmental universals was proposed by Jakobson in 1941 (Jakobson, 1941/1968). Appealing to typological universals, he suggested that whether a sound would be acquired early could be explained in terms of the distribution of speech sounds among the world's languages. Therefore, nasals, front consonants, and stops, which are found in virtually all languages, would be acquired early. His claim was subsequently challenged by counter-examples on two fronts: individual variations within one language and language variation in the acquisition of the same sounds. Similarly, the predominance of monosyllables among early word productions of English-speaking monolingual children, that has been assumed as typical for the early stages of phonological development irrespective of language, does not apply to the production of children acquiring French, Japanese, or Swedish (Vihman, 1996). These examples illustrate how developmental universals are proposed in the context of currently available information. Multilingual research provides evidence for or against specific developmental phonological universals.

Data from the studies reported in this book reveal similarities and differences in developmental patterns across languages. The rate of acquisition of a particular phoneme or syllable component can be different across languages, and the same phoneme may be associated with different error patterns[1] across languages. The coda provides a summary of the similarities and differences described, that bears on the notion of phonological universals.

Theoretical Accounts of Phonological Acquisition

Theoretical accounts of phonological acquisition, apart from Jakobson's (1941/1968) 'law of irreversible solidarity', include markedness (Edwards, 1974; Dinnsen, 1992), biological and articulation constraints (Locke, 1980, 1983b; Kent, 1992), and functional load (Pye *et al.*, 1987).

Markedness

The concept of markedness, which originated in the context of typological universals, has often been resorted to in the studies of language acquisition as an explanatory theory for the ease or difficulty associated with the learning of some features. (For its role in phonological acquisition, see Anderson, 1983; Eckman, 1977; Jakobson, 1941/1968; for syntax, see Rutherford, 1983.) It was hypothesised that those sounds or features that appear early in a child's inventory were maximally unmarked, while those occurring late were marked. Therefore, children would use unmarked sounds as substitutions for marked sounds. Edwards' (1974) study of English-speaking children aged 1;8–3;11 found that children usually substituted the unmarked member for those marked contrasts (e.g. [s] for /ʃ/), but details varied from one child to another and from one developmental stage to another. While the notion of markedness appeals to intuition, the way the markedness is decided has been criticised for being circular in that the cause-and-effect relationship seems to be used arbitrarily – a feature is acquired early because it is unmarked and a feature is considered as unmarked because it is acquired early (Lindblom, 1998).

As an alternative concept to markedness, Dinnsen (1992) proposed a feature hierarchy stating that there might be a universal hierarchical structure with a highly limited set of ordered features applicable to the phonetic inventories of all languages. Each feature in the hierarchy has a number of default specifications (i.e. unmarked values). Children's acquisition would therefore be a process of replacing a default value with a language-specific value. The order of phoneme acquisition of a particular language would correspond with the hierarchical relationships and default values: features ranked high in the hierarchy would be acquired early; default features would be acquired before non-default features. Dinnsen's model offers an alternative account for cross-linguistic similarities and differences in the order of phoneme acquisition. However, the explanatory power of his model has so far rarely been tested with the phonological acquisition of languages other than English (cf. Wong & Stokes, 2001).

Similar to the feature hierarchy, Clements (1990) proposed a sonority hierarchy that states that the more sonorous a sound, the easier its acquisition. The sonority index of a sound is affected by two factors: the degree of opening of the oral cavity in producing the sound and the sound's propensity for voicing. The more open the articulation of a sound, the greater its sonority level. If two sounds have the same degree of opening, the voiced one will have greater sonority than its voiceless counterpart. Following this definition, vowels, glides, and nasals are more sonorous and are therefore acquired earlier than stops, fricatives, and affricates which are at the bottom end of the hierarchy. In terms of cluster acquisition, the greater the sonority distance is between the first and the second member in the coda cluster, the more natural (easier to acquire) it would be. Evaluation of the application of sonority hierarchy can be found in Chapters 8 and 9 of this volume.

Biological model and articulatory complexity

Locke (1980, 1983b) proposed a biological model to emphasise the role of articulatory and perceptual constraints on children's acquisition of phonology. It was stated that children's phonetic repertoires are essentially the same and hence universal, subject to 'the size and shape of infant vocal tract and the relative complexity of neuromotor control required for various articulations' (Vihman, 1996: 68). The acquisition of sounds takes the form of maintenance, learning and loss: once children have passed the babbling stage and started to acquire a target phonological system, certain sounds are maintained from their babbling repertoire; sounds not present in the babbling repertoire are then learned through interactions in the linguistic environment; extra-systemic sounds (sounds existing in the babbling repertoire but not in the target phonological system) will be removed from the system. Further to Locke's biological model, Kent (1992) proposed an articulatory complexity model to link the degree of motor control required and that of ease or difficulty in articulation.

While the role of articulation and perceptual constraints on phonological acquisition in the babbling stage and early words (Vihman, 1996) is well demonstrated, these biological factors seem to play a lesser role in phonological development after speech onset. This is supported not only by the reported individual differences in acquiring a particular sound in one language but also by differences in the age and order of acquisition of sounds by children learning different target phonologies.

Functional load

Functional load, first proposed by the Prague School, refers to the relative importance of each phoneme within a specific phonological system. Pye *et al.* (1987) proposed that discrepancies between the age of acquisition of the same sounds in different languages are the result of different functional loads of the same sounds in the different languages. However, functional load is difficult to measure across languages (Catford, 1988). Pye *et al.* measured the functional load of syllable-initial consonants in Quiche by counting the frequency of syllable-initial consonants occurring in the 500 most commonly used words of five- and six-year-old children. This method of determining functional load is problematic (Zhu & Dodd, 2000a; So & Dodd, 1995). Firstly, there is no guarantee that sounds frequently used by children are significant for a phonological system. Secondly, the rank-order of frequencies for syllable-initial consonants common to Quiche and English does not support the similarities and differences found in the children's order of acquisition. For example, the sound /w/ was ranked as the second most frequently used in Quiche and seventh in English, indicating that /w/ should be acquired earlier in Quiche than in English. In fact, it was acquired at the same age in both languages. Thirdly, other aspects of phonology that may contribute to the functional load, such as vowels, syllable structure, and tones in tonal languages have not been considered.

None of these theories account for language variation or individual variation in the order and age of phoneme acquisition, suggesting a need for a model that is both universally applicable and sensitive to language-specific parameters, as well as taking into consideration phonological acquisition at various levels. Against this background, the concept of phonological saliency is proposed in Zhu and Dodd (2000a) and Zhu (2002) based on Putonghua data.

The concept of 'saliency' is well-defined in speech perception. It refers to the relative control a particular acoustic parameter (duration, intensity, formant frequency, pitch, etc.) has in discriminating phonemes, syllables, words, and phrases (Weitzman, 2004). The role of phonological saliency in acquisition has been alluded to by others (Peters, 1983; Vihman, 1996), but there is no agreement on its definition. Here, phonological saliency is defined as a language-specific and syllable-based concept. Given that children's speech and language acquisition is primarily driven by the need to communicate (Pinker & Jackendoff, 2005), phonological saliency takes into account the role of each syllable component in carrying and differentiating lexical information. Components with higher phonological saliency would be acquired earlier than components with lower saliency.

Phonological saliency is determined and affected by:

- The capacity of a component to differentiate lexical meaning of syllables; a component that is more capable of distinguishing lexical information is more salient than one which carries less lexical information.
- The status of a component in the syllable structure, especially whether it is compulsory or optional; a compulsory component is more salient than an optional one.
- The number of permissible choices within a component in the syllable structure. A component with more choices would be considered *less* salient compared to one with fewer choices.

For example, tones in Putonghua have the highest saliency because they are compulsory for every syllable. Change of tones varies lexical meaning, and there are only four alternative choices. The effect of the high saliency value of tones on the process of phonological acquisition of Putonghua-speaking children was evident in that tonal acquisition is complete before syllable-initial and -final phonemes and vowels. Tones are also resistant to phonological impairment and hearing impairment, as reported in Zhu (this volume). In contrast, syllable-initial consonants in

Putonghua have the lowest saliency since their presence in a syllable is optional and there is a range of 21 syllable-initial phonemes that can be used. Putonghua-speaking children aged above 4;6 still made errors on syllable-initial consonants. In addition, children with phonological impairment and hearing impairment are most likely to experience difficulties with syllable-initial consonants compared with tones, vowels and syllable-final consonants.

Since the concept is defined at the syllable level, it is not applicable to the acquisition of phonemes. We cannot say that one phoneme is acquired earlier than the other because it is more salient – at least not in the current definition. Although growing empirical evidence supports the concept of phonological saliency (see this volume), the concept needs to be refined so that it is more capable of capturing cross-linguistic differences in phonological acquisition and development. Two important questions need to be addressed. Do other factors need to be considered apart from the lexical information carried by the components currently considered? Is there a ranking order among the constraining factors? Data described in this volume bear on these issues.

Bilingualism

Theories of phonological acquisition need to be validated with evidence from the language acquisition of bilingual and multilingual children. More than half of the world's population is bi- or multilingual (Crystal, 1995). In fact, many researchers argue that bilingualism and multilingualism, not monolingualism, are typical of society today (Cook, 2003). Yet most of the current theories and models of speech and language acquisition are based on monolingual populations. The study of bilingual and multilingual children's acquisition of phonology is challenging, however, because their linguistic systems may not develop in the same way as those of their monolingual peers due to the interaction and/or interference between the phonological systems of the languages learned.

Children confronted with the challenge of learning two or more phonological systems are not a homogeneous group in terms of their language learning situation or the degree of similarity between the phonological systems they must acquire. While some researchers claim that no child can be considered bilingual unless they are exposed to two languages within hours of birth, others define bilingualism as some functional use of more than one language. While facility in each language used by an individual might affect the results of any research study, disallowing research on people who might have better language skills in one language than the other would result in only partial knowledge of the effects of exposure to, and use of, more than one language. What is important, then, is for researchers to provide precise information about their population's language skills, and to use that information to interpret their findings.

Research in bilingualism has rarely investigated its recurring questions with reference to phonological data. The studies in this book provide novel data on the following issues: successive versus simultaneous acquisition, unitary or differentiated systems, bilingual versus monolingual acquisition, interactions between languages, and effect of specific language combinations.

Simultaneous versus successive acquisition

A confounding issue in bilingual acquisition research is the age of first exposure to the two languages. For example, a normally developing child's phonological system is definitely well established by 30 months of age, therefore exposure to another language at 30 months will presumably yield quite different results than that of a child exposed to two languages from birth: they will have a phonological system already in place as opposed to developing one or two systems simultaneously. The resultant differences between simultaneous and successive acquisition on bilingual children's language have not been identified (De Houwer, 1995) despite many children acquiring at least minimal competence in one language (their mother tongue) before exposure to the second language (Karniol, 1990). Researchers have often ignored this demographically significant group of children, particularly in countries with large immigrant populations such as Australia and Britain (Karniol, 1990; Genesee, 1993). Yavaş (1998: 217) suggests that these children, who 'grow up in the home environment with their first dominant language and start acquiring the target community language when they begin (pre) schooling', are representative of many situations around the world. Chapters in this book specifically investigate children who are *successive bilinguals*.

One or two systems?

Phonological evidence regarding the use of single or separate systems is minimal, but may be affected by simultaneous or successive language learning. Some studies reported initial periods of a single phonological system for simultaneous learners (Burling, 1959/1978; Leopold, 1939–1949; Schnitzer & Krasinski 1994, 1996; but also see Johnson & Lancaster, 1998). In contrast, both Wode (1980) and Watson (1991) suggested that successive bilinguals are more likely to superimpose an unknown system on the known: using one system as a base, and differentiating the second system by altering or adding to the first system. Fantini (1985) described some aspects of the phonological development of his son Mario, a successive bilingual in Spanish, then English. The evidence presented supports Watson's hypothesis: Mario appeared to initially use a phonological system based on Spanish when he began to speak in English.

Another study reported the longitudinal development of two Cantonese–English successive bilingual two-year-old children who were assessed on a monthly basis from shortly before the introduction of their second language (Holm & Dodd, 1999a). The data presented provides evidence that the children had separate phonological systems for each language. Their speech development indicated that:

- shared phonemes were often used in one language before the other;
- different phonological error patterns were used for each language;
- language-specific phonemes were not used in the *wrong* language;
- the same phonemes were simplified differently in each language; and
- errors always obeyed the phonotactic constraints of the appropriate language.

Both of the children in the longitudinal study also used some phonological error patterns that are atypical of monolingual developmental patterns in each language, after exposure to English, though not before that exposure. Some preliminary group data on the phonological skills of bilingual Cantonese–English speaking children, compared to monolingual children, has also suggested that there may be some differences, in the phonological error patterns used by normally developing bilingual children (Dodd *et al.*, 1996).

Bilingual versus monolingual phonological development

The effects of simultaneous and successive language learning environments have also given rise to different research findings when it comes to different types of developmental error patterns. For example, De Houwer (1995) claims that her subject made errors that were typical and age-appropriate for monolingual peers in both English and Dutch. The evidence from successive language learners differs. The longitudinal (Holm & Dodd, 1999a) and group studies of Cantonese–English bilingual children (Dodd *et al.*, 1996) indicate that the phonological development of bilingual children may be qualitatively different to that of monolingual children. In Dodd *et al.*'s study, the pre-school children had been exposed to English following an initial period of exposure only to Cantonese. The children's error patterns were different for their two languages – supporting Watson's claim that bilingual children use two separate phonological systems. However, there were also differences in the *types* of error patterns that were common across the group. The bilingual children were using a number of phonological error patterns that are associated with phonological disorder in monolingual children (e.g. initial consonant deletion, backing, aspiration). The data suggest that exposure to a bilingual Cantonese–English environment may result in the development of speech error patterns that would be considered unusual for a monolingual child.

Another group study of bilingual phonological acquisition has been conducted by Navarro *et al.* (1995). They analysed the phonology of 11 successive bilingual Spanish–English pre-school children. They also concluded that bilingual and monolingual children 'might be following different paths to reach the same goal' (Navarro *et al.*, 1995: 4). However, in contrast to the Cantonese–English studies, they did not find the bilingual children were using unusual error processes. In fact, they concluded that the bilingual children in their study were *less* likely to use uncommon error processes.

Although the findings on the use of unusual error patterns among bilingual children seem to be contradictory between these studies, the concept of phonological interference, phonological mixing, or what is sometimes referred to as a form of accent, is reported consistently in the bilingual literature. That is, the pair of languages being learned may affect the type of phonological errors made. These differences suggest that exposure to two specific phonological systems leads to specific developmental error patterns.

Interaction and interference

There has been little systematic research on the presence of transfer or interference effects in bilingual children's phonology. Watson (1991) reported a relative developmental delay in the perception and production of voice-onset time in French–English bilingual children, attributing these differences to specific voicing contrasts within the two phonological systems. There is also considerable evidence of interference from case studies (Burling, 1959/1978; Fantini, 1985; Itoh & Hatch, 1978; Leopold, 1939–1949; Schnitzer & Krasinski, 1994; Vogel, 1975) that include use of language-specific elements in the wrong language, shared phonemes being used in the wrong phonotactic position, simplification of clusters in English by inserting an epenthetic vowel when such clusters were not shared by both languages.

The literature indicates that although bilingual children usually appear to develop two phonological systems that are separate and differentiated, each phonological system may not develop in the same way as in monolingual children. Watson (1991: 37) concluded that 'one system, or at least aspects of it, will dominate the other, so that the child fails to make some oppositions in one language, or at least produces some sounds in a *foreign* way, due to interference'. Genesee (1993: 63) highlighted the possibility of 'specific interaction effects between particular language combinations'. Ingram (1981: 105) also suggests (in relation to the question of identification of separate systems within the bilingual child) that it is important to investigate children 'who are learning highly different languages'. However, there are very few specific references to these cross-linguistic effects in the bilingual literature. Most research on bilingual children's acquisition of language has focused on children acquiring two languages from the same language family. While these languages may have different sets of phonemes and different predominant syllable structures, they are often similar. For example, Germanic languages do not possess lexical tone contrasts as do Chinese languages. As yet, little is understood about how the degree of relatedness of the two phonological systems being learned affects their acquisition by a bilingual child, irrespective of whether they are learned simultaneously or successively.

Differences in development stem from the characteristics of the ambient phonology of the language as well as from interactions between the two systems. This fact indicates that different language combinations need investigation. The research studies presented here investigate the specific interaction effects between the two languages, the within-language processes common to all bilingual children, and identify the characteristics that reflect the nature of the specific phonological system.

Clinical Populations

Over 6% of otherwise normal children are referred to speech and language therapy clinics for investigation of spoken phonological difficulties (Broomfield & Dodd, 2001). Bilingual children, however, are conspicuously under-referred (Broomfield & Dodd, 2001; Winter, 2001). Explanations for this shortfall include lack of parental understanding of available speech and language therapy services, referrers attributing children's limited language, including phonological errors, to bilingualism and lack of normative data for bilingual children on which clinicians can base diagnosis.

Apart from the obvious problem of children in need of intervention for phonological disability not benefiting from available services, bilingual children's phonological difficulties provide an opportunity to address significant issues into the nature of phonological acquisition and disorder. For example, one way of validating any classification system for speech disorders is to examine its usefulness cross-linguistically. A classification system should be able to account for all children with speech disorders in any language. The proportion of children belonging to particular subgroups of speech disorder should be approximately the same (given reasonable subject numbers and random sampling). Other important questions are whether phonological disability is always present in both languages, and if so, whether the two phonological systems are similarly affected. Answers to these questions would provide insight into the nature of the deficits underlying phonological disability and evidence concerning the classification of subgroups of phonological disability. Holm and Dodd's (Chapter 12) data suggest that children always have difficulties in both their languages and that while errors are not identical in both, they share the same diagnostic subgroup classification. Another significant issue concerns cross-language generalisation of intervention. Treatment studies (Holm & Dodd, this volume: chap. 12) indicate that subgroup diagnostic classification predicts cross language generalisation.

The answers to the questions posed above are important theoretically. They would bear on the issue of the separateness of the mental representation of children's phonological systems, and on the effect of the nature of a phonological system on the types of developmental errors made. Clinically, data on a range of different language learning situations and languages would provide normative information with which bilingual children suspected of being at risk of experiencing difficulties in phonological acquisition could be compared. Data from children with speech difficulties would help illustrate on the nature of phonological disorder and provide treatment indicators.

About This Book

This edited volume brings together a collection of cross-linguistic studies on the phonological acquisition of monolingual children speaking different languages (English, German, Putonghua, Cantonese, Maltese, Telugu, Colloquial Egyptian Arabic, and Turkish) and bilingual children speaking different language pairs (Spanish/English, Cantonese/English, Mirpuri/Punjabi/Urdu–English, Welsh/English, Arabic/English and Putonghua/Cantonese), in both typically and atypically developing children. This book seeks to define similarities and differences between different groups of children: those speaking English or another language, monolingual or bilingual, and those who are developing phonology typically or atypically. Differences between these groups will contribute to teasing out feasible developmental universals and the effect of specific languages' phonology on acquisition. This book also aims to inform clinical decision-making by providing baseline information. It is also hoped that the methodological and theoretical issues explored in the book will inspire more researchers to carry out multilingual studies on phonological acquisition.

Note

1. Error patterns and phonological processes are used interchangeably in different chapters in this volume to refer to the consistent differences between adult targets and children's erroneous realisations. Phonological processes, originated in natural phonology (Stampe, 1969), have been criticised as lacking in psychological reality since the concept assumes errors as the result of a set of mental processes by which the child consciously changes or deletes phonological units. Despite this criticism, the general consensus is that the phonological process does provide the most economical way of describing the relationship between adult targets and children's erroneous realisation of them.

Chapter 2

The Need for Comparable Criteria in Multilingual Studies

ZHU HUA

Given that one of the aims of multilingual studies is to contribute to our understanding of language universals by comparing developmental patterns across different languages, the research cycle for multilingual studies usually consists of the following stages:

Stage 1: Identification of typical developmental patterns of children speaking a particular language or language pair.

Stage 2: These developmental patterns are compared with atypically developing groups of children acquiring the same language or language pairs: speech disorder, hearing impairment, etc., to derive common developmental patterns shared by various groups of children.

Stage 3: The developmental patterns identified in Stages 1 and 2 are compared with those of other languages or language pairs to test existing hypotheses on developmental universals and put forward new hypotheses.

Stage 4: Hypotheses are confirmed or revised, or new hypotheses are devised to generate the next cycle of research with the same or different languages, language pairs or groups of children. Alternatively, experimental studies are set up to test hypotheses and explore the underlying mechanisms in language acquisition which, in turn, motivate new multilingual studies.

As indicated in the four stages outlined above, data from multilingual studies are often compared. The essential prerequisite for these studies is that the criteria used in data collection and analyses are clearly defined. If possible the methodology used should be comparable, if not identical, to that of other multilingual studies so that comparison can be made on a 'like-for-like' basis. Unfortunately, this need is not always recognised, resulting in difficulties in making comparisons and, in some cases, resulting in misleading generalisations and time-wasting arguments.

The purpose of this chapter is to establish clear criteria for comparative analysis in multilingual research with specific reference to phonological acquisition and disorders.

Criteria in Acquisition of Sounds

Since the acquisition of sounds occurs gradually and evolves over time, studies need to clarify the age of acquisition and the criterion for the degree of mastery. Several paradigms have been used in the past.

- Phonetic versus phonemic acquisition. This set broadly differentiates the ability to articulate a sound and to use a sound in a word context with a certain degree of production accuracy. Therefore, following this distinction, a phonetic inventory consists of all the sounds that the child can use either in a word, irrespective of whether it occurs at the correct place, or in isolation through elicitation. A phonemic inventory should include all the sounds that a child can use correctly in most production opportunities. An example is the English data reported in this volume.
- 'Phoneme emergence' versus 'phoneme stabilisation'. This distinction emphasises the phonemic nature of acquisition. 'Phoneme emergence' refers to the ability to produce a sound in a word context irrespective of whether it is used correctly. 'Phoneme emergence' does not include speech sounds produced in isolation. 'Phoneme stabilisation' refers to all the sounds that a child can produce correctly on at least two out of three opportunities. An example is the Putonghua data reported in this volume.

There are differences, then, in the criteria used in the construction of speech sound inventories, and in determining whether or not a speech sound has been acquired. Given that acquisition takes place gradually rather than across-the-board, and the limitations of picture-naming tasks (described later), clearly stated criteria need to be agreed by researchers.

Criteria for Defining Sound Acquisition in Relation to Word and Syllable Position

Different ages of acquisition have been reported for some phonemes in different word positions. For example, Olmsted (1971) found that /ɪ/ was acquired in syllable-initial position earlier than in syllable-final position. In contrast, /θ, z, dʒ/ were acquired earlier word-medially than word-initially and word-finally and /l, tʃ/ were acquired at a later stage word-medially than in the other two word positions. Consequently, Sander (1972) generated the term 'customary' production to refer to those sounds produced correctly in at least two of three word positions, while 'mastery' indicates that a sound is produced correctly in all word positions.

Criteria for Group Acquisition

For deriving age of acquisition at a group level, there is a need for an 'arbitrary' minimum percentage for the number of children of a particular age who can produce a sound correctly. In the past, various criteria have been used for English-speaking children: 75% in Wellman *et al.* (1931), Templin (1957), Prather *et al.* (1975); 100% in Poole (1934); 90% in Dodd *et al.* (2002).

Amayreh and Dyson (1998) defined three types of age of acquisition combining the criteria for minimum percentage of group acquisition and that for word position. The three types are:

- *age of customary production*: at least 50% of children in an age group produce the sound correctly in at least *two* positions;
- *age of acquisition*: at least 75% of children in an age group produce the sound correctly in *all* positions;
- *age of mastery*: at least 90% of children in an age group produce the sound correctly in *all* positions.

While the minimum percentage criterion for a group of children varies from study to study, the choice of 90% has a clinical basis in the sense that it takes account of the upper range of children who may have speech difficulties. Prevalence figures for developmental speech disorders are reported to range from 3% to 10% of the pre-school population in English-speaking children (Kirkpatrick & Ward, 1984; Enderby & Philipp, 1986; Broomfield & Dodd, 2004).

Some chapters in this book report the age of acquisition derived using both 90% and 75% criteria for the purpose of cross-linguistic comparison. Alternatively, Sander (1972) suggested that instead of one single age, age ranges of phoneme acquisition for each phoneme (i.e. upper and lower percentage) should be reported. For example, the age range for acquisition of the sound /l/ is {3;0, 5} using 50% and 90% as group criteria. This means that while 50% or more of three-year-olds are able to produce /l/, it is not until children are five years old that 90% or more of that group can produce /l/.

Criteria for Sustainability Across Age Groups

The process of phonological acquisition is not linear, but involves regression. Smith (1973) documented incidence of loss of phonetic and phonemic contrasts (i.e. the child fails to produce sounds which s/he has been able to use correctly on previous occasions) during the course of his subject's development. This phenomenon occurs not only at an individual level, but also at a group level, though other factors (such as statistical probability and representativeness) may complicate the situation more when it comes to a group trend. Sometimes, more than 90% of one age group are found to be able to produce a sound, while only 80% of an older age group can produce the sound correctly. Figure 13.3 in Chapter 13 is a good example of this type of 'regression'. When this happens, a minimal number of consecutive age groups which have satisfied the acquisition criteria needs to be set up to maintain consistency across different sounds. Dodd et al. (2003) followed this practice.

Criteria for Inclusion of Children with Atypically Developing Conditions in a Cross-Sectional Normative Study

To ensure representativeness of the sample, there are a number of variables that need to be considered in sampling children for a normative study. These are age, socio-economic variables (including family background), gender, language background, sibling order, etc. One decision the researchers on normative studies have to make is whether children with atypical developing conditions such as phonological disorders, hearing impairment, dyspraxia, etc. will be included in the sample. This population is often excluded because these children do not represent normally developing children. However, Law et al. (2000) argued that by excluding these children, who fall at one end of bell-shaped normal distribution, the 'normal' average derived is inflated, i.e. higher than the real value and thus reflect a misleading picture. However, a fine balance needs to be struck between the number of children included in a sample (hence the scale of a study) and the representativeness of the children. The more children a study examines, the less the effect of inclusion of children with difficulties and the more representative the description of phonological acquisition.

Criteria for Selecting Words for Picture-Naming and Description Tasks

Many of the early data on phonological acquisition relied on observational diary studies of speech samples collected in unstructured sessions in a naturalistic setting, usually in mother–child interaction (for a summary, see Ingram, 1989a). Current studies usually use picture-naming and picture-description tasks to elicit data. The tasks are designed to assess all possible speech sounds and sound combinations. Firstly, children's productions are recorded. By providing opportunities for the production of all sounds, the tasks reduce the effect of phonological selectivity inherent in naturalistic observation (i.e. the absence of a particular sound in data collected in an unstructured approach can be either due to the child's inability to produce the sound in question or due to the lack of opportunity). Secondly, picture naming and description used in a cross-sectional design can increase consistency across the data and thus make it feasible for comparison and generalisation.

However, the tasks need to be carefully designed and administered. The following criteria need to be met while designing the tasks:

(a) opportunities for all the phonemes or phonological features (such as clusters, mutation, tones, if applicable or relevant to research questions);
(b) opportunities for all the phonemes in each 'legal' word or syllable position;
(c) a balanced but not equal frequency of occurrence of phonemes;
(d) words likely to be known by young children and able to be presented as a picture;
(e) the length of the task needs to be short due to the child's short attention span.

The frequency of occurrence of phonemes may affect the size of inventories and needs to be controlled to some extent. For example, frequent occurrence of a particular phoneme in a task may give a child more opportunities to produce it and as a result, the sound is more likely to be included in the phonetic inventory. However, equal distribution of all the phonemes in a task is neither feasible, due to the constraints listed above, nor theoretically justified. As studies on functional load show, phonemes in a phonological system carry different loads in terms of contrastiveness, and therefore some occur more frequently than others in a lexicon (Catford, 1988). Consequently there is no need to pursue equal distribution of the phonemes in the sampling of speech data.

Criteria for Inclusion of Imitation or Spontaneous Speech

This is an issue that all the studies on child phonology have to address. When a child fails to produce the target word spontaneously, there are three scenarios apart from the test factor:

(a) the child may not know the word;
(b) the child has a temporary lexical retrieval problem and thus is unable to fulfil the phonological task. In this case, giving the child a semantic cue may overcome the lexical retrieval difficulty. Presenting the child with a forced choice (e.g. *Is it a glass or an elephant?*) will help the child to provide a speech sample;
(c) the child knows the word but is using an avoidance strategy to evade the phonological task (Macken & Ferguson, 1983).

The question of whether to include imitated productions in a normative study has generated considerable debate. Common practice is that although imitation will be used to elicit a speech sample, imitated responses are only taken into account when the age of phonetic acquisition is considered, since in phonetic studies the focus is on the child's ability to articulate the sound. When age of phonemic acquisition is concerned, imitated data are often excluded. In some studies (e.g. Dodd *et al.*, 2003), imitated data were included in the analysis of age of acquisition for the youngest age group of 2;0 due to scarcity of spontaneous data collected through the picture-naming task from this group of children.

Criteria in Defining an Age-Appropriate Error Pattern/Phonological Processes

Error patterns are defined as consistent differences between child and adult realisations. Similar to the calculation for age of phoneme acquisition, group criteria and the minimal frequency of occurrence at an individual level need to be considered in defining an age-appropriate error pattern. Preisser *et al.* (1988), Hodson and Paden (1981) and Roberts *et al.* (1990) judge only one occurrence of an error pattern as evidence that the pattern is used consistently. In contrast, Dodd *et al.* (2003) used the minimal occurrence of five observations of use of an error pattern for each child in their normative studies on English-speaking children. For the group criterion, for an error pattern to be categorised as age appropriate, more than 10% of children in an age group had to exhibit the error pattern at least five times (twice in the case of weak syllable deletion due to the low frequency of occurrence of weak stress in target words).

Criteria in Defining Consistency of Errors

Children's speech is often characterised by multiple mismatches between the realisation and the target. These mismatches are of two types: intra- and inter-word inconsistency or variability (Ingram, 1979). Inter-word variability refers to the situation when a child produces a target segment in different ways across words and contexts, while intra-word variability takes place when a child produces a given word in different ways in the same context. While variability between correct and error forms may indicate the developmental nature of the child's phonology in some cases, a high percentage of intra-word variability (a variability score of 40% or above) may indicate that the child has difficulties in assembling plans for word production (Dodd, 1995).

Procedures to calculate variability rating and to identify those with inconsistent phonological disorders using Dodd's 25 word consistency test are as follows (Dodd, 1995):

(1) Children are asked to name pictures of 25 words three times, each trial being separated by another activity.
(2) Variability rating = the number of words which have variable productions (either consonants or vowels)/the number of words which have been produced three times × 100%.
(3) A score of 40% would indicate a diagnosis of inconsistent phonological disorder.
(4) Some examples of inconsistency are:
 - kangaroo: [tæŋæwu], [tæŋæku], [tæŋæwuk]
 - elephant: [ɛnzɛnt], [ɛləðɪnk], [ɛləsɪnk]
 - teeth: [tif], [tis], [tit], [tɛf], [tæf], [tɪf]

In addition to these nine essential criteria, another empirical issue deserves consideration in multilingual studies, i.e. categorisation of the target phonology. While English phonology has received a great deal of research attention, and its description is relatively uncontroversial, other languages require systematic work so that agreement can be reached about the characteristics of some phonological features. For example, there is disagreement about whether /i/ and /u/ should be considered as 'medial' sounds (as in traditional Mandarin phonology) or as semi-vowels when they are the first vowels in triphthongs in Putonghua (Zhu, 2002). Another example is /kw, k^{h}w/ in Cantonese (So, this volume: Chap. 6). The debate is on whether these phonemes should be considered as labialised velar clusters or as labialised velar stops.

The list of criteria discussed above reflects the complex and multifaceted nature of phonological acquisition. Some criteria have theoretical implications; some are related with data robustness, and others arise out of practical concerns and constraints. The following checklist summarises the fundamental issues discussed above and each researcher is welcome to add issues specific to his/her individual study.

Checklist for Designing a Cross-Linguistic Study

- Sound inventory:
  (a) Phonetic versus phonemic
  (b) The extent of phonemic stability and consistency
  (c) Word and syllable position
  (d) Minimum percentage of an age group
  (e) Sustainability across age groups

- Subject inclusion criteria: representativeness of the sample
  (a) Age
  (b) Socio-economic variables (including family background)
  (c) Gender
  (d) Language background
  (e) Sibling order
  (f) Typically or atypically developing condition
- Selection of words for picture-naming and -description tasks
  (a) Opportunities for all the phonemes and phonological features
  (b) Word or syllable position
  (c) Frequency of all the phonemes and phonological features
  (d) Familiarity of words and ease of presentation
  (e) Length of the task
- Imitation or spontaneous speech
- Error patterns
  (a) The minimal frequency of occurrence versus opportunity
  (b) Consistency of error pattern use
  (c) Group criteria

Part 2
Monolingual Context

Chapter 3

English Phonology: Acquisition and Disorder

B. DODD, A. HOLM, ZHU HUA, S. CROSBIE and J. BROOMFIELD

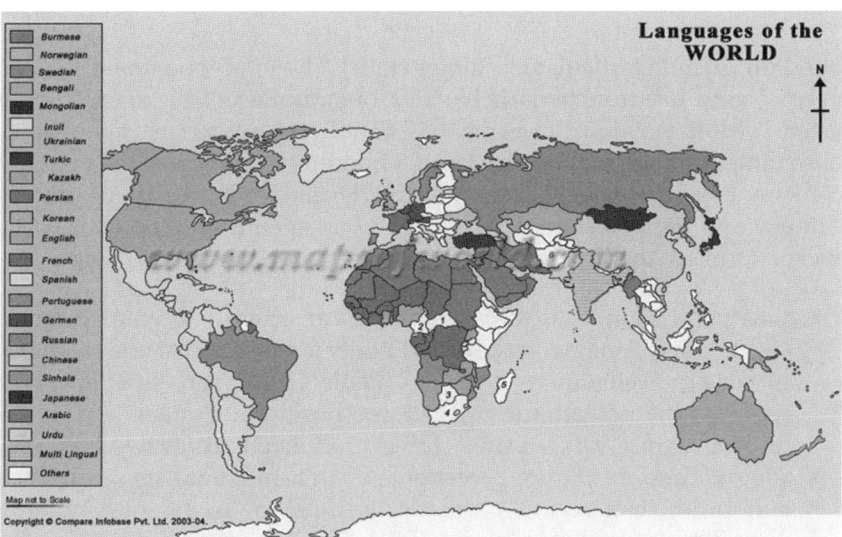

Figure 3.1 Languages of the world

English is spoken as a first language by between 320–380 million people worldwide (see Figure 3.1) but more people speak English as a second language than as a first language (Crystal, 1995). English belongs to the Indo-European family of languages and is most closely related to the Western Germanic languages such as German, Flemish, and Dutch (Crystal, 1995).

The characteristics of the English phonological system are shown in Table 3.1.

Acquisition

Children's speech sound development can be analysed in two ways: phonetic versus phonemic acquisition. The term 'phonetic' refers to speech

Table 3.1 Characteristics of English phonology

Vowels and diphthongs	21
Triphthongs	5
Consonants	24
Clusters	49
Syllable shapes	(CCC)V(CCC)
Stress	Complex
Lexical tones	None
Word length	Many multi-syllabic words

sound production (articulatory/motor skills). The term 'phonemic' refers to speech sound use (functions/behaviour/organisation of the speech sound system). Most previous research has conducted phonemic analyses on consonants. In a phonemic approach, children's production of sounds in word contexts are usually examined in terms of degree of production accuracy and the percentage of children of an age group who reached the level of accuracy in phoneme production. Researchers need to decide:

- whether a sound has to be produced correctly in all word positions (word-initial, -medial, and -final) or only in word-initial and -final position (e.g. Wellman *et al.* (1931), Poole (1934) and Templin (1957) required correct production in three positions. Prather *et al.* (1975) and Smit *et al.* (1990) required correct production in only two positions);
- the required minimum percentage of children of an age group who can produce a sound correctly as defined in the first criterion (e.g. 75% in Wellman *et al.* (1931), Templin (1957), Prather *et al.* (1975); 100% in Poole (1934)).

Table 3.2 summarises the criteria used, demographic characteristics and age of sound acquisition in some of the well-cited studies. Variations exist between the sample size, age range of the subjects, elicitation techniques, criteria used and data presentation. For example, Olmsted (1971) classified the sounds into two groups according to whether they were acquired before four years of age and listed different age of acquisition of sounds at different word positions. In contrast, Smit *et al.* (1990) presented separate and different age of acquisition of some sounds for girls and boys. Not surprisingly, these differences, especially in the criteria used, resulted in differences in the stated age of acquisition of sounds.

A comparison of these studies reveals significant anomalies.

- The age of acquisition of the same sounds in Poole's study (1934) was systematically later than the findings of Wellman *et al.* (1931),

Templin (1957), and Prather *et al.* (1975), probably because she used more stringent criteria in deciding the age of acquisition.
- Among the six studies, the findings of Wellman *et al.* and Templin are most similar: the same age of acquisition was reported for seven sounds, with a difference of one year on 11 sounds and a difference of two years on two sounds. The resemblance may reflect use of the same criteria. The differences in age of acquisition of some sounds, however, could reflect a difference in the two tests in the complexity of target words (Ingram *et al.*, 1980). Syllable length, together with familiarity of the lexical items, may have affected phoneme production. Ingram *et al.* (1980) found that accuracy of word-initial fricatives is reduced in words with greater syllable length while Badar (2002) found that phoneme production consistency also tends to deteriorate with increasing syllable complexity. This factor may also account, in part, for differences in the reported age of acquisition in different studies.
- Prather *et al.* (1975) consistently found earlier age of acquisition for the same sounds than other studies. This may reflect the inclusion of a lower age group of children in their study.
- Smit *et al.* (1990) were the only ones to include children who were receiving intervention for articulation in the cohort in an effort to more closely represent the population on which to base norms. Their criteria for determining age of acquisition are unclear. They used a 90% accuracy level (i.e. correct production of a sound against the number of attempts to produce a target sound) when deciding the age of acquisition. However, they do not specify the percentage of each age group required to be able to use the sound correctly to assign age of acquisition. Smit *et al.* found gender exerted a significant influence on the age of acquisition. They reported a different age of acquisition for girls and boys for 11 sounds. The most striking gender difference was reflected in the acquisition of the voiced dental fricative /ð/: girls acquired the sound by the age of 4;6 while boys were aged 7;0.

Despite differences in their sample size, elicitation methods, criteria used in the analysis, and findings, these studies have consensus on the status of some sounds. As shown in Table 3.2, children tend to acquire /m, n, p, b, w/ earlier than other sounds while /θ, ð, z, ʒ, dʒ, ŋ/ seem to be among the last group of sounds they acquire. This is consistent with findings of some studies using a distinctive feature approach.

Several studies in the 1960s, 1970s, and 1980s described normal phonological development in terms of distinctive features (Hodson & Paden, 1978; Irwin & Wong, 1983; Menyuk, 1968: Prather *et al.*, 1975). These studies used the analytical model of the distinctive feature theory by Jakobson *et al.* (1969). It examined sound acquisition in a set of binary

Table 3.2 An overview of studies on phoneme acquisition

	Wellman (1931)	Poole (1934)	Templin (1957)	Olmsted (1971)	Prather (1975)	Smit (1990)
Subject no.	204	65	480	100	147	997
Age range	2;0–6;0	2;6–8;6	3;0–8;0	1;3–4;6	2;0–4;0	3;0–9;0
Area	Iowa	Michigan	N/A	N/A	Seattle	Iowa/Nebraska
Speech mode	S and I	S and I	S and I	S	S	S
Word-position	I, M, F	I, M, F	I, M, F	I, M, F	I, F	I, F
% age group	75%	100%	75%	50%?	75%	N/A
Acquired first	m, n, b, f, w, h	m, p, b, w, h	m, n, ŋ, p, f, w, b	–	m, n, ŋ, p, h	m, n, p, b, d, w
Acquired last	ŋ, θ, ð, ʒ, dʒ	θ, s, z, ɹ	ð, z, ʒ, dʒ	ŋ, ð, ʒ, tʃ, dʒ	v, θ, z, dʒ	ŋ, s, z, ɹ
m	3	3;6	3	<4	2	3
n	3	4;6	3	<4	2	3;6f, 3m
ŋ	>6	4;6	3	>4	2	7–9
p	4	3;6	3	<4	2	3
b	3	3;6	4	<4	2;8	3
t	5	4;6	6	<4 I, F; >4 M	2;8	4;6f, 3;6m
d	5	4;6	4	<4	2;4	3f, 3;6m
k	4	4;6	4	<4	2;4	3;6
g	4	4;6	4	<4	3	3;6f, 4m
f	3	5;6	3	<4	2;4	I: 3;6; F: 5;6

v	5	6;6	6	<4	>4	5;6
θ	>6	7;6	6	<4 M, F; >4 I	>4	6f, 8m
ð	6	6;6	7	>4	4	4;6f, 7m
s	5	7;6	4;6	>4	3?	7–9
z	5	7;6	7	<4 M, F; >4 I	>4	7–9
ʃ	No info	6;6	4;6	<4	3;8	6f, 7m
ʒ	6	6;6	7	>4	4	No info
tʃ	5	No info	4;6	<4 F; >4 I, M	3;8	6f, 7m
dʒ	6	No info	7	<4 M; >4 I, F	>4	6f, 7m
l	4	6;6	6	<4 I; >4 M, F	3;4	I:5f, 6m; F:6f, 7m
ɹ	5	7;6	4	<4	3;4	8
w	3	3;6	3	<4	2;8	3
j	4	4;6	3;6	No info	2;4	4f, 5m
h	3	3;6	3	No info	2	No info

Notes:
1. I, M, and F refers to word-initial, -medial, and -final positions.
2. % age group refers to the minimum percentage of children of an age group required in deciding the acquisition of phoneme.
3. In the Speech mode row, S and I refer to spontaneous production or imitation.
4. In the results section, Olmstead (1971) and Smit *et al.* (1990) list different age of acquisition for some of the phonemes at different word positions. Smit *et al.* (1990) also list different ages of acquisition for some of the phonemes by girls (indicated by f) and boys (indicated by m).
5. The number of sounds listed for the rows 'sounds acquired first' and 'sounds acquired last' is limited to about five sounds.

acoustic, perceptual and articulatory features that distinguish one phoneme from another. Menyuk (1968) and Prather *et al.* (1975) found that there seemed to be an order of acquisition of features within a language: consonants containing [+nasal] and/or [+grave] features appeared early while those containing [+continuant] and/or [+strident] came later. However, these two studies did not give any information on the age of feature development.

Hodson and Paden (1978) examined the feature production of 60 normally developing American English-speaking children aged four years. They found most of the features, with the exception of Coronal and High, relatively established at the age of four. Irwin and Wong (1983) confirmed the early development of features. They described the production of sounds and features of children aged 1;6, 2, 3, 4, and 6 years using the Chomsky–Halle feature system and their own feature system. They found that by the age of two children had generally acquired all the features in the Irwin–Wong system except for the place feature of 'linguadental'.

These normative studies represent first attempts to analyse the phonemic repertoire and development of children of various age ranges. However, it is important to review the weaknesses or concerns associated with these studies. Most concerns are related to methodological issues, particularly, the criteria used. First, studies usually adopted a cross-sectional design in which a large sample of children was selected across several age bands. In essence, the norms developed this way provide only probabilistic statements regarding the rate and pattern of development. They do not trace the sequential developmental pattern of a particular child and minimise individual differences. Individual variations in early phonological development are well-documented (e.g. Vihman, 1996), therefore, they should be taken into account when deriving and applying norms.

The second issue of concern with these studies is related to the first one. Since the cross-sectional study cannot trace sequential development of phonemes and different groups of children were examined in different age ranges, some sounds might be produced correctly by more children in a younger age group than those in an older age group. For example, Poole (1934) reported that the sounds /s, z/ appeared in the five-and-a-half-year-old age group, then disappeared in later age groups and did not reappear until the seven-and-a-half-year-old age group. This phenomenon, referred to as 'reversal' by Wellman *et al.* (1931), may partly reflect a child's inconsistent production (i.e. a child may vary between correct and incorrect production). Therefore, fluctuation in a sound inventory is unavoidable even in a longitudinal study where phoneme development is recorded sequentially (Zhu, 2000). Researchers have to decide, therefore, how to assign an age of acquisition to sounds whose production is not stable across age groups.

Thirdly, the acquisition of sounds occurs gradually and progressively. It is not all or nothing (Olmsted, 1971). Normative studies, therefore, need to clarify the level of acquisition targeted in analysis. Unfortunately, this information was missing in most of the studies. For phonetic acquisition, a distinction can be made between phonetic development in words and phonetic development prior to word learning (Winitz, 1969). The latter has a physiological basis. It involves learning sounds in and out of one's ambient language. The former may be a physiological process to a lesser degree in the sense that it involves a stable sound-meaning relationship.

In phonemic acquisition, a distinction can be made between 'customary production' (e.g. sound produced correctly in at least two of three word positions) and 'mastery' (e.g. sound produced correctly in all word positions) (Sander, 1972). A distinction can also be made between 'phoneme emergence' (e.g. producing a sound correctly at least once) and 'phoneme stabilisation' (e.g. producing a sound correctly on at least two of three opportunities) (Zhu, 2002).

Taking into consideration both individual variation and group trend, Amayreh and Dyson (1998) defined three types of age of acquisition: 'age of customary production' (i.e. at least 50% of children in an age group produce the sound correctly in at least two positions); 'age of acquisition' (i.e. at least 75% of children in an age group produce the sound correctly in all positions); and 'age of mastery' (i.e. at least 90% of children in an age group produce the sound correctly in all positions).

Most of the studies reviewed earlier (except Smit *et al.*, 1990) considered a phoneme or feature acquired when 75% or 90% of children of an age group met the criteria. Sander (1972), however, suggested age ranges of phoneme acquisition for each phoneme should be given. He reanalysed the data of Wellman *et al.* (1931) and used both lower percentage (i.e. 50% of the children) and upper percentage (i.e. 90% of the children) in deciding the age of acquisition. His results showed that the age of acquisition of sounds such as /s/ differed as much as five years depending on the percentage of children used as minimum requirement.

Any normative study on the age of sound development needs to address these three issues of concern in its design to ensure theoretically valid and practically meaningful norms.

Development of Error Patterns

Error patterns (sometimes referred to as phonological processes) are another measure frequently used to describe a child's phonological system. Originating in Natural Phonology (Stampe, 1969) and widely adopted in the field of child phonology (Ingram, 1976), phonological processes are defined as a set of mental operations that change or omit phonological units as the result of the natural limitations and capacities of human vocal production and perception. Despite criticisms from some researchers that the original concept of phonological processes lacked psychological reality or explanatory power (for a review, see Bankson & Bernthal, 1998), the general consensus is that phonological processes are the most economical way of describing the relationship between adult targets and a child's production. This paper refers to error patterns rather than phonological processes to avoid theoretical assumptions associated with phonological processes.

Error patterns in English-speaking children's speech have been identified and categorised at several levels. At the first level, error patterns are categorised into two groups: syllable error patterns (errors that affect the syllabic structure structures of the target words) or substitution error patterns (errors involving substituting one sound for another) (Bankson & Bernthal, 1998).

At the second level, syllable error patterns are divided into eight sub-categories. Variations exist in the terms used. The primary sources for the following listing are Stoel-Gammon and Dunn (1985), Dodd (1995), Bankson and Bernthal (1998): final consonant deletion; weak syllable deletion; reduplication; consonant cluster reduction; assimilation; epenthesis; metatheses; coalescence. Substitution error patterns can also be classified into eight sub-categories: velar fronting; backing; stopping; gliding of liquids; affrication; deaffrication; vocalisation; voicing.

At the third level, each error pattern is realised by one or several rules (Edwards, 1992; Dodd, 1995). Specifically, an error pattern is a general tendency that affects a group of sounds. In comparison, a rule is a statement of the specific contexts under which the error pattern occurs (Holm, 1998). For example, the syllable error pattern of cluster reduction could include a range of different realisation rules (e.g. 'deleting /s/ preconsonantally' /spaɪdə/ → [paɪdə] and 'deleting /ɪ/ postconsonantally'/bɹɛd/ → [bɛd]).

Although the categorisation of error patterns described above has been well documented, very few studies have tried to determine the age, or age range, at which the various error patterns are present in the speech of normally developing children (Stoel-Gammon & Dunn, 1985).

- Preisser *et al.* (1988) examined the occurrence of error patterns in the speech of 60 children aged 1;6–2;6 years. They found that the most common error patterns used were cluster reduction, liquid deviations, stridency deletion, velar deviation, and nasal/glide deviation (such as deletion of nasal or glide in clusters).
- Hodson and Paden (1981) observed the use of error patterns in the speech of 60 children aged 4;0–4;11 years. They found that although articulation performance of the children of this age group closely approximated the adult models, some error patterns occurred once or several times by more than 12% of the children. In the

order of their frequency of occurrence these error patterns were: devoicing of word-final consonants; anterior strident substitutions for /θ, ð/ (e.g. /θ/ → [f] or [v]); vowelisation of postvocalic or syllabic /l/, frontal lisp; depalatalisation of /ʃ, tʃ, dʒ, ʒ/ (e.g. shoe → [su]); metathesis; assimilation; and gliding.
- Roberts et al. (1990) conducted a quasilongitudinal study in which they annually assessed common error patterns in the speech of the 145 children aged 2;5–8;0 years. They used a standardised articulation test and found that error patterns resolved rapidly between 2;5 and 4;0 years. While error patterns of cluster reductions, deletion of final/medial consonants, liquid gliding, fronting, stopping, and deaffrication were dominant in the speech of children under four years, only error patterns of cluster reductions, liquid gliding and deaffrication persisted after four years of age.

The information reported by these studies is useful but not comprehensive because of the way they identified error patterns. Each study required only one occurrence for judging whether an error pattern existed. Whether a single occurrence of an error can warrant the existence of a particular error pattern is questionable. As discussed earlier, an error pattern is a general tendency that affects a group of sounds. A distinction should be made between one instance of an error, which may take place by chance or occur due to developmental fluctuation, and the frequent occurrence of a type of error that represents a certain tendency in a child's speech.

Apart from these studies, most information on the development of error patterns comes from either longitudinal studies of one or several children (Dodd, 1995; Smith, 1973), or a collation of previous findings in several case studies (Ingram, 1976; Stoel-Gammon & Dunn, 1985). Grunwell (1981b) reported widely used norms on error patterns derived largely from data recorded by Ingram (1976) and Anthony et al. (1971). These norms are based on a very small group of children.

Study of Normal Development: Aims and Hypotheses

The research study reported in this chapter aimed to provide valid and reliable normative data for the phonological development of British English-speaking children. Previous research has focused on small numbers of children, limited age ranges or has been flawed by methodological issues such as the criterion number of occurrences for identification of an error type. The study was designed to address the methodological issues reviewed here or in the introductory chapter of this book. It was hypothesised that:

- Phonological skills will develop with age so older children will have more accurate speech and fewer error patterns in their speech.

- Girls will display higher levels of phonological accuracy than boys.
- Children from higher socio-economic families will have superior phonological skills than their peers from lower socio-economic families.

Method

The participants

This study assessed 684 mono-lingual English-speaking British children aged between 3;0 and 6;11 years. The sample contained 326 boys and 358 girls (see Table 3.3). A letter explaining the purpose of the study and inviting participation was sent to schools and nurseries. All children in participating schools and nurseries were given an explanatory letter and a consent form, to be signed by parents, to take home. Parents were invited to attend the assessment. To reach their quotas in terms of age, gender and SES in particular geographic areas, assessors randomly selected children whose parents had agreed to participate in the study.

An additional 32 children aged 2;0–2;11 were tested to allow the identification of developmental patterns used before 36 months. The children attended a nursery in a lower/middle SES area of Newcastle upon Tyne.

The assessors

Three paediatric speech and language therapists, eight undergraduate and postgraduate speech and language therapy students, and two clinical linguists in the Speech and Language Sciences Section, University of Newcastle upon Tyne tested children for the normative sample. The assessors were trained to ensure consistency of test administration.

Table 3.3 UK normative sample by age

Age group	n	Mean age (year; month)	SD (months)	% of sample
3;0–3;5	51	3;2	1.83	7.5
3;6–3;11	85	3;8	1.79	12.4
4;0–4;5	98	4;2	1.62	14.3
4;6–4;11	100	4;8	1.75	14.6
5;0–5;5	93	5;2	1.72	13.6
5;6–5;11	93	5;8	1.75	13.6
6;0–6;5	97	6;2	1.51	14.2
6;6–6;11	67	6;7	1.05	9.8
Total	684	5;6	12.68	100

They received precise instructions on sampling, phonetic transcription (particularly of dialectal variations), elicitation techniques, equipment and scoring. Assessors collected data in their own home counties, and were instructed to accept dialectal variations as correct.

Procedure

Each child was seen individually. The assessor established rapport with the child prior to testing in a quiet room. Assessor and child were seated side by side at a table appropriate for the child's height. The stimulus book was clearly visible to both. The assessor transcribed the child's responses on-line but also audio recorded the assessment. This recording was used to check and complete the transcription after the assessment session. It was also used for reliability sampling. The assessor provided positive feedback to encourage children to cooperate. Appropriate cues were used to elicit test items (e.g. 'The man gives the lady some flowers. What does she have to say?' Following the administration of the test, assessors analysed the data and entered scores on the record forms for each individual assessment.

Materials

Two subtests from the Diagnostic Evaluation of Articulation and Phonology: DEAP (Dodd *et al.*, 2002) were used to assess the children's speech abilities.

The Articulation Assessment

The Articulation Assessment examined a child's ability to produce individual speech sounds, either in words or in isolation, by establishing the child's phonetic inventory.

The assessment consists of two parts:

- Articulation picture naming. In this task, the child is asked to name 30 pictures. Most of the syllable shapes of the target words in the picture-naming task are CVC. The sounds elicited cover all the consonants at syllable-initial and -final positions (except ð) and almost all vowels (see Appendix 1). The test is the first step towards determining whether a child can articulate a sound in the context of a syllable. Frequency distribution of phonological features in the picture-naming task is given in Appendix 1.
- Speech sound stimulability. This task looks at the child's ability to produce a consonant in CV/VC syllable context or in isolation. If a child fails to produce a consonant correctly in the picture-naming task, the examiner asks the child to imitate it in a syllable, allowing three attempts. A stimulus list is given. If a child fails to imitate the

sound correctly in a syllable, the examiner attempts to elicit the sound in isolation.

The Phonology Assessment

The Phonology Assessment from the DEAP (Dodd et al., 2002) was used to determine the use of surface speech error patterns (e.g. fronting, stopping, cluster reduction, final consonant deletion). Children were asked to name 50, 20 × 14 cm colour pictures (see Appendix 2 for items). The target words elicited all consonants in syllable-initial and -final positions and all vowels and diphthongs (except/ʊə/as in cure). The distribution of the phonological features of the picture-naming test is given Appendix 2. An error occurs when there is a difference between the child's and adult's realisation of a word. The identification of an error pattern was based on five occurrences of an error type (e.g. cluster reduction). Appendix 3 provides definitions and examples of typical and atypical error patterns used in analysis. The word list allows ample opportunity for five productions of all predictable error patterns except those involving weak syllable deletion. The criterion for weak syllable deletion was two occurrences.

Measures and Analyses

Phonetic inventory

The assessor established each child's phonetic consonant and vowel inventory. A consonant was included in an individual child's inventory if it was produced either spontaneously or in imitation. Imitated sounds were accepted as evidence of articulatory competence. The speech sounds were spontaneously produced correctly or imitated by 90% of the children in each age group. Non-dialectal phonetic variation (e.g. lisp) was counted as an error. A 90% criterion was used because estimates of children with speech disorders generally fall between 3% and 10% of the normal population (Enderby & Phillipp, 1986). Normative data, derived from an unselected population, will include data from children with speech disorder.

Error patterns

The assessor identified error patterns, i.e. consistent differences between child and adult realisations on the Phonological Assessment. Error patterns (i.e. where there were five examples of a particular error type, e.g. cluster reduction, or two examples of weak syllable deletion) were classified as age-appropriate, delayed or unusual:

- Age-appropriate error patterns: error patterns used by at least 10% of the children in the same age band in the normative sample.

- Delayed error patterns: error patterns not used by 10% of the children in the same age band in the normative data, but used by more than 10% of younger children.
- Unusual error patterns: error patterns *not* used by more than 10% of children of any age in the normative sample.

Note that in some varieties of English, syllable final /l/ is vocalised. This has been regarded as an allophonic variation rather than an error.

Quantitative measures

Three quantitative measures were made:

- Percent consonants correct (PCC): the percentage of consonants pronounced correctly divided by the total number of consonants elicited in the Phonological Assessment.
- Percent vowels correct (PVC): the percentage of vowels pronounced correctly divided by the total number of vowels elicited in the Phonological Assessment.
- Percent phonemes correct (PPC): the percentage of phonemes (consonants + vowels) pronounced correctly divided by the total number of phonemes elicited in the Phonological Assessment.

Inter-rater reliability between different examiners for transcription and analysis was examined. The tape recordings of 69 children (10.2% of the sample, all age ranges sampled, mean age: 5;3 years, around 10 for each assessor) were transcribed. Each tape was reanalysed by an additional assessor. Point to point agreement was calculated, including both errors and correct realisations. The correlations between scores were: PCC 0.886, $p < 0.001$; PVC 0.315, $p < 0.01$; PPC 0.876, $p < 0.001$.

Age grouping statistical analysis

The initial statistical testing examined the combined effect of age (in six-month bands), gender, and SES. As expected the effect of age was such that neither gender nor SES was significant in this analysis. The decision was made to create larger age subgroups of subjects according to their phonological development. To do this an ANOVA of age alone was conducted to determine which subjects were developmentally at the same phonological stage (at least statistically).

The data were divided into three age groups based on the one-way ANOVA results comparing the children's results on the phonological accuracy measures (PCC, PVC, PPC) of the children in six-month age bands. The results indicated significant differences between the children in the following groups: 3;0–3;11 years; 4;0–5;5 years; 5;6–6;11 years. Table 3.4 provides information about the age groups' characteristics.

Table 3.4 Three age group subject characteristics

Age group	n	Mean age (year; month)	SD (months)	% of sample	Girls (n)	Boys (n)
3;0–3;11	135	3;6	3.36	19.7	75	60
4;0–5;5	291	4;8	5.27	42.5	150	141
5;6–7;0	258	6;1	4.82	37.7	133	125
Total	684	5;6	12.68	100	358	326

Post hoc Bonferroni comparisons revealed that each age group differed significantly to the other two on each measure except for one: the older two age groups showed no significant difference on vowel accuracy. All further analyses used this grouping.

Results

Phonological accuracy

Age

The mean scores and standard deviations of each age group for each measure are shown in Table 3.5. The older children performed more accurately than the younger children on all phonological accuracy measures.

Gender

Table 3.6 provides the means and standard deviations of the boys and girls on each of the measures. One-way ANOVA results showed no differences between the two gender groups in the younger age groups. However, the girls' phonological accuracy on each measure was better than the boys' in the oldest age group.

Socio-economic status

Table 3.7 provides the means and standard deviations of each of the socio-economic groups on each of the phonological accuracy measures. One-way ANOVA comparisons of the socio-economic groups' phonological

Table 3.5 Mean correct percentage (SD) by age group on phonological accuracy measures

	Whole group	3;0–3;11 (n = 135)	4;0–5;5 (n = 291)	5;6–7;0 (n = 258)
PCC	90.81 (10.14)	82.11 (13.0)	90.37 (9.05)	95.86 (5.2)
PVC	98.72 (2.45)	97.39 (3.96)	98.93 (1.63)	99.19 (1.89)
PPC	93.63 (7.02)	87.54 (9.34)	93.44 (6.07)	97.03 (3.59)

Table 3.6 Phonological accuracy (% and SD) of each age group by gender

		3;0–3;11 (n = 135)	4;0–5;5 (n = 291)	5;6–7;0 (n = 258)	Whole group (n = 684)
PCC	Girls	81.9 (12.65)	90.29 (9.66)	96.89 (3.67)	91.05 (10.33)
	Boys	82.37 (13.51)	90.46 (8.40)	94.74 (6.29)	90.55 (9.94)
PVC	Girls	97.97 (2.56)	98.84 (1.87)	99.45 (1.08)	98.88 (1.88)
	Boys	96.72 (5.08)	99.02 (1.32)	98.92 (2.47)	98.55 (2.95)
PPC	Girls	87.60 (8.77)	93.37 (6.59)	97.76 (2.45)	93.84 (7.06)
	Boys	87.47 (10.04)	93.51 (5.48)	96.23 (4.38)	93.40 (6.98)

accuracy measures overall and for each age group did not reveal any significant differences.

Phonological patterns

Phonological error patterns are defined as consistent differences between child and adult realisations of the target words. They are a general tendency that affects a group of sounds. Table 3.8 lists the error patterns that occurred frequently in the normative sample. To be categorised as age appropriate, more than 10% of children in an age group had to exhibit the error pattern at least five times (twice in the case of weak syllable deletion). For clinical usefulness the qualitative error pattern data is presented in the original six-month age bands instead of the larger age groupings.

Age

One-way ANOVA analysis revealed significant differences in error pattern use across the three age groups. Table 3.9 provides the

Table 3.7 Phonological accuracy and socio-economic status

	PCC		PVC		PPC	
SES group	Mean	SD	Mean	SD	Mean	SD
1. (n = 68)	92.67	7.35	99.23	1.32	95.04	4.97
2. (n = 57)	91.57	9.15	99.05	1.47	94.31	6.15
3. (n = 77)	90.50	9.33	98.97	1.54	93.48	6.29
4. (n = 99)	90.78	12.45	98.56	3.52	93.54	8.87
5. (n = 90)	88.63	9.95	98.52	1.84	92.19	6.55
6. (n = 163)	91.09	9.14	98.80	2.09	93.81	6.26

Table 3.8 Phonological error patterns used by 10% of normal population ($n = 684$)

Age group	Gliding	Deaffrication	Cluster Reduction	Fronting*	WSD	Stopping	Voicing
3;0–3;5	■	■	■	■	■	■	
3;6–3;11	■	■	■	■	■		
4;0–4;5	■	■	**				
4;6–4;11	■	■	**				
5;0–5;5	■						
5;6–5;11	■						
6;0–6;5							
6;6–6;11							

*Fronting of velars /k, g/ was not present after 3;11. More than 10% of the sample fronted /ŋ/ to /n/ in fishing until the age of 5;0 despite being able to produce it correctly in other test items.
**Tricluster: three consonant cluster (e.g. /stɹ/).

Table 3.9 Mean (SD) error pattern use and posthoc analyses ($p < 0.05$) of pattern use by age group

		Mean	SD	1	2	3
Cluster reduction	1	0.28	(0.45)	–		
	2	0.08	(0.28)	*	–	
	3	0.02	(0.14)	*	*	–
Stopping	1	0.11	(0.32)	–		
	2	0.03	(0.16)	*	–	
	3	0.01	(0.08)	*	NS	–
Fronting	1	0.30	(0.46)	–		
	2	0.13	(0.33)	*	–	
	3	0.10	(0.31)	*	NS	–
Gliding	1	0.40	(0.49)	–		
	2	0.23	(0.42)	*	–	
	3	0.09	(0.28)	*	*	–
Voicing	1	0.05	(0.22)	–		
	2	0.00	(0.00)	*	–	
	3	0.0	(0.06)	*	NS	–
WSD	1	0.24	(0.43)	–		
	2	0.05	(0.22)	*	–	
	3	0.00	(0.06)	*	NS	–

mean (SD) error pattern use and posthoc analyses of pattern use by age group.

Gender

The girls in the oldest age group had higher phonological accuracy scores than the boys. To explore this finding we compared girls and boys use of error patterns in the 5;6–6;11 age group. The only significant difference in phonological error pattern use was cluster reduction (F (1,257) = 5.587 $p < 0.05$). The boys (4%, SD 2.0) were reducing more clusters than the girls (0%).

Phonetic acquisition

Age

The assessors established each child's phonetic consonant and vowel inventory. A consonant was included if it was produced either spontaneously or in imitation. Table 3.10 shows the development of the

Table 3.10 Phonetic acquisition: 90% of children

Age	Present	Absent
3;0–3;5	Plosive p, b, t, d, k, g	
	Nasal m, n, ŋ	
	Fricative f, v, s, z, h	Fricative θ ð, ʃ, ʒ
		Affricate tʃ, dʒ
	Approximate w, l-, j	Approximate ɹ
3;6–3;11		Fricative θ, ð, ʃ, ʒ
		Approximate ɹ
	Affricate tʃ	Affricate dʒ
4;0–4;5	Fricative ʒ	Fricative θ, ð, ʃ
	Affricate dʒ	
		Approximate ɹ
4;6–4;11		Fricative θ, ð, ʃ
		Approximate ɹ
5;0–5;5	Fricative ʃ	Fricative θ, ð
		Approximate ɹ
5;6–5;11		Fricative θ, ð
		Approximate ɹ
6;0–6;5	Approximate ɹ	Fricative θ, ð
6;6–6;11		Fricative θ, ð
7;0 above	Fricative θ, ð	

children's phonetic repertoires for each age band. For clinical usefulness the data is presented in the original six-month age groups. All children in the sample were able to spontaneously produce or imitate all vowels. The speech sounds were correctly spontaneously produced or imitated by 90% of the children in each age group. A subgroup of children ($n = 63$) were examined to determine whether they could produce sounds in isolation that they failed to imitate correctly in CV words. For most speech sounds there was little difference between imitation of the single sound in isolation and CV syllable. However, 30% of the children assessed, who failed to imitate /θ/ in thigh were stimulable for /θ/ in isolation.

Gender

The girls in the oldest age group had higher phonological accuracy scores than the boys. To explore this finding we compared the acquisition of phonemes for girls and boys in the 5;6–6;11 age group. The only significant difference in phone acquisition was /θ/ (F (1,256) = 5.828 $p < 0.05$) and /ð/ (F (1,256) = 9.260 $p < 0.01$). The boys were making more errors than the girls on these sounds (/θ/: 25% of girls (SD 4.3); 39% of boys (SD 4.9); /ð/: 5% of girls (SD 2.2); 17% of boys (SD 3.8)).

Discussion

The speech samples of 684 British English-speaking children, aged between 3;0 and 6;11 years, were analysed to obtain normative data. Two aspects of speech development were considered: the age of acquisition of sounds (phonetic acquisition) and the age that error patterns were evident (phonemic acquisition). It was hypothesised that phonological skills would develop with age. The results supported this hypothesis. Older children had more accurate production and fewer error patterns were evident in their speech. Gender was hypothesised to influence speech sound development. Girls were predicted to display higher levels of phonological accuracy than boys. No gender differences were found in the younger age groups. However, in the oldest age group, the girls' phonological accuracy measures were better than the boys. Socio-economic status was hypothesised to affect speech development with children from higher socio-economic families predicted to have superior phonological skills compared to their peers from lower socio-economic families. No significant differences were found on any of the phonological accuracy measures. The effect of age, gender and socio-economic status on speech sound development will be discussed separately.

Age

Children's speech becomes more accurate as they get older. They articulate more sounds correctly and use fewer error patterns. Analysing performance in six monthly age bands revealed a gradual progression of speech accuracy. Significant differences were identified between groups of children aged 3;0–3;11 years, 4;0–5;5 years, and 5;6–6;11 years. Differences were found between the three age groups on the number of consonants (PCC) and sounds (PPC) that they produced correctly. Accuracy increased with age. The youngest group differed from the two older groups on the percentage of vowels (PVC) they produced correctly. Ceiling effects meant that the two older age groups did not differ on vowel accuracy (PVC).

The acquisition of vowels is assumed to be complete by the age of three, therefore it is not assessed explicitly in most normative studies (Bankson & Bernthal, 1998). However, James (2001) argued that the acquisition of vowels continues after the age of three. Allen and Hawkins (1980) found that children mastered vowels in stressed syllables by three years of age but did not master vowels in unstressed syllables until they were four to five years old. Further research is required to describe how normally developing children acquire vowels and the effects of context on accuracy.

The sequence of sound acquisition reported in this study was consistent with previous studies: /m, n, p, b, d, w/ were among the first sounds acquired while /ɹ, θ, ð/ were the last sounds acquired. The age of acquisition for sounds was similar to Smit *et al.* (1990) with two exceptions /v, s/. The earlier age of acquisition for /v/ and /s/ reported in this study was comparable to the ages reported by Prather *et al.* (1975).

Earlier ages of acquisition may be due to different criteria used in other analyses. Smit *et al.* (1990) analysed sounds in word initial and final position. They used a 90% accuracy criterion (child had to produce the sound accurately at least 90% of the time) but it is unclear what proportion of children in an age band had to have 90% accuracy for an age of acquisition to be assigned to a sound.

The current study implemented a phonetic approach. The assessors included a sound in a child's inventory if it was produced spontaneously or in imitation. Phonetic acquisition would be expected to occur prior to phonemic mastery. When children are first exposed to a word they may imitate it correctly (e.g. chicken) once the word is a lexical item they may then go on to use a system-level sound substitution (e.g. chicken is pronounced /tɪʔən/. Phonetic acquisition of /tʃ/ has occurred but not phonemic mastery.

Error patterns decreased with age. Ninety percent of the assessed children over six years of age had error-free speech. Voicing had resolved by 3;0 years; stopping by 3;6; weak syllable deletion and fronting by 4;0 years. Deaffrication (change of a feature of the affricate) and cluster reduction was resolved by 5;5 years. Liquid gliding persisted up to six years. The results of this study are consistent with Roberts *et al.* (1990) who reported that the majority of error patterns resolved rapidly between 2;5 and 4;0 years.

Gender

This study found that gender did not exert an influence on speech accuracy until children were 5;6 years. In the oldest age group girls performed better than boys on all of the speech accuracy measures. Phonetic and phonemic differences were evident in the older age group. Girls mastered the interdental fricatives (/θ/, /ð/) earlier than boys and were less likely to reduce clusters. These findings are consistent with one of the earliest studies that reported an interaction between gender and age in speech sound acquisition. Poole (1934) claimed that gender differences would only become apparent after 5;6 years with girls having a more rapid growth rate and completing sound acquisition one year earlier than boys. A more recent study by Smit *et al.* (1990) found gender differences in 4;0, 4;6, as well as 6;0 years.

The finding (i.e. superior speech skills of girls in the older age group) is consistent with clinical studies reporting that a higher number of boys are referred for speech and language therapy (Law *et al.*, 1998; Weindrich *et al.*, 1998). A systematic review by Law and his colleagues (2000) reported that speech and language delays were more common in males than females. Petheram and Enderby (2001) reviewed the demographics of clients referred to speech and language therapy at 11 centres over nine years. They reported a consistent gender bias with two females referred to every three males.

Socio-economic background

Socio-economic background did not affect the phonological accuracy measures of any age group in this study. Smit *et al.* (1990) similarly found no significant effect of socio-economic background on the age of acquisition of speech sounds. However, socio-economic background has been reported to affect other areas of language development: vocabulary (Bates *et al.*, 1994); phonological awareness (Burt *et al.*, 1999); cognitive, linguistic, and pre-reading measures (Robertson, 1998). Factors associated with low socio-economic background are reduced quality of the linguistic environment, poor interpersonal interactions and decreased exposure to books. Other aspects of language may be more susceptible to impairment under circumstances of increased deprivation. However, the link between socio-economic background and speech and language impairment is weak (Bishop, 1997; Law, 1992).

Clinical implications

Results of this investigation have significant implications for the assessment of developmental speech disorders. Speech and language therapists are required to assess and decide whether a child's speech skills are developing normally. It is essential that reliable and representative normative data are available to make clinical decisions.

The normative data reported were based on a large representative sample. The data included all children to reflect the true population and avoid over-identification of speech difficulties (i.e. children whose speech skills are at the bottom end of the normal range). It was designed to include different groups of children acquiring English so that the norms would be sensitive to socio-linguistic variations. Speech and language therapists can use this information to assess speech sound acquisition (phonetic inventory), accuracy (linked to intelligibility), and whether the path of speech development is typical (error patterns). Effective clinical decisions should be based on the assessment of multiple aspects of a child's speech sound development.

However, while speech difficulties are the commonest difficulty faced by young children (Law, 1992), there is limited information about the nature of speech difficulties presenting in clinical settings. The remainder of this chapter describes children with speech disorder who were referred to a paediatric speech and language therapy service between January 1999 and April 2000.

Speech and Language Therapy in the UK

Estimates of the prevalence of speech disability in the literature range from 2–3% to 24.6% (Law *et al.*, 2000). The wide range reflects various definitions, classifications and means of identification of children with speech disability. Classification of types of speech disability poses a particular problem, since these children are a heterogeneous population. Stackhouse and Wells (1997) discussed three classification systems that have been applied to speech disability, one based on the medical model (e.g. Shriberg, 1984), the second of a psycholinguistic nature (Stackhouse & Wells, 1997), and the third of a broad linguistic nature (Dodd, 1995).

Dodd and McCormack (1995: 66) matched specific surface speech error patterns to particular areas of psycholinguistic breakdown, stating that 'the search for a single deficit in the speech-processing chain that explains phonological disorder must be abandoned in favour of differential diagnosis of sub-groups of phonological disorder which have different underlying deficits'. Dodd (1995) identified four sub-types of functional developmental speech disorders.

(1) *Articulation disorder* is the inability to produce a perceptually acceptable version of particular phones. No specific deficit in the speech processing chain has been found, but the disorder seems to reflect specific difficulties in phonetic planning.
(2) *Phonological delay* occurs when children make errors characteristic of younger normally developing children. No specific deficit in the speech processing chain has been found.
(3) *Consistent phonology disorder*. Children consistently use one or more error patterns that are atypical of normal phonological development. The children may also evidence use of phonological delay. Based on their poor performance on phonological awareness, metalinguistic and literacy tasks and normal performance on oro-motor and speech motor planning tasks, these children have been hypothesised to have a cognitive-linguistic impairment in abstracting the phonological rules governing language (Bradford & Dodd, 1996; Dodd & McCormack, 1995).
(4) *Inconsistent phonology disorder*. Children whose speech is characterised by inconsistent errors (in the absence of oro-motor difficulties) are hypothesised to have a deficit at the level of constructing,

storing and/or retrieving a phonological output plan. Some inconsistency, for example between the correct target phoneme and a consistently used error form, is positive: it indicates that the phonological system is developing. However, inconsistency characterised by multiple error types is atypical and poses the theoretical problem of how to account for such a surface error pattern and the clinical problem of choosing what to target, and what to contrast, in therapy.

In this section of the chapter we describe a large group of children ($n = 320$) referred for assessment of a functional speech disability, in terms of presenting subgroup, population factors, case history issues, and co-occurring communication impairments.

Methods and Procedures

Initial assessment was offered within eight weeks of referral. Speech subgroup, severity and co-occurring communication impairment was determined by standardised assessment of a range of speech and language skills. A different set of assessments was used for each of five age bands, in order that uniformity was maintained, for each grouping, across the service (see Appendix 4). The presence of a difficulty was determined by performance below -1 SD and/or a profile of speech disability as observed through clinical symptoms. A detailed case history was also taken at the initial appointment. Assessment findings were computed into a severity score using the therapy outcome measure (TOM) impairment measure (Enderby & John, 1997). Identification of the nature of the presenting speech difficulty was made using Dodd's classification system (1995: 55–57).

Results

Incidence

Of the appropriate referrals (for all types of functional speech and language disability) received who attended for assessment, 43.8% (320 children) had a primary speech disability. A further 25.5% had a primary expressive disability that in most cases also involved speech difficulties. Phonological delay was the most common subgroup (57.5%). Thirty percent of children had atypical phonology, with 20.6% consistently using some atypical error patterns and 9.4% having inconsistent phonological disorder. The remaining 12.5% had an articulation disorder. No child was identified as having developmental verbal dyspraxia. Incidence of referred and attending cases for the locality was calculated from the number of referrals in a single year and the average number of annual live births (4000). The overall incidence (i.e. new cases referred) of speech disability was 6.4%.

Referral source

Health visitors referred 43.1% of children with speech disability; they tended to refer children with phonological disability rather than articulation disorder. Teachers and parents each referred 15.9%, with teachers referring equal proportions across the subgroups, but parents referring articulation disorder and inconsistent phonological disorder. GPs referred 6.9%, with the majority being articulation disordered.

Gender

Table 3.11 identifies both the age and gender of speech disability subgroups. Referrals under two years of age are grouped together, as were children between seven and 11, and those over 11 years of age, due to limited numbers. The overall gender ratio for speech disability was around 2:1, and this was the ratio of phonological delay. The gender ratio varied in the other subgroups, with consistent phonological disorder being 3:2, inconsistent phonological disorder being more than 3:1, with articulation disorder being more balanced at 4:3.

Socio-economic status

Table 3.12 identifies the socio-economic strata by speech disability subgroup. Based on the index of multiple deprivation and enumeration districts, four strata were identified. These were affluent, mild deprivation, moderate deprivation and severe deprivation. Table 3.12 shows different patterns of subgroup frequency of occurrence with articulation disorder being the primary referral category for children from affluent

Table 3.11 Age and gender shown as a percentage of each subgroup

Years	Articulation ($n = 40$)	Delay ($n = 186$)	Consistent ($n = 66$)	Inconsistent ($n = 30$)	Total ($n = 320$)	%
0 < 2	0.0	1.6	0.0	0.0	3	0.9
2 < 3	0.0	7.1	18.2	0.0	25	7.8
3 < 4	12.5	32.1	37.9	60.0	107	33.4
4 < 5	12.5	30.4	22.7	30.0	85	26.6
5 < 6	17.5	18.5	13.6	6.7	52	16.3
6 < 7	10.0	6.5	6.1	0.0	20	6.2
7 < 11	32.5	3.3	1.5	3.3	21	6.6
11+	15.0	0.5	0.0	0.0	7	2.2
Boys	57.5	63.0	59.1	76.7	201	62.8
Girls	42.5	37.0	40.9	23.3	119	37.2

Table 3.12 Socio-economic status (SES) by subgroup

SES	Articulation (n = 40)	Delay (n = 186)	Consistent (n = 66)	Inconsistent (n = 30)	Total (n = 320)	%
Affluent	45.0	37.5	24.2	26.7	111	34.7
Deprivation						
Mild	32.5	27.7	36.4	13.3	92	28.7
Moderate	7.5	14.1	16.7	23.3	47	14.7
Severe	15.0	20.7	22.7	36.7	70	21.9

backgrounds and phonological disorder being more commonly referred in socially deprived populations.

Severity

Table 3.13 shows the degree of severity of speech disability subgroups and indicates that moderate difficulty is the most common level of impairment. Children with disordered phonology, however, are more likely to be classified as having severe or moderate-severe impairment.

Co-morbidity

Table 3.14 details the percentage of children showing co-occurring difficulties, indicating that speech disability is likely to be associated with difficulties in other aspects of language (e.g. 63.3% of children with inconsistent phonological disorder also perform poorly on vocabulary measures). Chi-square statistics indicated that co-morbidity between impaired aspects of language functioning increased with level of severity.

Table 3.13 Severity (TOM impairment level) by percentage of each subgroup

Severity	Articulation (n = 40)	Delay (n = 186)	Consistent (n = 66)	Inconsistent (n = 30)	Total (n = 320)	%
Profound	0.0	0.0	0.0	6.7	2	0.6
Severe	0.0	2.2	21.2	60.0	36	11.3
Mod–severe	2.5	8.7	63.6	30.0	68	21.3
Moderate	65.0	57.1	15.2	3.3	142	44.4
Mild	32.5	32.0	0.0	0.0	72	22.5

Severity was determined by number of standard deviations below the mean on standardised tests: profound -3, severe $-2 < -3$, moderate-severe $-1.5 < -2$, moderate $-1 < -1.5$ SD, mild $-0.5 < -1.0$ (in normal range, but with clinical symptoms).

Table 3.14 Co-mobidity shown as a percentage of each subgroup

Assessed area	Artic (n = 40)	Delay (n = 186)	Consistent (n = 66)	Inconsistent (n = 30)	%
Comprehension	17.5	23.4	30.3	40.0	25.6
Expression	22.5	34.2	45.5	66.7	38.1
Vocabulary	30.0	50.5	59.1	63.3	50.9
Processes	65.0	100.0	100.0	100.0	95.6
Consistency	20.0	50.3	75.0	100.0	55.9
PCC	80.0	84.2	93.9	100.0	87.2

Artic: articulation disorder.

Discussion

Children with speech disability formed the largest group of referrals received. Of these, over half had a phonological delay, one-fifth consistently used atypical error patterns, almost one tenth had inconsistent phonological disorder, and one-eighth had an articulation disorder. No children with developmental verbal dyspraxia were identified, suggesting that this disorder occurs rarely.

A significant association between age of referral and speech type was observed. Few children were identified under three years, since both expressive language and speech sound systems are limited at this age. Articulation disorder was typically referred at school-age, perhaps because in earlier years phonological processes mask its occurrence. All types of phonological disability were referred between three and six years. The fact that the majority of inconsistent children were referred between three and four years demonstrates the impact of this subgroup of speech disorder on intelligibility and therefore on referrer concern.

While the gender bias was upheld (Law et al., 1998; Weindrich et al., 1998), the distribution was more even for articulation than phonology. The bias in phonological disability matches that of language disability, confirming the linguistic nature of these speech difficulties. The distribution of speech disability across socio-economic status was similar to that of the local population, although there was a slight increase for affluent children. This particularly related to the increased proportion of articulation disorder and phonological delay in this population. In contrast, the consistent use of atypical error patterns was associated most with mild deprivation, while inconsistency was most associated with severe deprivation.

Children with articulation disorder had mild/moderate disability, as few phonemes are affected and phonological systems were often intact. Phonological delay was rarely severe or profound. The two subgroups of phonological disorder were the most pervasive speech disability. Isolated speech impairments were rare. Many children with phonological delay or disorder had broad communication impairments, also performing poorly on measures of expressive and receptive language. Articulation disorder was often isolated, although language difficulties did co-occur for around 20% of these children.

Conclusions

The key conclusions about speech disability were:

- Incidence of speech impairment was 6.4%.
- Of the children with speech disability, 57.5% had phonological delay, 12.5% had an articulation disorder, 20.6% had consistent phonological disorder, and 9.4% had inconsistent phonological disorder.
- Developmental verbal dyspraxia seems very rare – no cases were found in 256 children with speech disability in one year.
- Age, gender, and socio-economic status vary according to subgroup diagnosis.
- Comorbidity was common.
- The choice of classification system used, i.e. based on surface phonology with linguistic underpinnings, was supported.
- Broad-based assessments are essential in order that all elements of a communication disability are identified. Detailed investigation of the nature of variability is essential in order that accurate diagnoses can be made.

The description of a large group of speech disordered children referred for assessment to one paediatric speech and language therapy service indicates the need for differential diagnosis of subgroup of speech disorder. They vary not only in terms of the presenting surface error pattern but also in terms of referral source, age of referral, gender ratio, severity, and co-occurrence of other language difficulties. Other research suggests that they also differ in terms of their response to specific therapeutic intervention approaches (Dodd & Bradford, 2000). Given that delayed phonological development is the most common subgroup of speech disorder, it is essential that clinicians have reliable norms for diagnosing delay (as opposed to the lower end of the normal range), not only for children acquiring English phonology, but for all languages.

Appendix 1: Frequency Distribution of Phonological Features in the Articulation Picture-Naming Task

Consonant (24 in total)	Frequency		Syllable	Frequency
	Syllable-initial	Syllable-final	Shape	
p	1	1	CV	9
b	3	1	CVC	19
t	2	1	V	2
d	1	1	CVCC	2
k	2	2	CCVC	2
g	1	2	CCV	1
m	1	2		
n	2	3		
ŋ	–	1		
f	3	1		
v	2	1		
θ	1	1		
ð	1	0	Number in word	
s	2	1	1 syllable	26
z	1	1	2 syllables	3
ʃ	1	1	3 syllables	–
ʒ	1	–	4 syllables	1
tʃ	1	1		
dʒ	1	1		
l	3	1		
ɹ	4	0*		
w	1	–		
j	1	–		
h	1	–		

*Occurs in some dialects in English.
–Does not occur in English.

Appendix 2: Frequency Distribution of Phonological Features in the Phonological Picture-Naming Test

Consonant (Total = 24)	Frequency		Syllable Shape	Frequency
	Syllable-initial	Syllable-final		
p	1	3	V	4
b	4	1	CV	26
t	6	3	VC	2
d	2	1	CVC	24
k	4	3	CCVC	9
g	1	3	CVCC	2
m	2	2	CCV	5
n	1	5	CCVCC	2
ŋ	–	4	CCCVC	1
f	4	2	CCVCCC	1
v	1	2	CCCV	2
θ	1	2		
ð	2	–	Number in word	
s	3	5	1 syllable	27
z	2	2	2 syllables	20
ʃ	2	2	3 syllables	2
ʒ	–	–	4 syllables	1
tʃ	1	1	Initial consonant clusters	
dʒ	1	2	plosive + approximant	9
l	5	2	fricative + approximant	2
ɹ	3	–	/s/ + approximant	1
w	2	–	/s/ + plosive	3
j	1	–	/s/ + nasal	1
h	2	–	/s/ + plosive + approximant	3

Appendix 3: Definitions of Typical Error Patterns

Pattern	Description	Examples
Gliding	Replacement of liquids /l, ɹ/ with glides [w, j]	/ɹabɪt/ → [wabɪt] /lam/ → [jam] /jɛli/ → [jɛwi]
Deaffrication	Modification of the affrication feature	/wɒtʃ/ → [wɒʃ] /bɹɪdʒ/ → [bɹɪdz]
Fronting	Place of articulation is moved to a more anterior position	Velars: /mʌŋki/ → [mʌnti] /ɛg/ → [ɛd] Fricatives: /ʃip/ → [sip]
Cluster reduction	Deletion of one consonant from the cluster	/spaɪdə/ → [paɪdə] /bɹɛd/ → [bɛd] /skwɛə/ → [swɛə] /ɛləfənt/ → [ɛləfən]
Weak syllable deletion	Deletion of an unstressed syllable	/tə'matoʊ/ → [matoʊ] /ʌm'bɹɛlə/ → [bɹɛlə] /dʒɜ'ɹaf/ → [dɹaf] /ɛləfənt/ → [ɛfən]
Stopping	Replacement of fricatives with stops	/van/ → [ban] /ðɪs/ → [dɪs] /zɛbɹə/ → [dɛbɹə]
Voicing	Prevocalic voicing & postvocalic devoicing	/pɹam/ → [bam] /pɪg/ → [pɪk]

Other normal error patterns, identified in the speech of the two-year-old sample were:

Pattern	Description	Examples
Assimilation	Influence of another phoneme in the target word	/jɛləʊ/ → [lɛləʊ] /bɹɛd/ → [bɛb]
Final consonant deletion	Deletion of word final consonants (most commonly plosives, l, s and z)	/dʌk/ → [dʌ]
Reduplication	Complete or partial duplication of a stressed syllable	/taɪgə/ → [taɪtaɪ]

Appendix 4: Assessments and Assessment Packs by Age Band

Age range	0;0–2;0	2;0–3;6	3;6–5;0	5;0–7;0	7;0–16;0
Pack	Pack A	Pack B	Pack C	Pack D	Pack E
Main assessments					
Language comprehension	REEL	REEL/ RDLS	RDLS	RDLS/ CELF	CELF
Expressive language	REEL	REEL/ RDLS	RDLS/ RAPT	RAPT/ CELF	CELF
Expressive vocabulary	Word list	Word list	WFVT	WFVT	CELF
Speech	Transcript	Transcript	25 words	25 words	25 words
Supplementary assessments					
Phonological awareness	N/A	N/A	PIPA Sub-tests	PIPA Sub-tests	PIPA Sub-tests
Pragmatics	Rating scale	Rating scale	Rating scale	Rating scale	Rating scale
Oromotor skills	Rating scale	Rating scale	Ozanne	Ozanne	PAT
Non-verbal skills	Griffiths	Griffiths	Draw-a-man	Draw-a-man	Draw-a-man

Key: REEL, Receptive Expressive Emergent Language Scales; RDLS, Reynell Developmental Language Scales III; RAPT, Renfrew Action Picture Test; WFVT, Word Finding Vocabulary Test; CELF, Clinical Evaluation of Language Fundamentals (UK); PIPA, Pre-school and Primary Inventory of Phonological Awareness; 25 words, 25 word Consistency Assessment; Ozanne, Oromotor Assessment; Griffiths, Griffiths Mental Development Scales; Draw-a-man, Goodenough Drawing Assessment (Aston Index); PAT, Phonological Abilities Test, speech rate sub-test.

Chapter 4
Evidence from German-Speaking Children

A.V. FOX

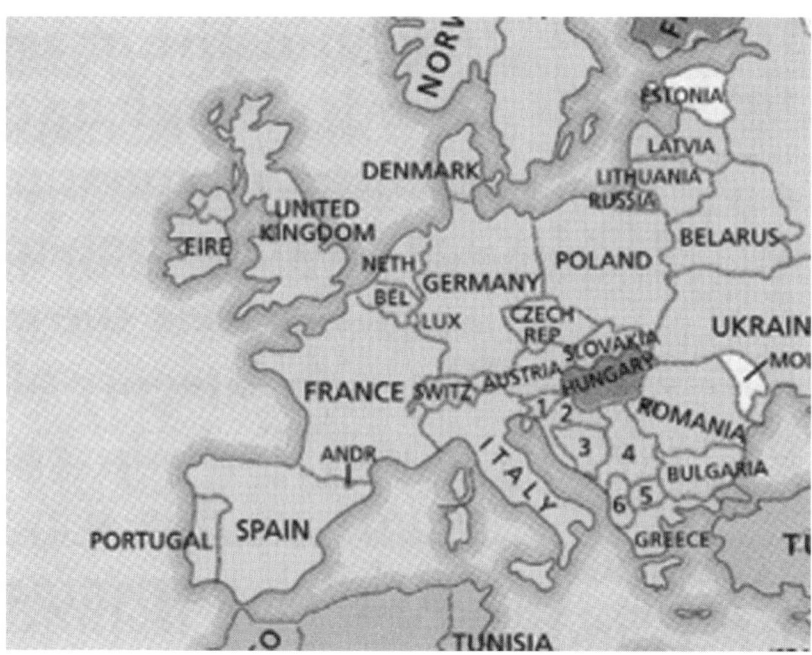

Introduction

German belongs to the Germanic languages and has about 121 million native speakers in 15 countries, the largest communities being in Western and Central Europe. It is the official state language in Germany, Austria, parts of Switzerland, Liechtenstein, and Luxembourg (Barbour & Stevenson, 1990; Crystal, 1997; Durell, 1992; Lyovin, 1997). Strong regional variations in pronunciation, from accents to dialects, of the official language High German (Hochdeutsch), which is based on a North German pronunciation of the written language, can be found (Barbour & Stevenson, 1990; Durell, 1922; Goltz & Walker, 1961). Over the past years, however, at least in Germany, the use of dialects has diminished although accent often makes it possible to identify the regional origin of a speaker. Children growing up in Germany use High German as their everyday language, since it is the official language spoken in kindergartens and schools. In general, the spelling of standard German gives a clear guide to pronunciation.

The Phonetic and Phonological System of German

High German contains 23 consonants [p b t d k g f v s z ʃ x ç h m n ŋ l ʁ j ʔ pf ts]. In addition, the sound [ʒ] is found in words of foreign origin but since it is not necessarily part of a child's phonological inventory, it will not be not considered here. The sounds [pf] and [ts] will be presumed to be affricates following Ternes (1987), and not two-element clusters even though there is disagreement about this in the literature (Kohler, 1995; Ternes, 1987; Wiese, 1996). In word final position the contrast between voiced and voiceless consonants is neutralised, with all consonants being voiceless. In word initial position there are 22 two-element clusters and two three-element clusters. There are also many word medial and word final clusters. Table 4.1 describes the consonant system of German according to place and manner of articulation.

The vowel system contains 13 monothongs [i y e ø o u ɪ ʏ ɛ œ ɔ ʊ a] and 3 diphthongs [aɪ au ɔɪ], which, in the North, have a tendency to be over stressed (referred to as Lenisierung by Goltz & Walker, 1961).

The shortest possible syllables are the structures CV e.g. [kuː] = *Kuh* (cow) and VC e.g. [ap] = *ab* (off) Structures of the combinations C_{1-3} VC_{1-3} in mono-syllabic nouns: C_{1-3} e.g. [ʃtʁ] in *Strumpf* (sock) and $C_{1-3} VC_{1-5}$ in mono-syllabic verbs are possibly due to verb inflection: C_{1-5} e.g. [mpst] in *du schrumpfst* (you shrink).

German is an agluttinating language where, by addition of nouns, words can be made up to about eight syllables or more e.g. *Hallenhandballweltmeisterschaft* (indoor handball world championship) (Meinhold & Stock, 1980).

All children assessed for the following studies grew up in Northern Germany in Hamburg and Schleswig-Holstein. They, therefore, showed some specific characteristics of a Northern accent, such as the vocalic substitution of the sound /ʁ/ before consonants and in word final position (*Berg* (mountain): [beek]; *Tiger* (tiger): [tiːgɐ]) or the word initial realisation of [f] instead of [pf]: *Pferd* (horse) [feːɐt]).

Table 4.1 The German consonant system

	Bilabial		Labiodental		Interdental		Alveolar		Palato-alveolar		Palatal		Velar		Uvular		Glottal	
Voice	−	+	−	+	−	+	−	+	−	+	−	+	−	+	−	+	−	+
Nasal		m						n						ŋ				
Plosive	p	b					t	d					k	g				ʔ
Fricative			f	v			s	z	ʃ		ç		x			ʁ	h	
Affricate	pf						ts											
Approximant												j						
Vibrant								r										

Phonological Development in German-Speaking Children

Until the 1990s very little and unreliable information about the phonological development in German-speaking children existed. The most important studies were the following:

Grohnfeldt (1980) investigated the order of sound acquisition, assessing 312 normally developing children aged 3;0–6;0. In his 'sound-diagram' isolated sounds and clusters were grouped depending on their 'grades of difficulty' i.e. the later a sound is acquired the more difficult it is. A sound was judged to be acquired when it was at least 75% or 90% correctly produced by all children within a six-month age range. Unfortunately, some sounds were only described as part of consonant clusters and the subjects were three years old at the start of the investigation.

As yet, there are only three studies that describe phonological acquisition in normal speech development in terms of phonological processes. Elsen (1991) described her own daughter's speech development. Unfortunately information about the criteria used to assess phonetic and phonemic inventories and her discrimination between the two inventories was unclear.

Fongaro-Leverin (1992) assessed 24 German-speaking children between the ages of 2;1 and 5;0 for her cross-linguistic study of German and Brazilian-Portuguese. The phonological inventories and phonological processes observed in each of her six age groups showed very broad variations.

Romonath (1991) assessed 34 German-speaking children between the ages of 5;3 and 7;2, focusing on the phonological processes that were still apparent. Unfortunately, she did not report the chronological age at which phonological processes were still observable.

Due to this unsatisfactory situation a study was designed in order to gain a more complete picture on the topic (Fox & Dodd, 1999).

Subjects

One-hundred and seventy-seven monolingual German-speaking children aged 1;6–5;11 years were assessed by a German speech and language therapist in their normal crèche, kindergarten or home environment. The children were divided into nine age groups with an age range of six months each. There were approximately 10 boys and 10 girls in each group. The parents or the nursery nurses had reported that none of the children showed any intellectual or hearing impairment or any history of speech and language disorders. The kindergartens chosen for assessment reflected a range of socio-economic status.

A picture-naming assessment procedure was used to elicit data. The assessment included 99 items (see Appendix 1) assessing all German phonemes in all possible word positions as well as most word initial clusters and a sample of word medial and final clusters. For the first age group, children's spontaneous speech was included in the sample, because of their restricted vocabulary and young children's reluctance to name pictures. A Sony Professional Micro Stereo Recorder including a stereo microphone was used to record all sessions.

Data analysis

All utterances were audio-taped and immediately transcribed by the assessor using the International Phonetic Alphabet (IPA) revised 1993. The utterances were transcribed again later from audio-tape to check on the original transcription and a second rater (a native German-speaker who was a phonetician) additionally transcribed 10% of the data. The inter-rater-reliability was 96.5% when sibilant differences were excluded and 94.8% when they were included.

The material was analysed to provide normative data on the acquisition of phonetic and phonemic inventories and phonological process use in German-speaking children. Criteria set for each sub-analysis will be described in the results section. Two further analyses were carried out: the overall error rate for phonemes (PPI) and for consonants (PCI) was calculated in order to describe a very broad acquisition pattern of speech and to provide some evidence concerning phoneme acquisition in different word positions. These figures will also be used as a baseline (z-scores) for comparing data from children with speech disorders to the norm.

Results

Overall error rate

The overall error rate of phonemes for each age group is given in Table 4.2. In row 1 the mean of incorrect phonemes across all children (PPI = Percent Phonemes Incorrect) for each age group are shown, with standard deviation values shown in row 2. Rows 3–4 present the mean error percentage for single consonants compared to the total number of consonants (PCI) occurrences per word position. A phoneme was accepted as correct when it was used correctly in its target word position environment.

Phonetic inventory

In order to describe the acquisition of the phonetic inventory, two criteria were used: when 75% of the children in an age group produced

Table 4.2 Percentage Phoneme/Consonants Incorrect (PPI/PCI) in different age group (WI/WF = word initial and word final % incorrect consonant production)

Age	1;6– 1;11	2;0– 2;5	2;6– 2;11	3;0– 3;5	3;6– 3;11	4;0– 4;5	4;6– 4;11	5;0– 5;5	5;6– 5;11
$\bar{X}$PPI	26.05	21.19	12.59	9.011	5.75	4.86	3.80	2.57	1.92
+/−SD	11.1	10.5	8.1	5.1	4.1	3.5	4.0	2.4	2.3
PCI WI	28.05	26.14	15.40	9.93	5.98	5.56	3.85	2.77	2.31
PCI WF	25.71	31.73	14.93	11.39	7.51	10.06	6.55	4.67	4.88

Table 4.3 Phonetic acquisition according to 75% and 90% criteria

Age group	Age	75% criterion	90% criterion
1*	1;6–1;11	m b p v f d t n l g k h	m b d t n
2	2;0–2;5	pf	p f v l
3	2;6–2;11	j ŋ ç x ʁ	x g k h ʁ pf
4	3;0–3;5		j ŋ
5	3;6–3;11	ʃ	
6	4;0–4;5		ç
7	4;6–4;11		ʃ
8	5;0–5;5		
9	5;6–5;11		

*For age group 1 the appearance of a phone once was accepted as the phone being acquired, since the data in this age group were limited.

this phone at least twice throughout the speech sample in any word position, whether correct or not. A phone was counted as having been mastered by an age group when 90% of the children produced the phone at least twice throughout the sample. Table 4.3 displays the results found.

Phonemic inventory

Two criteria were used to evaluate phoneme acquisition: when 75% and 90% of the children within one age group were able to produce a phoneme at least two out of three times correctly in its correct word position environment[1] (see Table 4.4).

Table 4.4 Phonemic acquisition according to 75% and 90% criteria

Age group	Age	75% criterion	90% criterion
1	1;6–1;11	m b p d t n	m p d
2	2;0–2;5	v h s/z*	b n
3	2;6–2;11	f l j ŋ x ʁ g k pf	v f l t ŋ x h k s/z*
4	3;0–3;5	ç ts*	j ʁ g pf
5	3;6–3;11	ʃ	ts*
6	4;0–4;5		ç
7	4;6–4;11		ʃ
8	5;0–5;5		
9	5;6–5;11		

*Both an interdental and a correct realisation of the target phones /s/ and /z/ were accepted.

Vowels

The investigation of the vowel system indicated that vowel errors were a very rare phenomenon at an early stage of development and mainly diphthongs were affected. However, vowel errors occurred so rarely that they did not fulfil the criterion of a phonological process and thus must be seen as a non-developmental process in German-speaking children.

Consonant clusters

The acquisition of consonant cluster was investigated and it was found that children of 3;0 years started to realise both cluster elements. The first group of clusters acquired consisted of those containing a plosive or /f/ plus /l/ or /ʁ/. The second group contained /ʃ/+x and finally three element clusters were acquired (see Table 4.5).

Developmental phonological processes

The phonological process analysis was carried out twice. The following criterion was used in the first round of analysis: a phonological process must be observed twice in a child and further in 10% of the children of an age-group (Fox & Dodd, 1999). This criterion was used in order to use the identical criterion as used by Zhu Hua and Dodd (2000a) and by So and Dodd (1995). However, clinical experience indicated that this criterion was not strict enough and some non-developmental processes might be identified as developmental. Therefore, the analysis was repeated using a stricter criterion: A phonological process needed to be observed three times in a child (Fox, 2003). The reasons for this decision are twofold. Firstly, it will be argued that a substitution or omission that is found twice within about 100 utterances of one child might be coincidence and does not necessarily reflect a pattern. Secondly, it is difficult to justify why a pattern that occurs within a group of 20 children in two or three children but only in each child twice can be called a developmental phonological process. Additionally, clinical experience and an interpretation of the normative data according to the number of items affected by this pattern demonstrated that in some processes not only the occurrence but also the frequency of occurrence was of importance. Thus the number of occurrence was added as a factor. Table 4.6 describes the

Table 4.5 Cluster-acquisition according to 75% and 90% criteria

Age	75% criterion	90% criterion
3;0–3;5	bl bʁ fl fʁ dʁ tʁ gl kl	fʁ kl
3;6–3;11	gʁ kʁ kv ʃm ʃn ʃʁ ʃp ʃv	bl bʁ fl gl gʁ
4;0–4;5	kn ʃl ʃpʁ ʃtʁ ʃt	dʁ tʁ kʁ kn kv ʃl ʃm ʃn ʃʁ ʃp ʃv ʃt
4;6–4;11		ʃpʁ ʃtʁ

Table 4.6 Developmental phonological processes in German-speaking children

Process	2;0–2;5	2;6–2;11	3;0–3;5	3;6–3;11	4;0–4;5	4;6–4;11
Weak syllable deletion*	■					
Cluster reduction	■	■				
Final consonant deletion*	■					
Assimilation*	■	■	■	■		
Fronting /k g/ → /t d/	■	■	■	■		
Fronting /ŋ/ → /n/	■	■				
Fronting /ʃ ç/ → /s/	■	■	■	■	■	
Backing /ʃ s/ → /ç/	■	■	■			
Stopping*	■					
Glottal Replacement /ʁ/	■					
Voicing/Devoicing*	■	■	■	■	■	
Cluster devoicing	■	■	■	■		
Deaffrication*	■	■				
Interdentality /s z/ → /θ ð/	■	■	■	■	■	■

*These processes occurred only in a very limited number of items per child (3–5 items out of 100). It will thus be assumed that a higher frequency of occurrence is an indication for a non-developmental pattern.

types of developmental phonological processes in German, and their importance and frequency of occurrence. The first age group (1;6–2;0) was excluded from the analysis because of their small vocabulary and their inconsistency in word production (Teizel & Ozanne, 1999).

Uncommon processes are listed and explained below:

Glottal replacement of /ʁ/: Children up to the age of 2;5 often replaced the phoneme /ʁ/ by /h/.
Backing of /ʃ/ and /s/: The only form of backing which could be considered as developmental was the replacement of /s/ and /ʃ/ by /ç/.
Voicing/devoicing/cluster devoicing: Regional accents and dialects have a strong influence on voicing/devoicing rules. Nevertheless, at an early stage children showed voicing errors.
Interdentality: Up to 35% of children aged 6;0 years and up to 25% of children aged six to 10 years (Fox, 2003) showed a complete substitution of /s z/ by /θ ð/.

Discussion

The results of the presented study on 177 monolingual German-speaking children agreed in general with earlier research findings on phonological acquisition by German-speaking children for order of phoneme acquisition and type of phonological processes used. Differences occurred when the age of acquisition was compared. Results from this study indicated that the phonemic inventory of German-speaking children was acquired by the age of 4;5–4;11. This age of completion of acquisition seemed to disagree with earlier studies, which reported earlier or later age of acquisition (Elsen, 1991; Fongaro-Leverin, 1992; Grohnfeldt, 1980). However, these differences and differences in the variation of some phonological processes could be explained by differences between the studies' methodologies (e.g. cross-sectional versus longitudinal and differing criteria concerning phoneme acquisition).

Methodological differences present a problem for cross-linguistic comparisons of phonological acquisition. Nevertheless, the phonological processes that have most frequently been described for all other languages so far investigated are highly similar to the ones found in this study: deletion of weak syllables and final consonants, fronting of velars and sibilants, consonant harmony (or assimilation), cluster reduction, and stopping and voicing (e.g. Yavaş, 1998; see also Chapter 17 for summary of results from all the studies investigated). This agreement supports the concept of universality especially since the languages compared belong to different linguistic families, English and German being West Germanic, Swedish being North Germanic, Spanish, Portuguese, and Italian being Italic, Turkish being Turkic, and Cantonese and Putonghua being Sinitic (Crystal, 1997).

On the other hand, some developmental processed observed for German children are not typical of development in some other languages providing evidence against a narrow concept of universality. For example, backing of sibilants was found to be a developmental process in German. Backing has also been described as a developmental process in Putonghua where alveolars were produced as post-alveolars and /x/ was substituted for a variety of front fricatives (X-Velarization) in normally developing children (Zhu Hua & Dodd, 2000a). In contrast to these findings, backing has been described as an idiosyncratic process for many other languages investigated (e.g. English). However, it needs to be stated that the form of backing observed in German-speaking children could also possibly be an articulatory slightly lateral substitution of /s/ and /ʃ/ by /ç/. Acoustic analysis in a further project will need to clarify whether this form of backing really needs to be considered as a developmental phonological process or as an articulatory substitution.

A further process that is idiosyncratic in English (Dodd, 1995) but developmental in German is the glottal replacement of /ʁ/, this being common also in Swedish-speaking children (Nettelblad, 1983). Further forms of glottal replacement need to be considered as non-developmental.

Finally, the replacement of /s/ and /z/ by /θ/ and /ð/ was found frequently in German-speaking children and similarly in Maltese-speaking children (Grech, 1998) but in no other language so far assessed. It will be argued that the interpretation of the replacement pattern needs to be evaluated differently for both languages. Most of Maltese-speaking children grow up bilingual (Maltese–English) and even if they do not do so sufficiently to be good bilingual speakers, English is pervasive. Thus for these children the sounds /θ/ and /ð/ are part of their phonetic and phonemic inventory, which could lead to a phonological confusion. However, /θ/ and /ð/ are not part of the German phonetic inventory and the substitution does not affect phonemic contrasts. Additionally it is a pattern that is not overcome by children over time and is not affected by phonological intervention (Fox, 2003). It will, therefore, be considered as an articulatory substitution and not as a developmental phonological process. Given that up to 40% of children evidenced interdentality, this is likely to reflect allophonic variation, which is increasingly acceptable.

A further language-specific finding is also related to the sounds /s/ and /z/ but additionally to the sounds /d/ and /v/. It does not concern a phonological process but the order phoneme acquisition. The three phonemes /d/, /v/, and /z/ are acquired earlier in German than in English (see Table 4.7). Since all three sounds are part of both languages' phonemic inventories the difference in order of acquisition contradicts the hypothesised universal phonological acquisition (e.g. Jakobson, 1969; Stampe, 1979).

Even though these findings provide evidence of cross-linguistic differences, such differences do not allow the rejection of the idea of

Table 4.7 Comparison of phoneme acquisition in English (Prather *et al.*, 1975) and German*

Age (years)	German	English
1;6–1;11	m b p d t n	No data
2;0–2;5	v h s/z	m n p h
2;6–2;11	f l j ŋ *x* ŋ g k *pf*	b f d t w j ŋ k
3;0–3;5	*ç ts*	l s *r* g
3;6–3;11	ʃ	ʃ tʃ
4;0–4;5		ð ʒ
>4.6		dʒ θ v z

*Shaded phonemes are those shared by both languages, but acquired at very different age stages, phonemes in italics are language specific phonemes.

universality. Most phonological theories admit the influence of the ambient languages in the language learning environment (e.g. Natural Phonology, Generative Phonology, Non-linear Phonologies, Biological, Cognitive and Behaviourist Approaches). However, the findings challenge Stampe's (1979) theory that phonological processes are innate, universal and natural, since the processes 'represent a natural response to phonetic forces implicit in the human capacity for speech' (Donegan & Stampe, 1979: 130). If this was indeed the case, children should show the same developmental phonological processes irrespective of the language they are learning. Additionally they should also show the same pattern of age and order of phoneme acquisition.

Speech Therapy Provision on Germany

Currently, in Germany a number of different groups of speech therapists work with patients with speech and language disorders, the two main groups being Logopedics and Sprachheilpaedagogist. The first group, Logopedics, treats people with all kinds of communication impairments (comparable with speech and language therapists/pathologists in Great Britain and the USA). Their training, at colleges or polytechnics, is practically orientated and apart from students of one university of applied sciences for speech and language therapy, they do not gain a university degree. Logopedics work in private practices or are employed by hospitals, rehabilitation centres and all types of special needs centres for children and adults. The second group, Sprachheilpaedagogists, is educated at university and may be employed in language units, nurseries, and schools for speech and language impaired children. Their focus lies on the educational aspects of children with speech and language problems. However, more Sprachheilpaedagogists also work in private practices. Speech therapy is generally seen as a medical problem and is thus covered by the national health insurances. All referrals to speech therapy are via a medical route and must come either from a paediatrician, ENT-specialist, phoniatrist or neurologist. So far, the number of speech and language therapy sessions for children is not restricted.

Speech Disorders in German-Speaking Children

Until recently, the majority of speech therapists in Germany were predominantly employed in clinical work, rather than universities where research is done. Consequently, research was rare and the theoretical knowledge base underdeveloped. However, especially during the past 10 to five years more research centres have started to investigate speech and language development and its disorders (e.g. Department of Patholinguistics at Potsdam University, Department of Child and Adolescent Psychiatry at Munich University, Department of Speech at Idstein University of Applied Sciences, Department of Teaching and Research Logopedics of Aachen University). Nevertheless, child speech disorders had received little attention so far.

Studies on Child Speech Disorders up to 1999

Until 1999 only two studies had assessed the distribution of phonological processes in speech disordered children. Hacker and Weiss (1986) studied 15 five to seven-year-old children with speech disorders. Most errors were substitutions, 9% were deletions and 4% were assimilation errors. The processes most frequently identified were cluster reduction, fronting, stopping and backing. Although their study sought to identify delayed or deviant acquisition, this could not be achieved since normative data were limited.

Romonath (1991) assessed 35 children aged 5;3–7;2 years and compared the number and types of phonological processes of children with speech disorders with an age-matched normally developing control group. Children with speech disorder used a greater number of processes and a quarter of their processes did not occur in the speech of normally developing children of the same age. Processes occurring frequently were: velar fronting, backing of consonants, prevocalic voicing, alveolar assimilation, stopping of liquids, obstruent devoicing, cluster reduction, and final consonant deletion.

Möhring (1938) investigated the vulnerability to error of each phoneme of German in 1000 children aged 6–10 years. He described a hierarchy of difficulty according to their percentage incorrect production. Three groups of different difficulty level were identified:

(1) 1.5–11.1%: m, n, b, d, p, l, t, f, v
(2) 17.9–28%: x, j, ʁ, ŋ, k, g
(3) 33.5–54.5%: ç, ʃ, s/z

Apart from these three studies, no studies investigated developmental speech disorders in German-speaking children. Classification within the German literature was based on severity or on etiological factors, with definitions varying from author to author, neither being based on research. Thus it seemed necessary to investigate whether current classification systems available in the literature for languages other than German were also applicable onto German speaking children. Additionally, for the purpose of cross-linguistic comparison in order to assess language universals and the identification of German-specific pattern more descriptive data were needed. Two studies (Fox & Dodd, 2001; Fox *et al.*, 2002) were carried out investigating the possibility of classifying developmental speech disorders in German-speaking children from either an etiological (e.g. Shriberg, 1997) or a psycholinguistic (Dodd, 1995) perspective. Results indicated that a unambiguous classification via etiological factors was not possible (Fox *et al.*, 2002). In contrast it was possible to successfully apply the psycholinguistic classification system which had been designed for English-speaking children (Dodd, 1995). The results of this study will be presented in the following section. A further analysis indicated that the subgroups of speech disorders suggested by Dodd (1995) could be connected with individual etiological factors.

Subjects

One-hundred and ten children between the ages of 2;7 and 7;7 years were assessed by a native German speech and language therapist. They had been referred to Speech and Language Therapy because of concerns about their speech. Most children ($n = 79$) were on the waiting lists at two private practices in Northern Germany and were randomly chosen for an assessment by the practice therapists. Thirty-one additional children were referred to the study by nursery nurses during the collection of data on normal speech development in kindergartens. Criteria for participation in the study were: aged between 2;6 and 8 years, referred for assessment of suspected speech disorder, no previous therapy, no sensory impairment, organic motor disorder, cranio-facial anatomical anomaly, or intellectual impairment, being monolingual in German and no hearing loss detected at assessment.

One-hundred children proved to be suitable for the study. Ten were excluded for the following reasons: one child did not speak; two children named too few pictures to obtain an adequate speech sample; seven children no longer evidenced speech problems. There were 63 boys and 37 girls in the population. This proportion of around 2:1 is reported to be commonly found in children with speech and language difficulties (Romonath, 1991).

Procedure

The children were assessed individually in a single session at the private practice to which they had been referred. The assessment took place in a quiet room with only the tester, the child and the mother (or parents) present. The session consisted of three parts: assessment tasks, free play, parental advice. The whole session was recorded on audiotape using a Sony Professional Micro Stereo Recorder for a second phonetic transcription of the assessment. During the assessment, the mothers were asked to fill in a questionnaire about the child's developmental and medical history and for their permission to use all data anonymously in the study. At the end of the session the mothers were informed whether treatment was indicated and were advised how to deal with the speech and language problem supportively in daily communication.

All children were assessed by a native German speech therapist using the PLAKSS (Psycholinguistic Analysis of Child Speech Disorders; Fox, 2002):

(a) Single Word Picture Naming Test. A picture naming assessment procedure (Single-Word-Test) was used to elicit data. The task was identical to the one used for our normative study (Fox & Dodd, 1999; see also Appendix 1). The aim was to investigate the child's phonetic and phonemic inventory and to derive the phonological processes used. The children were asked to name the pictures presented and were offered a sentence completion task in case of any difficulties. If this did not provide enough help they were offered a choice of possible answers. Direct imitation was avoided.

(b) The 25-Word-Consistency-Test. A German version of the 25-Word-Consistency-Test (Dodd, 1995) was created (Appendix 2). It is a picture naming task containing words of up to five syllables, with many consonant clusters or words that are, from clinical experience, difficult for German-speaking children to produce. Children are asked to name the pictures on three separate occasions within one assessment session, each occasion being separated by another activity. The words of this assessment could all be found in the Single-Word-Test. The child was asked to repeat these 25 words twice more throughout the session, which was either done as a straightforward picture-naming task or integrated in a game, depending on the child's age and co-operation. This task was carried out in order to assess whether the child was consistent in his pronunciation of phonemes in an identical phonetic context, when producing single words.

Analysis

Each child's transcript was analysed to derive the following measures: *Phonetic Repertoire, Phoneme Repertoire, Percent Phonemes Incorrect* (PPI: The percentage of phonemes incorrect was calculated by multiplying the number of incorrect phonemes by one hundred, and dividing by the total number of phonemes produced within the picture-naming task), *Inconsistency score*: an inconsistency score was derived by calculating the number of trials where a word was not produced identically on all three opportunities, multiplied by 100 and divided by the number of trials (out of 25) where a word was attempted at all three opportunities. Only spontaneous productions of the target word are included in the analysis. *Number and types of phonological processes:* a phonological process was counted as being present if it occurred more than twice in different lexical items of the picture-naming task. Utterances from the free play phase were only used in order to cross check whether additional or different phonological processes were used in comparison to the ones found in the picture-naming task. Children were classified into the four sub-groups with reference to the study of normal phonological development (Fox & Dodd, 1999).

Definition of idiosyncratic pattern

The data on normal speech development of German (Fox & Dodd, 1999) and clinical experience indicated that for a phonological process being identified as developmental not only the presence of the process is of importance but in some cases also the pattern of its occurrence. Thus three types of idiosyncratic (non-developmental) processes can be defined for German:

(1) A phonological process that never occurs during regular development.
(2) A phonological process occurring to the phonemes other than observed during normal development, e.g. backing was only observed for /s/ and /ʃ/ to /ç/. Any other form of backing must be described as idiosyncratic.
(3) A phonological process that occurs in an unusual frequency, e.g. stopping of fricatives was observed as occurring in very young children in few items. However, stopping of all fricatives must be considered as idiosyncratic.

Results

Classification analysis

The data were inspected to determine whether the subgroups of articulation disorder, delay, consistent and inconsistent phonological disorder were apparent.

Twenty children (20%) were classified as having an articulatory disorder, distorting the sounds /s/, /z/, /ts/, and /ʃ/. Fifty-one children (51%) were classified as having delayed phonological development. Seventeen children (17%) were classified as having consistent phonological disorder and 12 children (12%) were classified as having an inconsistent phonological disorder (see Table 4.8). This distribution of subgroup occurrence is similar to that found by further classification studies on English (Broomfield, 2003), Cantonese (So & Dodd, 1994); Putonghua (Zhu Hua & Dodd, 2000b), Spanish (Goldstein & Iglesias, 1996) and Turkish (Topbaş & Konrot, 1997) (for cross-linguistic comparison see also Chapter 17).

Linguistic analysis
Next to the classification analysis, the question whether the four subgroups differed in their linguistic pattern was investigated. Table 4.9 provides an overview on the results of the four subgroups.

Articulation disorder
Children who consistently distorted one or more particular phonemes in all phonetic environments, but made no other errors, were classified as having an articulation disorder. Twenty children fell into this subgroup. Nineteen children replaced /s/ and /z/ by [θ] and [ð] and /ts/ and [tθ], and one child replaced these phones by a lateral [s]. Four children lateralised the phone /ʃ/. The distortions identified were interdental and lateral production of sibilants. The percentage of phonemes distorted (when counted as incorrect) lay between one and two standard deviations above the mean for normally developing age-matched children (data from Fox & Dodd, 1999). No children in this group showed an incomplete phonemic inventory (since the phoneme was marked consistently although distorted). Their inconsistency rating was 0%.

However, interdental production of sibilants does not necessarily merit a classification of articulation disorder since the normative sample (Fox & Dodd, 1999) indicated that interdental production might be considered allophonic (see Discussion). Tables 4.8 and 4.9 therefore present data for the articulation disordered group in two parts: when all children initially identified as being articulation disordered are included and when the 16 children whose only speech difficulty was interdental production of sibilants are excluded. When these 16 children are excluded the percentage of articulation disorder falls to 5%.

Delay
Fifty-one children were classified as delayed. The percentage of phonemes incorrect lay between one and two standard deviations above the mean for normally developing age-matched children, but increased in children older than 5;3 years to two to four standard deviations above the age-matched appropriate mean. Thirty-seven children (73%) showed an incomplete phonetic inventory when the phones /s/, /z/, and /ts/ were included, but only 26 (51%) did so when these phones were excluded. Apart from /s/, /z/, and /ts/ the main missing phones were identical to the missing phonemes. Thirty-five of the delayed children (69%) showed an age inappropriate phonemic inventory, with

Table 4.8 Subject information

	Articulation	Delay	Consistent	Inconsistent	Total
No. and % of children	20	51	17	12	100
No. and % of children when isolated /s/ and /z/ distortions are excluded	4 = 4.8%	51 = 61%	17 = 20.2%	12 = 14.3%	84 = 100%
No. of children additionally classified as articulation excluding interdentality[2]	n.a.	5	1	0	
No. of boys	13	31	12	7	63
No. of girls	7	20	5	5	37
$\bar{X}$ age	5;9	5;1	4;9	4;2	5;0

Table 4.9 Subgroup results

	Articulation	Delay	Consistent	Inconsistent
Articulatory processes	★	★	★	★
Developmental processes		★		n.a.
Idiosyncratic processes		★	★	n.a.
$\bar{X}$ Inconsistency	0%	13%	19%	59%
$\bar{X}$ no. processes	1.15	2.55	5.06	n.a.
Range no. of processes	1 to 2	1 to 7	3 to 10	n.a.
$\bar{X}$ PPI	7%	9%	19%	22%
$\bar{X}$ z-score PPI	1.89%	0.74%	3.98%	3.97%
$\bar{X}$ PCI	10%	14%	29%	35%
$\bar{X}$ no missing phones	2.05	1.9	3.6	2.25
Most frequently missing phones	s/z ts ʃ	s/z ts ʃ g k	s/z ts ʃ ç ʁ t d n pf	s/z ts ʃ ʁ pf v x
$\bar{X}$ no missing phonemes	0	1.72	4.29	4.75
Most frequently missing phonemes		ʃ ç g k ŋ	ʃ ts s/z ç f v pf d t n k g j ŋ	All but m n ŋ p b ç

a mean of 1.72 (SD 1.6) missing phonemes per child (usually /k/, /g/, /ŋ/, /ç/, or /ʃ/). The mean inconsistency rate for this group was 13%. The phonological processes of the children classified as showing a delay had to reflect normal development but be inappropriate for chronological age. The most common delayed processes were cluster reduction, fronting of plosives and sibilants and interdentality as an additional articulatory distortion.

Phonologically disordered–consistent

Seventeen children were classified as having a consistent phonological disorder. Their mean inconsistency rate was 19% and the mean PPI was 19%. Even though this mean percentage was high there was considerable individual variation: while some children's PPI was only one or two standard deviation above the mean for normally developing children, others reached a PPI of six to eight standard deviations above the mean.

Fourteen children (82%) showed an incomplete phonetic inventory and 15 children (88%) an incomplete phonemic inventory. Unlike the delayed group there were no phones or phonemes (excluding /s/, /z/, and /ts/) that were particularly affected. Phonemes missing (that should have been acquired) in four to seven of the children were /d/, /t/, /n/, /f/, /v/, /pf/, /s/, /ts/, /ç/, /k/, /g/, and /ʁ/. All children showed developmental phonological processes as well as idiosyncratic ones. Furthermore, some children used a very unusual pattern of cluster reduction and were therefore classified as having consistent phonological disorder. The most common developmental and idiosyncratic processes were: fronting, backing of plosives, /f/→[s] or [θ], and cluster reduction. Interdentality as an articulatory phenomenon was also common.

Inconsistent

Twelve children were classified as inconsistent. The mean inconsistency rate lay at 59%. A one-way ANOVA comparing the rates of inconsistency between the four subgroups demonstrated that significant differences could be found: $F(3,96) = 52.336$ $p < 0.001$. Post-hoc analysis using Student–Newman–Keuls showed that the inconsistent disordered group proved to be significantly different from all other subgroups. The same was found for the articulation-disordered group, which was highly consistent. No significant differences were found between the delayed and the consistent phonological disorder subgroups.

The mean PPI in the inconsistent disordered group was 22% and the highest of all groups. Nine children showed incomplete phonetic and 10 incomplete phonemic inventories. However, if the phones /s/, /z/, and /ts/ are excluded, only seven children (58%) show incomplete inventories with fewer phones than phonemes missing. The most vulnerable phonemes were /k/, /ʁ/, /f/, /v/, /x/, and /pf/. Since the main feature of these children is inconsistency, phonological process descriptions would only reflect that one assessment and would differ on reassessment. Ball (1994) therefore argues that it is inappropriate to analyse inconsistent errors for phonological processes.

Further evidence on idiosyncratic phonological processes

The main characteristic of children with a consistent phonological disorder is the usage of non-developmental processes. The previous study (Fox & Dodd, 2001) had already shown that some children within this subgroup produced individual processes which could not be observed in any other child. A number of processes, however, seemed to be very frequent. A further study on a larger group of children classified as having consistent phonological disorder was, therefore, carried out in order to gain deeper insight whether regularities of idiosyncratic phonological process usage exists within this subgroup. The 52 children

Table 4.10 Most common phonological processes in children with a consistent phonological disorder

	Process	Definition	% and n children
(1)	Backing of Alveolars	/d t n/ → /k g ŋ/	25% (n = 13)
(2)	Substitution of Fricatives	(a) Stopping or (b) Replacement of all Fricatives or (c) Substituting all initial fricatives by /h/,/s/, /θ/,/f/	63% (n = 33)
(3)	Initial sound process	Replacement of all initial sounds apart from /m n b p d t/ by either /d/ or /h/	19% (n = 10)
(4)	Combination of two processes above		11.5% (n = 6)

assessed (Fox, 2003) followed the same criteria as the subjects assessed by Fox and Dodd (2001). They were all classified as having consistent phonological disorder. The phonological process analysis indicated that most children showed one of the three following processes (Table 4.10).

Discussion

Cross-linguistic research provides evidence concerning the validity of classification systems for speech disorders. As previous studies have shown for Cantonese, Turkish, Spanish, and Putonghua (see additional chapters of this book), this study of German speaking children has further supported Dodd's (1995) classification of speech disorders that was based on English-speaking children. The four subgroups: articulation disorder, delay, consistent, and inconsistent phonological disorder, were apparent in 100 German speaking children referred to speech and language therapy for assessment of a suspected speech disorder.

Twenty children (20%) were classified as having a specific articulation disorder, which is high in comparison to other languages studied. There are two possible reasons for the finding. Data for this study were only collected in private practices and kindergartens. Children with an articulation disorder are usually referred to a private practice because the disorder does not have priority for assessment or treatment in public clinics. Data for the other languages were collected in hospitals or outpatients day centres. The difference in sampling may explain the difference in distribution of articulation disorders. An alternative explanation is that parents are more likely to seek treatment for a lisp in Germany than in other cultures.

However, the phones /θ/ and /ð/ are not part of the German phonetic inventory and the study on typically developing children up to the age of 6;0 showed that 35% of the children in the oldest age group used /θ/ and /ð/ consistently as allophones of /s/ and /z/ (Fox & Dodd, 1999). The question arises, then, whether the interdental production of the phonemes /s/ and /z/ really describes an articulation disorder, or whether nowadays this kind of replacement needs to be accepted as a normal variation. If the latter is true, sixteen of these 20 children would need to be excluded from our study leaving only 5% of children with an articulation disorder which is similar to the findings for English (14%), Putonghua (3%), Cantonese (12%), and Spanish (10%).

Fifty-one children (61% after exclusion of the 16 articulation disordered children with an interdental lisp) were classified as showing delayed phonological acquisition. The percentage found is similar to findings on all other languages reported. These children used developmental phonological processes typical of a younger child. Some children's speech phonological processes were chronologically mismatched, a finding also reported by Grunwell (1987) and So and Dodd (1994). The majority of children in this category presented a speech delay of six to nine months, although some children showed delays of more than 18 months. This finding raises the question concerning the clinical implications of the extent of delay. Given that delay is the largest subgroup, research is needed in order to address this question.

Seventeen children (20.2% after exclusions) were classified as having a consistent phonological disorder, a percentage consistent with other languages. As expected all children showed three types of processes: age appropriate developmental processes, age inappropriate developmental processes and non-developmental, idiosyncratic processes. While the presence of some normal developmental phonological processes is positive, the consistent use of idiosyncratic phonological processes that restrict syllable structure (all final consonants delete, not just /t k l/) and reduce a class of consonants (e.g. fricatives) to one phoneme (e.g. [s]) cannot be adequately described in terms of severity or delay. These non-developmental speech phonological processes indicate phonological processing difficulties that impair the ability to deduce the constraints of spoken phonology and how speech sounds can be represented orthographically (Leitão et al., 1997).

Twelve children (14.3% after exclusions) were classified as inconsistent, similar to findings on other languages. These children present the youngest age mean of all subgroups, a finding also made for Putonghua (Zhu Hua & Dodd, 2000b). There are two possible explanations. Ingram (1989b) argues that very young children (vocabularies of up to 50 words) show an inconsistent pattern of word production, that, therefore, inconsistency is a normal part of the acquisition process. Since these children represent the youngest age group, their inconsistency might reflect very severe delay. However, the children who make inconsistent errors do not have small phonetic repertoires typical of very young children. Further, Teitzel and Ozanne (1999) found that even very young children (aged 20–24 months) show a very consistent pattern of word production.

Alternatively, the younger mean age of the inconsistent group might reflect their unintelligibility. These children are often unintelligible even to their parents who cannot acquire knowledge of how particular words are pronounced, and thus parents might refer children who make inconsistent errors earlier. Data from the other subgroups provides some support for the suggestion that degree of unintelligibility affects the age at which children are referred. Children with an articulation disorder are usually intelligible and this subgroup had the highest mean age (5.9 years, the youngest child being 4.8 years). Similarly, children in the delayed subgroup, who make fewer errors than the two disordered groups, had a mean age of 5.1 years. The argument that it is the type of errors that is important, rather than the absolute number, is emphasised by comparison of the two disordered groups. Although these two groups had similar PPI z-scores (3.98 and 3.97), the inconsistent group had a younger mean age (4.2 years). Parents with children who consistently make the same errors (mean age in the current study, 4.9 years) learn to translate. Inconsistency makes such translation impossible, and is likely to increase parental anxiety.

As mentioned in earlier studies, some children show an articulation disorder in addition to a phonological delay or disorder (Dodd & Bradford, 2000). So and Dodd (1994) described two children with consistent disorder who also had an articulation disorder. In this study, five of the children who were classified as being delayed and one child classified as having consistent disorder, were additionally classified as having an articulation disorder in that they were unable to produce acceptable versions of particular phonemes in any phonetic context. All distorted the phones /s/ and /z/ consistently as [ɬ]. This is not surprising, the co-occurrence of phonological and articulation (or phonetic) disorder has already been recognised (Fey, 1992; Kamhi, 1992). In all three phonological subgroups about half of all children showed an interdental production of /s/ and /z/. Given that up to 40% of children in the normative study also evidenced interdentality, this is more likely to reflect allophonic variation than an articulation disorder. The other subgroups – delay, consistent, and inconsistent phonological disorder – are mutually exclusive *by definition*.

For most children, classification into the four subgroups was obvious, given the strict criteria. There were only a few cases where children made errors that raised doubts. Two children from the delayed subgroup made up to three vowel errors. Vowel errors are atypical of normally developing children, and if consistently used would indicate disorder. Six children made errors on up to three lexical items that were atypical of normal development. In the current study these children were classified as delayed because these few errors were the only sign of phonological disorder as opposed to delay. In a clinical situation any ambiguity in data from a standardised assessment procedure could be explored in more depth to ensure correct diagnosis.

Clinical implications

Clinical implications deriving from the presented studies are the following:

- Sound knowledge about the developmental acquisition pattern of the phonological system of an ambient language provides the basis for the analysis and interpretation of the speech of children who have been referred due to a suspected speech disorder. The data presented provide the first guideline for German-speaking children for speech therapists.
- Additionally, knowledge about the normal acquisition of phonology in an ambient language can argue for early identification and remediation of speech problems. This is specifically of importance for a country like Germany where it is still generally the medical opinion that the acquisition of the sound system is completed by the age of six only and that intervention before the age of four is not sensible. The data indicate that the acquisition is completed at approximately four and a half years of age and it is also possible to identify deviant forms of development at a much earlier age.
- The psycholinguistic classification system proposed by Dodd (1995) seems universally applicable. In this psycholinguistic model, a specific underlying deficit is assumed for each subgroup (see Dodd, 1995). If this was the case deficit-orientated intervention should be highly effective in contrast to a general intervention approach for all children with speech disorders. The effectiveness of such an approach has already been demonstrated for English (e.g. Dodd & Bradford, 2000) and German (Teutsh & Fox, 2004; Fox, 2000, 2003). Therefore the classification of speech disorders into subgroup is highly beneficial for the provision of time and cost effective intervention and for the benefit of the child, the parents and the financial resources of a country in a longer term.

Notes

1. If a phoneme was assessed only by two items it was marked as acquired when it was produced correctly once.

Evidence from German-Speaking Children 79

2. Because of findings by Fox and Dodd (1999), interdentality may be a variation of the norm rather than an indication of articulation disorder. Therefore, numbers of children with and without interdentality are presented.

Appendix 1: Itemlist Picture-Naming Test 'PLAKSS'

Mond	[m]	Zitrone	[tʁ]	Schnecke	[ʃn]
Eimer	[m]	Jäger	[j]	Schrank	[ʃʁ]
Baum	[m]	Eichhörnchen	[ç]	Schwein	[ʃv]
Ball	[b]	Milch	[ç]	Spinne	[ʃp]
Gabel	[b]	Taucher	[x]	Spritze	[ʃpʁ]
Blume	[bl]	Buch	[x]	Stuhl	[ʃt]
Brille	[bʁ]	Roller	[ʁ]	Kiste	[st]
Brief	[bʁ]	Schere	[ʁ]	Nest	[st]
Pilz	[p]	Gießkanne	[g]	Strumpf	[ʃtʁ]
Wippe	[p]	Nagel	[g]	Rutsche	[tʃ]
Korb	[p]	Berg	[k,ç]	Fenster	[nst]
Pferd	[pf]	Glas	[gl]	Heizung	[ŋ]
Apfel	[pf]	Gras	[gʁ]	Gespenst	[ʃp], [nst]
Topf	[pf]	Grün	[gʁ]	Schornstein	[nst]
Pflaster	[pfl]	Schlange	[ŋ]	Zebra	[bʁ]
Vogel	[f]	Anker	[ŋk]	Bild	[lt]
Marienkäfer	[f]	Kuh	[k]	Punkt	[ŋkt]
Schiff	[f]	Jacke	[k]	Bank	[ŋk]
Flasche	[fl]	Sack	[k]	Arzt	[tst]
Frosch	[fʁ]	Kleid	[kl]	Hund	[nt]
Wurst	[v]	Krokodil	[kʁ]	Gitarre	
Löwe	[v]	Knopf	[kn]	Hund	
Lampe	[l]	Quak	[kv]	Erdbeere	
Teller	[l]	Sonne	[z]	kaputt	
Ball	[l]	Hase	[h], [z]	Unfall	
Nuß	[n]	Haus	[s]	Elefant	

Continued

Appendix 1 (Continued)

Dusche	[d]	Zange	[ts]		
Feder	[d]	Katze	[ts]		
Rad	[t]	Pilz	[lts]		
Drachen	[dʁ]	Schuh	[ʃ]		
Tasse	[t]	Tasche	[ʃ]		
Auto	[t]	Fisch	[ʃ]		
Bett	[t]	Schlüssel	[ʃl]		
Traktor	[tʁ]	Schmetterling	[ʃm]		

Appendix 2: Itemlist 25-Word-Inconsistency-Tests 'PLAKSS'

Träcker	Marienkäfer	Elefant	Krokodil	Schiff
Flasche	Eichhörnchen	Schwein	Gespenst	Zwerg
Fisch	Strumpf	Springt	Brief	kaputt
Unfall	Rutsche	Schlüssel	Drachen	Glas
Knöpfe	Gitarre	Spritze	Frosch	Tiger

Chapter 5
The Normal and Disordered Phonology of Putonghua (Modern Standard Chinese)-Speaking Children

ZHU HUA

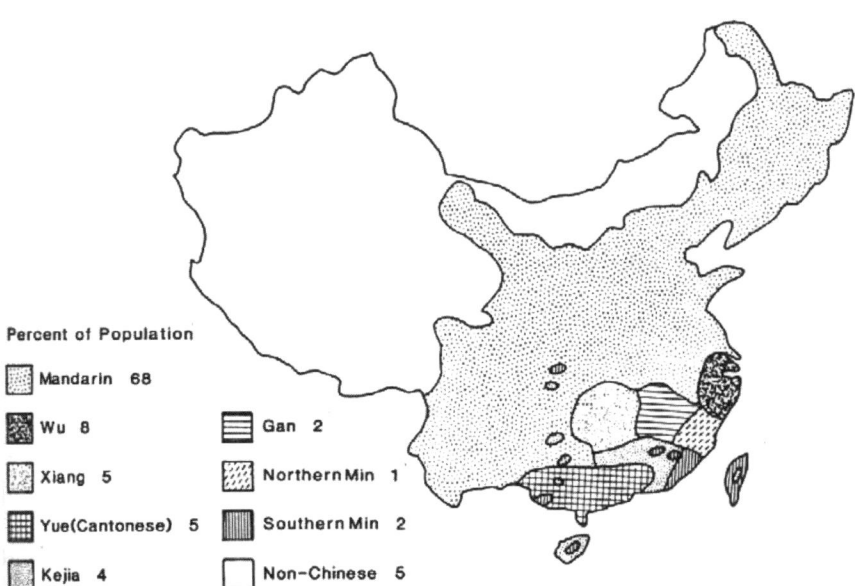

Figure 5.1 Language varieties in People's Republic of China (*Source*: Wang, 1973)

Putonghua (modern standard Chinese) is a standardised language variety based on the phonological and grammatical system of *Mandarin*, the native speech of about 70% of the Chinese population in mainland China. It has been promoted by the Chinese government since the 1950s and is widely used in the mass media and taught in schools in China. It has certain typological characteristics:

- Writing system: largely logographic, i.e. each symbol, or character is or originates from a logograph. Examples: 木 (wood), 林 (forest), 山 (mountain), 人 (person).
- Phonology: a lexical tonal language with a highly constrained syllable structure. No consonant clusters and only a restricted set of consonants are permitted at syllable-final position.
- It has very limited grammatical morphological markers such as case, number and tense markers.
- Syntax: topic-prominent in the sense that the topic, not the subject, always comes first in a Putonghua sentence.

This chapter first describes the phonological structure of Putonghua, focusing on those aspects that are relevant to the subsequent discussions of phonological acquisition and disorder in children, and then reviews findings on normally developing children and children with speech disorders in two separate sections.

Putonghua Phonology

A Putonghua syllable has the following structure:

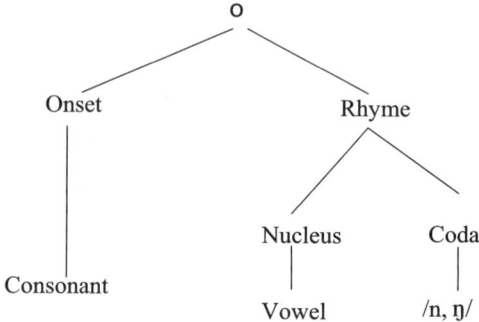

In a Putonghua syllable, the onset and coda are optional and the vowel in the nucleus is compulsory. There are 22 consonants in Putonghua (the place and manner of consonants are given in Table 5.1). All of these consonants can serve as an onset with the exception of /ŋ/, which can only occur in the coda. There are six pairs of aspirated and unaspirated consonants (i.e. /p, p^h, t, t^h, k, k^h, ts, ts^h, tʂ, $tʂ^h$, tɕ, $tɕ^h$/)

Table 5.1 Place and manner of articulation of Putonghua consonants

	Bilabial	Labio-Dental	Alveolar	Retroflex	Alveolo-Palatal	Velar
Stop	p pʰ		t tʰ			k kʰ
Nasal	m		n			ŋ
Affricate			ts tsʰ	tʂ tʂʰ	tɕ tɕʰ	
Fricative		f	s	ʂ	ɕ	x
Approximant			ɹ			
Lateral approximant			l			

and all of them are voiceless. There are three alveolo-palatal phonemes (i.e. ɕ, tɕ, tɕʰ), which seldom occur in other languages (Ladefoged & Maddieson, 1996). Only two consonants (i.e. /n, ŋ/) can occur in the coda. There is no consonant cluster.

Vowels can be classified into three groups: nine simple vowels, nine diphthongs and four triphthongs. The nine simple vowels are /i, y, u, ɤ, o, A, ə, ɛ, ɚ/ (see Putonghua vowel chart). The diphthongs can be divided further into offglides and onglides:

- /ae/, /ei/, /ɑo/, and /ou/ are offglides, the first element being longer and having more intensity;
- /ia/, /iɛ/, /uA/, /uo/, and /yɛ/ are onglides, the second element being sonorous.

In all of the four triphthongs (i.e. iɑo, iou, uae, uei), the middle element has the most intensity and is the longest.

Putonghua vowel chart

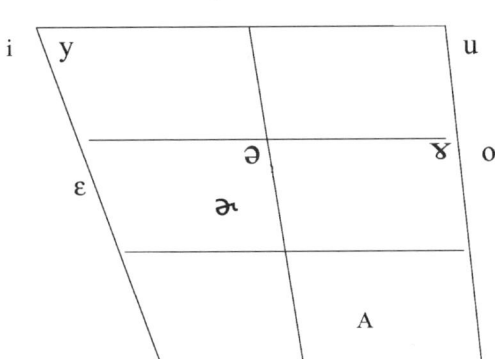

Tone, together with a vowel, is a compulsory component of syllable and differences in tones can change the meaning of a lexical item. There are four tones in Putonghua, i.e. high level, high rising, falling-rising, and high falling, primarily characterised by voice pitch but also by length and intensity. They are referred to as tones 1, 2, 3, and 4 respectively in this chapter. *Hanyu Pinyin* (known as 'Chinese phonetic writing system'), which was endorsed by the National People's Congress in 1958 in an effort to standardise pronunciation throughout China and to facilitate teaching and learning of Putonghua, uses diacritics to represent high level, rising, falling-rising and falling tones.

Examples:

Tone	Syllable	Tonal indicator	Hanyu Pinyin*	Meaning
High level	ba	1	bā	Eight
Rising	ba	2	bá	Pull out
Falling-rising	ba	3	bǎ	Target
High falling	ba	4	bà	Dad

The great majority of syllables in Putonghua begin with a consonant. The most important phonotactic rules are:

- the consonants /p, pʰ, m, f/ can combine with the vowel /u/, but not with any diphthong or triphthong beginning with /u/ (i.e. /uA, uo, uae, uei/);
- the consonants /t, tʰ/ cannot occur together with the vowels /y, yɛ/;
- the consonants /k, kʰ, x, s, ts, tsʰ, ɹ, ʂ, tʂ, tʂʰ/ cannot occur together with the vowels /i, ia, iɛ, iAo, iou, y, yɛ/;
- the consonants /ɕ, tɕ, tɕʰ/ can only occur with /i, ia, iɛ, iao, iou, y, yɛ/.

Altogether there are about 420 feasible combinations of onset and rhymes in Putonghua, and 1300 syllables if tonal variations are taken into account. The following are examples of Putonghua syllables:

ɚ3   'ear'
pA1   'eight'
kʰan4   'watch'
iɛn2   'strict'

Putonghua has often been described as 'monosyllabic', giving the false impression that Putonghua words are one syllable long. However, most words (with the exception of most particles, determiners, classifiers and

Table 5.2 Differences between Putonghua and English phonology

	Putonghua	English
Tones	Four tones	None
Syllable-initial consonants	p, p^h, t, t^h, k, k^h m, n f, s, ɕ, x, ʂ l, ɹ ts, ts^h, tɕ, tɕ^h, tʂ, tʂ^h	p, b, t, d, k, g m, n θ, ð, f, v, s, z, ʃ, ʒ, h, w, j l, ɹ tʃ, dʒ
Syllable-initial clusters	None	p b t d k g f T ʃ + l r j w s+ m n p t k l w s+ p t k +l r j w
Syllable-final consonants	n, ŋ	m, n, ŋ p, b, t, d, k, g θ, ð, f, v, s, z, ʃ, ʒ, l, ɹ
Vowels	i, y, u, ɤ, o, A, ə, ɛ, ɚ ae, ei, ɑo, ou, ia, iɛ, uA, uo, yɛ iAo, iou, uae, uei	i, ɪ, ɛ, æ, ʌ, ɑ, ɒ, ɔ, ʊ, u, ɜ, ə eɪ, əʊ, aɪ, aʊ, ɔɪ, ɪə, ɛə, (ɔə), ʊə (eɪə, əʊə, aʊə, ɔɪə)
Syllable structure	$C_{0-1}V C_{0-1}$ + Tone	$C_{0-3} V C_{0-4}$

prepositions) in Putonghua are disyllabic or more than two syllables long. DeFrancis (1984) suggested that the term 'morphosyllabic' is more suitable in describing the Putonghua syllable, since most morphemes in Putonghua consist of one syllable.

Differences between the phonology of Putonghua and that of English are summarised in Table 5.2. These differences will be referred to when the developmental phonological patterns of Putonghua-speaking children are compared to those of English-speaking children.

Phonology of Normally Developing Putonghua-Speaking Children

A small number of empirical studies have been carried out to characterise the phonological development of Putonghua-speaking children. Table 5.3 summarises the language varieties, the subject information and the main research questions addressed in these studies. In general, Mandarin-speaking children complete the acquisition of the four elements of Mandarin syllables in the following order: tones first (error-free by the age of two), then syllable-final consonants and vowels (almost error-free by the age of two); and syllable-initial consonants last (children younger than 4;6 would have most of the phonemes while some of them still make mistakes with the sounds /ʂ, tʂ, tʂ^h, ts, ts^h/).

Table 5.3 A review of studies on phonological acquisition of Mandarin/Putonghua

Study	Language	Subject info.	Main research questions and data
Chao (1951/1973)	Mandarin in USA	One girl aged 2;4	Phoneme inventory, tone inventory
Li (1977)	Mandarin in Taiwan	One boy aged 2;0–3;0 One girl aged 1;1–1;8	Order of acquisition of phonemes & tones
Li and Thompson (1977)	Mandarin in Taiwan	17 children aged 1;6–3;0	Order of acquisition of tones & tone sandhi Error patterns
Jeng (1979)	Mandarin in Taiwan	Two boys 0;2–1;8 1;3–2;7	Order of acquisition of phonemes & tones
Clumeck (1977)	Mandarin in USA	One boy aged 1;2–2;9	Process of tonal acquisition
Clumeck (1980)	Mandarin in USA	One boy aged 2;3–3;5 One girl aged 1;10–2;10	Order of acquisition of tones
Su (1985)	Mandarin in Taiwan	One boy 1;5–2;4 One girl 1;2–1;11	Order of acquisition of phonemes & tones Error patterns
Hsu (1987)	Mandarin in Taiwan	28 children aged 1;0–6;0	Age of acquisition of phoneme & tones
Shiu (1990)	Mandarin in Taiwan	One boy 1;0–3;0 One girl 0;7–2;4	Order of acquisition of phonemes & tones Error patterns
Zhu and Dodd (2000a)	Putonghua in Beijing	61 girls + 68 boys aged 1;6–4;6	Age of acquisition of phonemes Error patterns
Zhu (2002)	Putonghua in Beijing	One girl aged 1;1–2;1 One girl aged 1;2–1;8 One boy aged 1;0–2;0 One boy aged 0;10–2;1	Order of acquisition of tone & tone sandhi Order of acquisition of consonants Order of acquisition of vowels Error patterns

The following summary on the characteristics of developmental phonology of Putonghua-speaking children is mainly based on the cross-sectional and normative study reported in Zhu and Dodd (2000a) and the longitudinal study reported in Zhu (2002).

Tones

Source: The longitudinal study reported in Zhu (2002).
Background information of the longitudinal study:

- Subjects: four normally developing children from Beijing (age range in the table below):

Subject	Age range (year; month. day)	
	First recording	Last recording
J.J.	1;1.15	2;0.15
Z.J.	1;0.0	2;0.15
H.Y.	0;10.15	2;0.15
Z.W.	1;2.0	1;8.0

- Data: Child–parental conversation recorded every two weeks.

The longitudinal data provided an opportunity to examine the age at which the children were able to produce a feature once or several times in a word context irrespective of whether it is the correct target or at which the children were able to produce a feature consistently correctly. The main findings are:

- Tones versus segments: The acquisition of tones is completed by the age of 1;10, earlier than that of consonants and vowels.
- Order and age of emergence (a feature is considered to have emerged when it is produced correctly at least once in the speech): among the speech of four children under study, high level and high falling tones emerge first (as early as 1;2 or as soon as a child just begins to utter a recognisable meaningful word for the first time), followed by rising tones (usually one or two months later than high level and high falling tones). Falling-rising tones are the last to emerge (between 1;4–1;7) and subject to significant individual variations.

High level/high falling	>Rising	>Falling-rising
Age range: 1;2–1;4	1;3–1;4	1;4–1;7

- Order of stabilisation (a feature is considered stabilised when it is accurately and consistently produced on at least two of three opportunities): high level tones are stabilised first (by the age of 1;6), followed by high falling tones (by the age of 1;7). Rising and falling-rising tones are the last (by the age of 1;10).

High level	>High falling	>Rising/falling-rising
Age range: 1;2.15–1;5.15	1;4–1;7	1;4.15–1;10

- Error patterns: When errors occur to high level tones, the most frequent substitute is high falling tones. High level tones are the most frequent substitute for high falling, rising and falling-rising tones, although rising tones are also used to substitute falling-rising tones.

Target tones	The most frequent substitute(s)
High level	High falling
Rising	High level
Falling-rising	High level/rising
High falling	High level

Vowels

Source: The longitudinal study in Zhu (2002) (see previous section for background information).

The acquisition of vowels took place mainly between the age of 1;0 and 2;0 (Table 5.4). The specific patterns are:

- Simple vowels seemed to emerge earliest among the three types of vowels (simple vowels, diphthongs and triphthongs). Diphthongs and triphthongs emerged slightly later than simple vowels and were more prone to systematic errors.
- The central low vowel /A/ and back high vowel /u/ occurred earliest in the children's production in the first word stage. The retroflex vowel /2/ and the back vowel /o/ seemed to be among the last simple vowels to emerge in the children's production.
- Among the diphthongs, /ei/ tended to be acquired first and /yɛ/ last.
- Among the triphthongs, /iou/ tended to be acquired first and /uae/ last.

Table 5.4 Age of emergence of vowels in the longitudinal study

Age	J.J.	Z.J.	H.Y.	Z.W.
1;2	A		u, ɤ, A, ei,	
1;2.15	u, ei		iɛ, ua	i, ɤ, A, iɛ
1;3	i, ou		ɑo	u, ei
1;3.15	y, ia, iɛ, iɑo, iou			ia, ua, iou, uei
1;4	ɑo	i, u, A	ia	
14.15	uei	iou	ae	ou
1;5			i, ou	ɑo, uo
1;5.15	ɤ, ae, ua		iou, uae	ae, iɑo
1;6			uei	y, uae
1;6.15	uae	iɑo	iɑo	yɛ
1;7		y, ɚ, ɑo, ei		
1;7.15	o, ɚ, uo	ua		o
1;8		ae, ou, ia, uei	y, uo	No data
1;8.15		iɛ		No data
1;9		ɤ, o		No data
1;9.15		uo, uae		No data
1;10	yɛ			No data
1;10.15–2;0.15				No data
Missing/ no data		yɛ	o, ɚ, yɛ	2

Consonants

Source: The cross-sectional study reported in Zhu and Dodd (2000a). Background information of the cross-sectional study:

- Subjects: 129 children (61 girls + 68 boys) from Beijing, normal speech and language development
- Data: Spontaneous speech sampled in picture-naming and picture-description tasks. For the picture-naming task, 44 words were selected to sample all the tones and phonemes in each legal word position (Table 5.5).

The main findings:

- Age of emergence: Table 5.6 shows the norms on age of emergence of consonants derived from the cross-sectional study,

Table 5.5 Items used in picture-naming task

No.	English	Pinyin	IPA	No.	English	Pinyin	IPA
1	nose	Bizi	pi2·tsi0	23	light	deng	təŋ1
2	ear	erduo	ɚ3·tuo0	24	umbrella	yusan	y3·san3
3	mouth	Zui	tsuei3	25	sun	taiyang	tʰae4·iaŋ0
4	finger	shouzhi	ʂou3·tʂi3	26	moon	yueliang	ye4·liaŋ
5	hair	toufa	tʰou2·fʌ0	27	star	xingxing	ɕiŋ1·ɕiŋ(ɹ)0
6	foot	Jiao	tɕiɑo3	28	flower	hua	xuA(ɹ)1
7	shoe	Xie	ɕie2	29	bird	niao	niɑo(ɹ)3
8	skirt	qunzi	tɕʰyn2·tsi0	30	panda	xiongmao	ɕyuŋ2·mɑo(ɹ)1
9	apple	pingguo	pʰiŋ2·kuo3	31	plane	feiji	fei1·tɕi1
10	watermelon	xigua	ɕiɑ1·kua0	32	car	xiaoqiche	ɕiɑo3·tɕʰi4·tʂʰɤ(ɹ)1
11	banana	xiangjiao	ɕiɑŋ1·tɕiɑo1	33	ball	qiu	tɕʰiou2

12	meat	rou	ɹou4	34	piano	gangqin	kaŋ1·tɕʰin2
13	vegetable	cai	tsʰae4	35	girl	nühai	ny3·xae(ɹ)2
14	bowl	wan	uan(ɹ)3	36	boy	nanhai	nan2·xae(ɹ)2
15	chopsticks	kuaizi	kʰuae4·tsi0	37	red	hong	xwŋ2
16	knife	dao	tao1	38	heart	xin	ɕin1
17	table	zhuozi	tʂuo1·tsi0	39	thank you	xiexie	ɕie4·ɕie0
18	water	shui	ʂuei3	40	goodbye	zaijian	tsae4·tɕien4
19	wash face	xilian	ɕi3·lien3	41	stick	gunzi	kuən(ɹ)4·tsi0
20	brush teeth	shuaya	ʂua1·iA2	42	book	shu	ʂu1
21	bed	chuang	tʂʰuaŋ2	43	clip	jiazi	tɕia1·tsi0
22	gate	men	mən(ɹ)2	44	circle	yuanquan	yan2·tɕyan(ɹ)1

Note: Pinyin is the Chinese romanisation system. The numbers used in IPA transcription are tone indicators, representing high level, rising, falling-rising and high falling tones respectively. Weakly stressed syllables are marked by the number 0. Rhotacised features are marked by parentheses.

Table 5.6 Age of emergence of consonants in the cross-sectional study

	90% criterion	75% criterion
1;6–2;0	t, t^h, k, m, n, ŋ, x, tɕ, tɕ^h, ç	t, t^h, k, m, n, ŋ, f, s, x, tɕ, tɕ^h, ç, p^h, p
2;1–2;6	f, s, tʂ	ʂ, tʂ, tʂ^h, k^h
2;7–3;0	p, l	ts, l
3;1–3;6	p^h, k^h, tʂ^h	ɻ, ts^h
3;7–4;0	ʂ	
4;1–4;6	ts, ts^h, ɻ	

using 90% and 75% group criterion (i.e. 90% or 75% of the children in an age band are able to articulate the target sound at least once, irrespective of whether it was the correct target). The phonetic acquisition of the syllable-initial consonants (21 in total) was complete by 3;6 for 75% of children. Nasals and bilabials tended to emerge earlier than other sounds. In terms of features, unaspirated sounds tended to emerge earlier than aspirated sounds (e.g. /k/ earlier than /k^h/).

- Age of stabilisation: Table 5.7 shows the norms on age of stabilisation of consonants derived from the cross-sectional study, using 90% and 75% group criterion. By 4;6, 90% of the children were able to use all the syllable-initial consonants correctly on two-thirds of occasions with the exception of four affricates and a retroflex fricative (i.e. /tʂ, tʂ^h, ts, ts^h, ʂ/). Among the sounds stabilised early were bilabial nasal /m/, alveolar stop /t/ and bilabial stop /p/.

Table 5.7 Age of stabilisation of consonants in the cross-sectional study

	90% criterion	*75% criterion*
1;6–2;0	t, m, ŋ	t, t^h, m, n, ŋ, x
2;1–2;6	n	p, p^h, k, k^h, ç, tɕ, tɕ^h
2;7–3;0	p, t^h, f, x, ç	f
3;1–3;6	k, k^h	
3;7–4;0	p^h	
4;1–4;6	l, s, ɻ, tɕ, tɕ^h	l, s, ʂ, ɻ
>4;6	ʂ, tʂ, tʂ^h, ts, ts^h	tʂ, tʂ^h, ts, ts^h

- Emergence versus stabilisation: Some of the sounds (e.g. /t, m, p/) were stabilised as soon as the child was able to articulate them. These phonemes were basically error-free. Some of the sounds (e.g. /n, f, x/) took a relatively short period to become stabilised after the child was able to articulate them. Some of the sounds (e.g. /tɕ, tɕʰ, s/) took a long time to become stabilised after the child was able to articulate them.

Error patterns

The chronology of these error patterns (i.e. the age of onset, persistence, and disappearance of error patterns) is given in Table 5.8.

Fifteen error patterns, which can be generalised into three groups: assimilation, deletion, and systematic substitution, were present in the speech of more than 10% of the children in the youngest age group (1;6–2;0) in the cross-sectional study and five of these patterns (i.e. fronting alveolar-palatals as alveolars, stopping alveolar fricative as alveolar stop, affrication, aspiration, and gliding) disappeared in more than 90% of the children in the oldest age group (4;0–4;6).

The most typical realisations of these error patterns are outlined below:

- Assimilation. This occurs when one or more distinctive features of a sound are transferred to an adjacent sound. The transference can take place both within a syllable and across syllables. Twenty-one percent of the children harmonised a syllable-initial consonant with another consonant and 17% of the children nasalised syllable-initial consonants. Both progressive and regressive assimilation were found in the data.
- Deletion. Syllable-initial consonant deletion was very common in the youngest group. It happened most frequently before the vowels /i/, /y/, and /u/. For example, a number of the children deleted /l/ in the target word /liɛn/ and /ts/ in /tsuei/.
- Fronting. While the most typical fronting pattern is the realisation of target velar sounds as alveolars in English-speaking children, only 16% of the Putonghua-speaking children in this study used this pattern. The majority of the children (77%) fronted the retroflex sounds by realising them as alveolars and 36% replaced the alveolo-palatals with post-alveolars, which do not exist in Putonghua phonology.
- Backing. This occurs when the place of articulation moves backwards. This type of error is rarely reported in studies of other languages. However, in terms of the percentage of children, it is the second most frequent error pattern used by Putonghua-speaking

Table 5.8 Chronology of error patterns

Error patterns	Age (years)					
	1;6–2;0	2;1–2;6	2;7–3;0	3;1–3;6	3;7–4;0	4;1–4;6
Consonant assimilation	——	——	——	——	·····	
Syllable initial deletion	——	——	——	·····		
Syllable-initial*						
Fronting: /ş/ → [s]	——	——	——	——	——	——
/ɕ/ → [ʃ/ş]	——	——	——	——		
/k/ → [t]	——	——	——	·····	·····	·····
Backing: /s/ → [ş]	——	——	——	——		
Stopping: /ts/ → [t]	——	——	——	——	——	·····
/s/ → [t]		——	——	·····		
/x/ → [k]	·····	·····	·····	·····	·····	·····
Affrication: /ɕ/ → [tɕ]	——	——				
Deaspiration: /tʰ/ → [t]	——	——	——	——		
Aspiration: /t/ → [tʰ]	——	——	——	——	·····	
X-velarisation	——	——	——	——		
Gliding	——	——	——	——	·····	
Syllable-final						
Final /n/ deletion	——	——	——	——	——	——
Backing: /n/ → [ŋ]	——	——	——	——		
Final /ŋ/ deletion	——	——	——	·····		
Vowels						
Triphthong reduction	——	——	——	——	——	——
Diphthong reduction	——	——	——	·····		

········ Indicates that 10–20% of the children of an age group used an error pattern.
———— Indicates that more than 20% of the children of an age group used an error pattern.
*Typical examples are given next to error patterns.

children: 65% of the children substituted post-alveolars for alveolars. For example, /sua/ was realised as [ʃua].
- X-velarisation. X-velarisation is another frequent form of backing, and so frequent that it has been categorised as a group of its own for clarity: 48% of the children used [x], a velar fricative, to replace other fricatives and affricates. In most cases, X-velarisation occurred either before the vowel /u/ or before the vowels /i/ or /y/.
- Stopping. The most common type of stopping (63%) in the data was the substitution of stops from the same place or nearest place of articulation for affricates.
- Affrication. Opposite to stopping, affrication took place when stops were replaced by affricates. This type of error occurred in the speech of a relatively small number of the children (34%), compared with the error pattern of stopping.
- Deaspiration and aspiration. Deaspiration (56%) occurred significantly more frequently than the error pattern of aspiration (32%) and was often associated with other error patterns such as stopping and fronting. Among all the aspirated sounds, the aspirated retroflex /tʂʰ/ and alveolo-palatal /tɕʰ/ were most frequently deaspirated while /pʰ/ was rarely deaspirated.
- Gliding. /ɹ/ was replaced with [j] by 28% of the children. Apart from this type of substitution, 4% of the children replaced /ɹ/ with the liquid [l].
- Syllable final /n/ deletion: 57% of the children deleted /n/ at the syllable-final position. For example, /san/ → [sa].
- Syllable final /ŋ/ deletion: 29% of the children deleted /ŋ/ at the syllable-final position. For example, /pʰiŋ/ → [pʰi].
- Syllable final backing: 55% of the children replaced /n/ with [ŋ] at the syllable-final position, e.g. /san/ → [saŋ]. However, only 3% of the children used the opposite process: replacing /ŋ/ with /n/.
- Triphthong reduction: triphthongs were often reduced to diphthongs (in most cases) or sometimes to simple vowels. The middle vowel, the main vowel in Putonghua triphthongs, was maintained and one of the other vowels was deleted, for example, /iao/ [ia].
- Diphthong reduction: diphthongs were often reduced to simple vowels. The vowel retained was the more sonorant vowel of a diphthong. The children tended to produce the second element of ongliding diphthongs when the reduction took place, e.g. /ua/[A]. The first element of offgliding diphthongs was most often maintained, e.g. /ao/ [A].

Cross-linguistic similarities and differences

There are similarities and differences between the Putonghua-speaking children and children acquiring the phonology of other languages.

- In terms of error patterns, Putonghua-speaking children showed a tendency for structural and systemic simplifications in their production, which is similar to English-speaking children (Grunwell, 1981b). However, there are also some cross-linguistic differences in the error patterns. For example, syllable-initial consonant deletion and backing, which were considered atypical error patterns in English, were evident in the speech of the normally developing children acquiring Putonghua. In addition, substitution patterns and realisation rules of the same error patterns may vary from one language to another.
- In terms of phoneme acquisition, the features of aspiration, affrication and retroflex were acquired last. The late acquisition of affrication has been reported in English (Olmsted, 1971; Prather et al., 1975), Cantonese (So & Dodd, 1995), and Russian (Timm, 1977, cited in Locke, 1983a). However, the opposite pattern has been proposed in Japanese (Yasuda, 1970; Battacchi et al., 1964, both cited in Locke, 1983a). The late acquisition of the feature of aspiration is less controversial and it is supported by Cantonese data (So & Dodd, 1995).
- In terms of tonal acquisition, tones were found to be acquired earlier than segments by Putonghua-speaking children. The same pattern was found in Tse's study (1978) on the phonological acquisition of Cantonese. In addition, high level tones were acquired earlier than other tones by Putonghua-speaking children (possibly due to the fact that it only consists of the default feature – level tones). This is consistent with Tse's (1978) finding on Cantonese tonal acquisition, which suggested that all the level tones were acquired earlier than contour tones.

Putonghua-Speaking Children with Developmental Speech Disorders

Speech disorders in Putonghua-speaking children are rarely reported in the literature. This is partly because of the lack of normative data and partly because of a lack of awareness of such a developmental phenomenon. As a result, speech therapy resources are still to be developed in China and where resources are available, priority seems to have been given to hearing impairment. It was reported that among several speech and hearing clinics newly opened in China, almost all aim to provide an audiological service for the hearing impaired (Cheng, 2001). The lack of understanding on the nature of speech difficulties often lead to clinical misdiagnosis. Xu and Ha (1992) reported that children with speech difficulties in some clinics had been unanimously misdiagnosed as having a short frenum and their unintelligible speech did not improve after the frenum had been cut.

The following description of the characteristics of disordered phonology of Putonghua-speaking children is based on the study carried out by Zhu and Dodd (2000b). In their study, 33 children (nine girls and 24 boys, aged 2;6–7;6) were included in the phonology assessment. These children have normal hearing and language comprehension, but were referred by their nursery and school teachers for their 'atypical' speech. The speech data were assessed using the same picture-naming and picture-description tasks as in the cross-sectional study reported in Zhu and Dodd (2000a). (For picture-naming task, see previous section 'Consonants'.)

A number of quantitative and qualitative measures were used to analyse the children's speech:

- Phonetic inventory: All the sounds produced at least once in the speech sample, irrespective of whether they were the correct targets.
- Phonemic inventory: All the sounds produced both phonetically and phonologically correctly on at least two of three opportunities in different lexical items.
- Error patterns: Error patterns were classified as either age-appropriate, delayed or unusual. Age-appropriate error patterns are those used by at least 10% of the children in the same age band in the normative sample. Delayed error patterns are those used by fewer than 10% of the children in the same age band in the normative data, but appropriate for younger children. Unusual error patterns are those not used among more than 10% of the normally developing children in any age band.
- Percentage of Consonants in Error (PCE): The number of times phonemes are produced in error/the total number of phonemes in the sample × 100.
- Z-score for PCE: The difference between PCE and mean PCE of the children of the equivalent age band in the normative sample divided by standard deviation.
- Inconsistency rating: Comparison of the three productions of each of the 44 words. The number of words with two or three different productions was expressed as a percentage of the total number of words produced three times.

The main findings were as follows:

Despite the diversity of error types, the Putonghua-speaking children with speech disorder seldom made tone errors; only four (12%) children made vowel errors; and only four (12%) children used delayed error patterns affecting syllable-final consonants. Most errors affected syllable-initial consonants.

Four subgroups of children were identified, using Dodd's (1995) classification system (i.e. articulation, delayed development, consistent disorder, and inconsistent disorder). One child (3%) was diagnosed as having an articulation disorder; 18 (54.5%, mean age 4;8) had delayed phonological development; eight (24.2%, mean age 4;3) had consistent disorder, while six (18.2%, mean age 3;8) had inconsistent disorder. General information on the children's age, gender, PCE, z-score for PCE, inconsistency rating and diagnosis in terms of Dodd's classification system is summarised in Table 5.9. The error patterns used by the children in delay, consistent disorder and inconsistent subgroups are summarised in Tables 5.10 and 5.11. The characteristics of each subgroup are discussed in the following sections together with case examples.

Articulation disorder

This subgroup is characterised by mislearning of an articulatory gesture. A girl aged 7;6 was diagnosed as having articulation disorder. She had difficulty articulating /s/ both in word contexts and in isolation. She tended to substitute [θ], a non-Putonghua phoneme, for /s/. There was no apparent organic cause for her impairment: there was no anatomical anomaly and she passed oro-motor, hearing and VMI screening tests.

Delayed group

The largest subgroup had delayed phonological development. Almost all these children had one or several delayed error patterns in their speech, such as consonant assimilation, syllable initial deletion, fronting, stopping, affrication, X-velarisation, and gliding. These error patterns were not found among more than 10% of the children of the same age band in the normative data, but frequently used by more than 10% of the children of a younger age band. Since most error patterns are suppressed by the age of 5;0 in the normative data, the children older than 5;0 whose speech included several delayed error patterns were straightforward cases and often showed a severe degree of delay (see case study of Child 15).

Table 5.9 Quantitative data and diagnosis for speech disordered children

Child	Age	Gender	PCE	Z for PCE	Inconsistency	Diagnosis
1*	7;6	F	2	−0.13	14	Articulation
2	3;7	F	27	1.81	30	Delay
3	3;8	F	27.5	4.01	27	Delay
4	3;11	M	18	2.24	21	Delay
5	4;0	M	14	2.04	21	Delay
6	4;1	M	18	2.83	34	Delay
7	4;2	M	13	1.19	9	Delay
8	4;3	F	19.2	2.93	21	Delay
9	4;3	M	18	1.67	32	Delay
10	4;4	M	19	2.83	34	Delay
11	4;5	F	16	1.28	25	Delay
12	4;6	M	9	0.02	23	Delay
13*	4;7	M	16	1.98	28	Delay
14*	5;0	F	5	−0.25	30	Delay
15*	5;2	M	18	2.69	11	Delay
16*	5;6	M	9	0.92	16	Delay
17*	5;7	F	9	0.50	14	Delay
18*	6;1	M	5	0.21	18	Delay
19*	6;7	M	7	0.04	18	Delay
20	2;8	M	58	3.27	28	Consistent D
21	4;1	M	9	1.10	14	Consistent D
22	4;2	M	25	3.44	33	Consistent D
23	4;2	M	13	1.03	30	Consistent D
24	4;3	M	8	0.45	24	Consistent D
25	4;6	M	28	2.59	16	Consistent D
26*	4;8	F	29	4.38	32	Consistent D
27*	5;6	M	11	0.86	26	Consistent D
28	3;2	M	19	−0.19	58	Inconsistent D
29	3;6	M	39	3.18	49	Inconsistent D
30	3;7	M	64	8.88	76	Inconsistent D
31	3;11	M	43	8.01	49	Inconsistent D
32	3;11	M	39	6.77	60	Inconsistent D
33	4;0	M	2.05	2.05	55	Inconsistent D

Table 5.10 Error patterns used by the subgroup of delayed development

Child no.									Delayed development subgroup									
	2	3	4	5	6	7	8	9	10	11	12	13	14	15	16	17	18	19
Normal error patterns	*																	
Consonant assimilation														*			*	
Syllable initial deletion				*	*									*	*			
Fronting: /ɕ/ → [s]			*	*	*	*	*	*	*	*		*		*		*		*
/ɕ/ → [ʃ/ɕ]											*				*	*		
/k/ → [t]		*																
Backing: /s/ → [ɕ]		*							*	*		*	*	*				
Stopping: /ts/ → [t]	*	*	*		*		*	*	*	*				*			*	
/s/ → [t]	*																	

Error pattern															
/x/ → [k]											*				
Affrication: /ɕ/ → [tɕ]									*			*			
Deaspiration: /tʰ/ → [t]			*												
Aspiration: /t/ → [tʰ]				*											
X-velarisation		*													
Gliding					*	*			*				*		
Final /n/ deletion					*	*				*					
Backing: /n/ → [ŋ]			*							*					
Final /ŋ/ deletion											*				
Triphthong reduction															
Diphthong reduction															

Note: Shaded cells are delayed error patterns for a particular child. Typical examples are given next to each error pattern.

Table 5.11 Error patterns used by the subgroups of consistent and inconsistent disorders

	Consistent disorder										Inconsistent disorder			
	20	21	22	23	24	25	26	27	28	29	30	31	32	33
Normal error patterns	*													
Consonant assimilation		*	*	*				*		*	*			
Syllable initial deletion			*	*			*			*	*	*	*	*
Fronting: /ṣ/ → [s]					*		*				*	*		*
/ɕ/ → [ʃ/ṣ]	*													*
/k/ → [t]				*				*						*
Backing: /s/ → [ṣ]	*													*
Stopping: /ts/ → [t]	*								*	*		*		
/s/ → [t]			*							*		*		
/x/ → [k]		*									*			
Affrication: /ɕ/ → [tɕ]	*					*		*		*		*		*
Deaspiration: /tʰ/ → [t]	*		*							*			*	
Aspiration: /t/ → [tʰ]	*								*					
X-velarisation	*					*			*				*	
Gliding	*	*	*			*	*				*		*	*
Final /n/ deletion	*				*					*				
Backing: /n/ → [ŋ]	*									*				
Final /ŋ/ deletion	*										*			

Normal and Disordered Phonology of Putonghua

Error pattern													
Triphthong reduction	*												
Diphthong reduction		*											
Unusual error patterns													
Final consonant addition			*					*					
Syllable initial addition				*				*					
Vowel change					*								
/ŋ/ → [n]						*							
/ts, tʂ/ → [k]						*							
/k/ → /ts, tʂ/							*						
/tɕ/ → [ɕ]; /tʂ/ → [s]								*					
/k/ → [p]									*				
/ts/ → [tɕ]										*			
ɕ → t											*		
p → tɕ											*		
ʂ → l											*		
f → p												*	
tʂ → p												*	
t → p													*
t → p													*
p → f													*
p → tʂ													*
tɕ → n													*
t → k											*		
ʂ → k											*		
ʂ → f											*		

Note: Shaded cells are delayed error patterns.

> **Case Study: Child 15 (5;2, boy) – delayed development**
> - Four phones (/k, l, ɹ, tsʰ/) missing from his phonetic inventory.
> - Six phonemes (/k, l, ɹ, tʂʰ, ts, tsʰ/) missing from his phonemic inventory.
> - Four delayed error patterns:
>   (a) affricate-stopping (affricates realised as stops, e.g. /tsʰae/ [tae]);
>   (b) fronting velars as alveolars (/k/ realised as [t], e.g. /kua/ [tua]);
>   (c) gliding (/ɹ/ realised as [j], e.g. /ɹoʊ /[joʊ]);
>   (d) consonant assimilation (e.g. /pʰiŋ kuo/ [pʰiŋ puo]).
> - Three normal error patterns:
>   (e) syllable initial deletion (e.g. /liɛn/ [iɛn]);
>   (f) fronting retroflex as alveolar (/ʂ/ realised as [s], e.g. /ʂua/ [sua]);
>   (g) backing alveolar as retroflex (/s/ realised as [ʂ], e.g. /san/ [ʂan]).

Consistent disorder

A range of unusual error patterns were used by eight children diagnosed with consistent phonological disorder. They are syllable-final consonant addition, replacing the syllable-final velar /ŋ/ with alveolar nasal [n], substituting alveolar and retroflex affricates for the velar stop [k] and vice versa, reducing affricates to fricatives of the same place of articulation, etc. Apart from unusual error patterns, some of these children also used delayed error patterns (see case study of Child 21). Some of the children in this subgroup also had a restricted size of phonetic/phonemic inventories compared to normally developing children of the same age band. One child (no. 25, aged 4;6, boy) had four phones (/ɹ, ʂ, tʂ, ts/) missing from his phonetic inventory and seven phonemes (/ɕ, s, ɹ, ʂ, tʂ, tʂʰ, ts/) missing from his phonemic inventory.

> **Case Study: Child 21 (4;1, boy) – consistent disorder**
> - One phone (/ɹ/) missing from his phonetic inventory.
> - Five phonemes (/l, ɹ, tʂ, tʂʰ, ts/) missing from his phonemic inventory.
> - One delayed error pattern – gliding.
> - One unusual error pattern: /tʂ, tʂʰ/ realised as velar stops [k] or [kʰ] (e.g. /tʂəŋ/ [kəŋ]; /tʂʰuaŋ/ [kʰuaŋ]).
> - One normal error pattern: syllable initial deletion.

Inconsistent disorder

Six children classified with inconsistent phonological disorder had inconsistent production of more than 40% of the items when the same words were sampled in three separate trials. Their substitution patterns were unpredictable with the same target being replaced by different error sounds in the same environment. Vowels were also subject to error, while normally developing children rarely made vowel errors. Some sounds were used interchangeably (e.g. one child sometimes replaced/f/with [p] and sometimes replaced/p/with [f]). The case study of Child 30 shows the characteristics of an inconsistently-disordered phonology.

Case Study: Child 30 (3;7, boy) – inconsistent disorder

- Restricted phonetic and phonemic inventories.
- Eleven phones (/tʰ, k, kʰ, pʰ, s, tɕʰ, ʂ, tʂ, tʂʰ, ts, tsʰ/) missing from his phonetic inventory.
- Fifteen phonemes (/tʰ, x, ɕ, k, kʰ, pʰ, ɹ, s, tɕ, tɕʰ, ʂ, tʂ, tʂʰ, ts, tsʰ/) missing from his phonemic inventory.
- Restricted syllable structure: V or CV.
- Frequent occurrence of reduplications: substituting [tia], [tɕia] or [tɕɐ] for a large number of different syllables while retaining the original tones (e.g. /tʌŋ1/ [tia1]; /tʂʰuaŋ2/ [tia2]; /tɕʰyn2 tsi0/ [tɕia² ɕɐ0]).
- Frequent occurrence of assimilation: adjacent syllables sharing the same initial consonant and sometimes the same vowel (e.g. /ɕiaŋtɕiao/ [tiatiao];/nanxan/ [niania];/tsaetɕiɛn/ [tʂʌtʂiaŋ]).
- A number of deviant substitutions: [p] for /k/; [t] for /ɕ/; [l] for /ʂ/.
- Frequent variable productions. Examples:
  (a) /ɕin/ realised as [iŋ], [tia], or [tin];
  (b) /tsʰae/ realised as [sae], [xae], [tʰia], or [tsuo];
  (c) (/ɕywnmɑo/ realised as [iamɑo], [inmɑo], or [tʌmɑo]).

Similarities and differences between Putonghua-speaking children and children speaking other languages

Putonghua-speaking children shared the characteristics common to speech disordered children speaking other languages. These characteristics include persistent delayed error patterns, unusual error patterns, variability, restricted phonetic or phonemic inventory, and systematic sound or syllable preference. Despite these similarities, criteria used in diagnosing speech disorders should be language-specific. In other words, whether a specific error pattern is considered as delayed or unusual is relative to the normal patterns associated with the children acquiring that language. For example, an English-speaking child using a syllable-initial deletion error pattern would be considered disordered while a Putonghua-speaking child would not.

Cross-Populational Similarities and Differences and Phonological Saliency

The data reported here demonstrated that both normally developing and speech disordered Putonghua-speaking children showed similar sensitivity to the structure of the phonological system they were acquiring and the acquisition patterns across these two populations of Putonghua-speaking children were influenced by the saliency value of syllable components.

The notion of phonological saliency has been alluded to by others (e.g. Peters, 1983; Vihman, 1996), but there is no agreement on its definition. In the context of the current study, phonological saliency is used as a syllable-based, language-specific concept. It is determined and affected by a combination of several factors:

- The status of a component in the syllable structure, especially whether it is compulsory or optional; a compulsory component is more salient than an optional one.
- The capacity of a component in differentiating lexical meaning of a syllable; a component which is more capable of distinguishing lexical information is more salient than one which carries less lexical information.
- The number of permissible choices within a component in the syllable structure. For example, 21 syllable-initial consonants would be considered less salient compared to four tonal contrasts.

With regard to Putonghua, tone has the highest saliency: it is compulsory for every syllable; change of tone would change lexical meaning; and there are only four alternative choices. Lexical information of a word in Putonghua is conveyed by both tone and phoneme sequence. Therefore, tone is crucial in differentiating lexical meaning. In contrast, other syllable components are less vital: information lost by an incorrect phoneme within a phoneme sequence can be remedied to some extent by other phonemes in the sequence (e.g. in English we could guess that [lelou] means *yellow*). The phoneme sequence as a whole unit shares the task of conveying lexical meaning. Therefore, the significance of each phoneme in a sequence is less than tone.

The notion of phonological saliency accounts well for the acquisition patterns associated with tones. The studies reported in this book found that:

- Tonal acquisition was completed earlier than syllable-initial consonants, syllable-final consonants, and vowels in normally developing Putonghua-speaking children.
- Tone was resistant to impairment during the process of phonological acquisition. The study on 33 Putonghua-speaking children with speech disorders did not find any children who had difficulty with tones, even among the most severely disordered children. A boy aged 3;7 with inconsistent speech disorder presented an interesting case. He had preference for three consonant-vowel combinations: /tia/, /tɕia/, and /tɕɐ/. While these three combinations substituted for a number of different syllables (sometimes in reduplicated forms), the original tones of target syllables were maintained in the boy's speech.

In comparison, syllable-final consonants have a lower saliency value, because they are an optional component in a Putonghua syllable. However, their saliency value is higher than syllable-initial consonants, because there are only two syllable-final consonants (i.e./n, ŋ/) in Putonghua. The acquisition of syllable-final consonants was relatively error-free and less likely to be subject to impairment than syllable-initial consonants. For example,

- The phonetic acquisition of syllable-final consonants was completed by the age of two, while that of syllable-initial consonants was not completed until 4;6 for 90% of the children.
- Syllable-final consonants were less likely to be subject to impairment than syllable-initial consonants: only four children (12%) were found to have used delayed error patterns affecting syllable-final consonants.

Vowels have a higher saliency value, compared with syllable-initial consonants. Although vowels are a compulsory syllable component, the relatively large number of vowels lowers their saliency. The value of saliency of vowels influenced its acquisitional patterns:

- The vowels emerged early in the children's production, between the age of 1;0 and 2;0. The vowels were more resistant to impairment than syllable-initial consonants. One child (3%) used delayed error patterns affecting vowels and four children (12%) made unusual errors with vowels.

Syllable-initial consonants have the lowest saliency among the four syllable components, since their presence in a syllable is optional and there is a range of 21 syllable-initial phonemes that can be used. The low saliency value of the syllable-initial consonants resulted in their late acquisition and vulnerability to impairment. This is supported by the findings that

- syllable-initial consonants were the last syllable component to be acquired by the normally developing children in the cross-sectional study; and
- syllable-initial consonant errors had a remarkably higher proportion than other syllable components both in the speech of normally developing children and that of children with speech difficulties.

The role of phonological saliency in the acquisition of various syllable components is also supported by the previous research findings. So and Dodd (1995) reported that the consonant acquisition rate of Cantonese-speaking children was more rapid compared to that of English-speaking children. Cantonese-speaking children acquired their range of consonants by 3;6. English-speaking children's phoneme repertoires were not complete until they were five years old (Prather *et al.*, 1975). These discrepancies in consonant acquisition rates between Cantonese and English reflect different saliency ranking of the same syllable component in the two languages. Cantonese has only 17 consonants and two clusters, while English has 24 consonants and 49 clusters. Although consonants are optional syllable components in both languages, the larger number of consonants and clusters in English lowers the saliency of each consonant. Therefore, the rate of acquisition in English is slower than that of Cantonese.

Similarly, Mowrer and Burger (1991) found that Xhosa-speaking children acquired most consonant phonemes earlier than their English-speaking counterparts. although Xhosa has 41 consonants, it has a very simple syllable structure. A typical Xhosa syllable is structured as CV. In addition, Xhosa has very few consonant clusters. Their relatively indispensable status in a syllable and lack of clusters thus contribute to the higher saliency of consonants in Xhosa and explain their early acquisition, when compared to English.

It should be noted, however, that phonological saliency as defined here is a language-specific concept. The saliency value of a particular feature is primarily determined by its role within the phonological system of the language, not by reference to other languages. More cross-linguistic data was needed to test out the explanatory power of the concept of phonological saliency.

Chapter 6
Cantonese Phonological Development: Normal and Disordered

L.K.H. SO

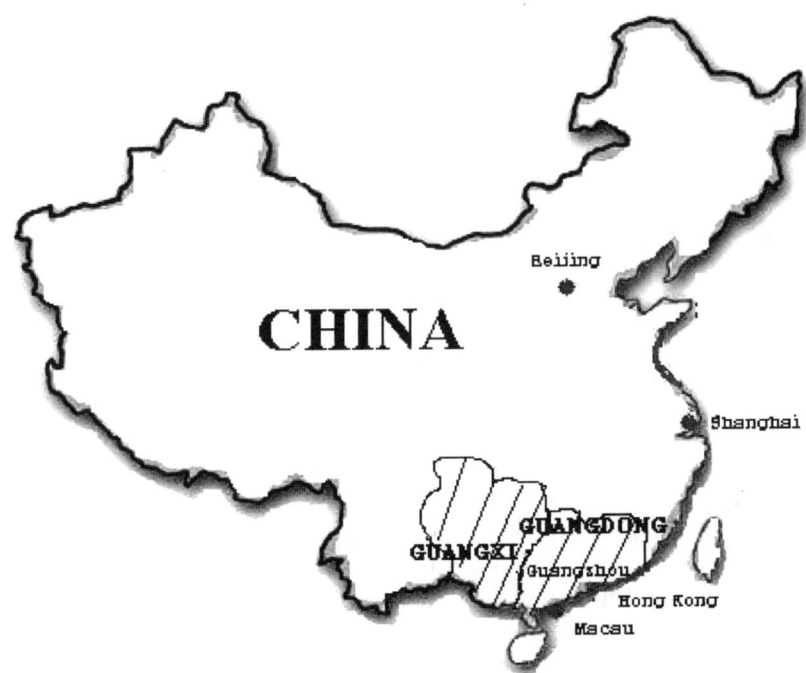

▨▨▨▨ Provinces in China where Cantonese is spoken

Figure 6.1

Introduction

Cantonese is spoken in the central and southwestern parts of Guangdong province and the southern parts of Guangxi province. In the literature, Cantonese is known as Yue Yu and refers to the dialect of the city of Guangzhou. In Hong Kong, 98% of the population speaks Cantonese. Li (1989) estimated that more than 40 million people used Cantonese as the primary language in Hong Kong, Guangzhou and the overseas Cantonese-speaking Chinese in Australia, America, Britain, etc. The variety of Cantonese spoken in Guangzhou and Hong Kong is regarded as the standard form of Cantonese and bears cultural and social prestige (Chao, 1947). In this study, the target language is the variety of Cantonese spoken in Hong Kong. Cantonese is a tone language. Most morphemes in Cantonese are monosyllabic and the structure of the syllable is relatively simple. Hashimoto (1972) proposed the following formula which can represent all Cantonese syllables except the two nasal nuclei [m̩] and [ŋ̍]

$$(C1)(G1) \ V \ (C2/G2).$$

Cheung (1986) proposed the following diagram to illustrate the structure of a Cantonese syllable:

$$\text{Syllable} \rightarrow \frac{\text{Tone}}{\text{(onset) vowel (coda)}}$$

In a Cantonese syllable tone is an obligatory element. Tone is a suprasegmental feature superimposed on the segmental units of a syllable. It is represented by a specific fundamental frequency pattern that is perceived as a pattern of varying pitch. In a tonal language, tone carries lexical meaning and is phonologically contrastive. Six of the nine Cantonese tones are contrastive whereas the other three are variants of the contrastive tones.

Consonants

There are 17 contrastive consonants and two consonant clusters in the Cantonese phonemic system. There are six plosives, three nasals, three fricatives, two affricates, two glides, a lateral and two labialized velar clusters.[1] Table 6.1 shows the Cantonese consonants.

Vowels

There are eight vowel phonemes in Cantonese, namely, /i, y, e, a, œ, ɐ, ɔ, u/.[2] Cantonese phonology differs from that of English in a number of important ways (Table 6.2).

Speech Language Therapy Practice in Hong Kong

Speech therapy is a young profession in Hong Kong. Although a speech therapy service started in 1970s, the scope of service and the knowledge of Cantonese-speaking clients' speech and language characteristics were

Table 6.1 Cantonese initials

	Bilabial	Labio-dental	Alveolar	Palatal	Velar	Labio-velar	Glottal
Stop/clusters	p pʰ		t tʰ		k kʰ	kw kʰw	
Nasal	m		n		ŋ		
Fricative		f	s				h
Affricate			ts tsʰ				
Approximant				j		w	
Lateral approximant			l				

Table 6.2 Differences between Cantonese and English phonology

	Cantonese	English
Tones	Six contrasting, three entering	None
Initial consonants	p pʰ t tʰ k kʰ	p b t d k g
	m n ŋ	m n
	f s h	θ ð f v s z ʃ ʒ h
	w j	w j
	l	l r
	ts tsʰ	tʃ dʒ
Clusters	kw kʰw	p b t d k g θ+l r j
		s+p t k l w
		s+p t k+l r j w
Final consonants	p t k	p b t d k g
	m n ŋ	m n ŋ
	w j	θ ð f v s z ʒ ʃ tʃ dʒ
		l r
Vowels	i ɐ u œ ɔ o ɛ a	i ɪ ɛ æ ʌ ɑ ɒ ɔ ʊ u ɜ ə
		eɪ oʊ aɪ aʊ ɔɪ ɪə ɛə ɔə ʊə
Syllable structure	[C]-[G*]-V-[C/G]	[C_{0-3}]-V-[C_{0-4}]

*G = glide.

very limited. Assessment, diagnosis and intervention strategies were based on knowledge about the English-speaking population. Knowledge on the developmental norms and speech/language error patterns of Cantonese is essential for assessment, diagnosis and treatment of speech/language problems of the Cantonese-speaking clients. With the establishment of the Speech and Hearing Sciences education programme in the University of Hong Kong in 1988, there has been a significant increase in the number of speech therapists in Hong Kong. The speech language therapy service has become more comprehensive and based on research findings from the Cantonese-speaking population. Assessment tools for assessing the Cantonese-speaking population are available too, for example, Reynell Developmental Language Scale (Reynell, 1987) and Cantonese Segmental Phonology Test (So, 1993).

In Hong Kong, speech therapy services are available in hospitals, child assessment centres, health services clinics, the Education department, special schools and voluntary agencies such as early education training centres and integrated child Centres. Private services are also available. Assessment and intervention covers all aspects of communication including all children and adult problems in areas such as speech and languages disorders, voice problems, hearing problems, neurological impairments, etc. A wide range of delivery modes has been used including individual and group therapy, an interdisciplinary team approach and a collaborative approach.

Aims of the Chapter

This chapter will provide background knowledge on the phonological acquisition of Cantonese-speaking children with normal or disordered phonological development.

Previous studies on the phonological acquisition by normally developing Cantonese-speaking children

There have been some studies on the segmental and tonal acquisition of Cantonese. Tse (1982) collected six speech samples from a girl between 19 and 32 months, plus cross-sectional samples from two children aged 20 months and 24 months. These samples were analysed to describe the children's phonetic inventories and phonological processes. At least two of the subjects had acquired the following segments – /m, n, ŋ, p, t, k, ts, ts^h, s, h, j/ by age two. No consistent patterns emerged from Tse's phonological process analysis.

Tse's (1991) longitudinal case study of a Cantonese-speaking boy between 15 and 30 months found evidence for universal trends in the sequence of phoneme acquisition. The acquisition of the language-characteristic feature of aspiration bore a strong resemblance to the acquisition of the voicing contrast in English. The types of phonological errors identified included assimilation, cluster reduction and systemic simplication (e.g. stopping, fronting). Most of these errors can be found in the developmental errors of English-speaking children. While Tse concluded that his findings confirmed Jakobson's (1941/1968) law of implicature, which states that the presence of one phoneme implies the presence of another, he also identified the use, by children acquiring Cantonese, of some phonological rules usually associated with disorder in English-speaking children, e.g. affrication of fricatives.

There are two studies on Cantonese tone development. Light (1977) studied his Cantonese-speaking daughter longitudinally from age 1;4 when the family moved from Hong Kong to the United States. He also provided data on the tone disintegration of his daughter at 1;7 or 2;7. The High Rising tone was substituted by the High Level tone and the Low Rising tone was substituted by the Mid-low tone.

Tse (1978) studied the tonal development of his son, Patrick. He kept a written diary during special observation sessions. He reported on the pattern of his son's tonal development and observed that the perceptual discrimination of linguistic tones began as early as the tenth month. The time span of Patrick's acquisition of the nine Cantonese tones was only eight months from the age of 1;2 to 1;9. This resembles Li and Thompson's (1977) findings for Mandarin children. Tse concluded that the acquisition of tones is completed earlier than that of segmental phonemes.

The few studies of Cantonese phonological development (Light, 1977; Tse, 1991; Tse, 1978; Tse, 1982), all report on the acquisition of Cantonese phonology by normal children. Their studies provide data on the phonological acquisition of only three children or fewer. As there are vast individual differences in children's phonological acquisition (Macken & Ferguson, 1983; Menn, 1976), it is important to study the phonological acquisition of more children to understand the normal developmental patterns.

So and Dodd (1995) studied the phonological development of 268 Cantonese-speaking children and the tonal development of four children. They concluded that the acquisition of tone was completed earlier than vowels which in turn were acquired earlier consonants. The rate of acquisition and the error patterns observed will be reported in this chapter.

Stokes and To (2002) studied the feature distinctions of the phonetic inventories of 112 normally developing Cantonese-speaking children aged 0;10 to 4;7. They also studied ten of these children longitudinally over a year, at three monthly intervals between the age of 1;4 and 2;9. From the children's performance, Stokes and To proposed an implicational feature hierarchy for Cantonese-speaking children. They claimed that the hierarchy could predict the route of sound changes of the children's phonetic inventories.

Stokes and Wong (2002) studied the feature development of 40 children aged 10 to 27 months. They proposed that the factors affecting vowel development are frequency of occurrence and feature complexity. The complexity of feature played a more important role than frequency of occurrence in vowel development between 15 and 18 months.

Previous studies on phonologically disordered Cantonese-speaking children

There are only a few studies on the phonologically disordered children. So and Dodd (1994) studied 17 Cantonese-speaking phonologically disordered children and found that these children could be classified into four different categories: namely articulation disorder, delayed phonological development, consistent phonological disorder and inconsistent phonological disorder. These children exhibited different error patterns. The details will be reported in this chapter.

Cheung and Abberton (2000) described the speech production of 251 phonologically disordered Cantonese-speaking children and concluded that these children's consonant production were more affected than vowels and that tone production was least affected.

Stokes (2002) reported a feature analysis of the longitudinal data from 10 phonologically disordered Cantonese-speaking boys. Dinnsen et al.'s (1990) implicational hierarchy was applied to the data and successful categorization was made for nine of the 10 children, with respect to the phonetic inventory. Eight of 10 children's phonological contrast could be captured by the phonemic inventory based on Dinnsen et al.'s (1990) phonetic inventory. Children with patterns different from the hierarchy were categorised as having deviant rather than delayed phonology.

The phonological acquisition of Cantonese-speaking children: normal development (So & Dodd, 1995)

Most studies of Cantonese phonological development focused on few subjects. So and Dodd (1995) studied the phonological development of 268 Cantonese-speaking children and the tonal development of four children. The method, acquisition rate and the error patterns are summarized below.

Method

Subjects: Cross-sectional study

Two-hundred and sixty-eight Cantonese-speaking children who attended child-care centres or kindergartens in Hong Kong were recruited as subjects. There were altogether eight groups of children in six-month age bands between two and six years: 2;0–2;5 ($n = 26$); 2;6–2;11 ($n = 33$); 3;0–3;5 ($n = 38$); 3;6–3;11 ($n = 33$); 4;0–4;5 ($n = 34$); 4;6–4;11 ($n = 34$); 5;0–5;5 ($n = 34$); and 5;6–5;11 ($n = 36$). Nearly equal numbers of boys and girls were tested in each age group. Children were from a range of socio-economic backgrounds. This was achieved by sampling in four different areas of Hong Kong, Kowloon and the New Territories. None of the children had any intellectual or hearing impairment, or any history of a speech or language disorder and all were acquiring Cantonese as their first and only language. Consent was obtained from all parents.

The test materials

The Cantonese Segmental Phonology Test (So, 1991) was the instrument used in this study. The test presents children with two tasks: naming pictures and re-telling stories; these two tasks comprise the sub-tests of the Test. The picture-naming sub-test employs 57 pictures selected for naming. The names of the objects in the pictures are words that collectively sample two examples of all Cantonese vowels, tones, and initial and final consonants. At least one representative of each class of medial sounds was also sampled. The words chosen name common objects likely to be known by preschool children. High-quality colour four-by-five-inch photographs of real objects were glued onto a separate white card and then laminated in clear plastic. The story re-telling sub-test employs two sets of five five-by-seven-inch photographs glued onto separate cards. Each set illustrates a narrative a child is asked to re-tell. The picture sequences have proved effective in eliciting samples of continuous speech including the pronunciation of words that include all Cantonese vowels, tones, and initial and final consonants. A child sees the two sets of pictures one after the other. One narrative concerns a trip to the park, the other concerns activities related to getting ready for school. A child was judged to have acquired a phoneme if it was produced correctly twice in the single-word naming test. If only one of these two items was correct, the continuous speech from story re-telling was examined to check whether the child had spontaneously produced the phoneme correctly in a second example. The continuous speech data are not otherwise drawn upon in this study.

Longitudinal study

An additional four children took part in a study on the acquisition of tones. At fortnightly intervals, between the ages of 14 and 24 months, two girls and two boys were assessed longitudinally. The children had been born at full term, were healthy and had reached developmental milestones at the appropriate chronological ages. None had any hearing impairment. Cantonese was the primary language spoken in their homes, where the language samples were recorded. Each visit consisted of a period of free play, then play with specific toys and looking at pictures in order to elicit all tones. The data were audiotaped using a high-quality tape recorder and microphone and transcribed immediately after the session. Reliability checks by another transcriber on 10% of the data, covering the total age range, revealed an agreement of 90%.

Results

An overview of the data from the large cross-sectional study is given in Table 6.3. Most errors affect consonants in the syllable-initial position. The percentage of vowel and syllable final errors was small and rose across the age span as the number of syllable initial errors decreased. The total number of errors declined over the age span.

Table 6.3 Overview of speech errors made in the cross-sectional study*

Age	2;0–2;5	2;6–2;11	3;0–3;5	3;6;–3;11	4;0;–4;5	4;6–4;11	5;0–5;5	5;6–5;11
Total errors	501	372	210	158	82	105	27	29
Mean error	19.3	11.3	5.5	4.8	2.4	3.1	0.8	0.8
% SI errors	89.8	76.3	88.6	88.0	82.9	78.1	48.2	75.9
% SF errors	5.0	17.0	8.0	8.2	15.9	10.5	37.0	24.1
% Vowel errors	4.4	5.1	2.9	3.8	1.2	8.6	14.8	0
Unclassifiable	0.8	1.6	0.5	0	0	2.8	0	0

*The above table appeared in So and Dodd (1995).

Table 6.4 Age of acquisition of syllable-initial and -final consonant phonemes (criterion: 90% of subjects)

Age	Male		Female	
	Initial	*Final*	*Initial*	*Final*
2;0	n ŋ	j w	p m n h w j t	j w
2;6	p t j	m	k ŋ l	p k m
3;0	m w k	p n ŋ	f pʰ	
3;6	h	t k	kʰ kw	
4;0	pʰ tʰ kʰ ts kw l f tsʰ		tʰ ts	n ŋ
4;6	s		s kʰw	t
5;0	kʰ w		tsʰ	

Age of acquisition of syllable-initial and -final consonant phonemes

A phoneme was judged acquired if 90% of the children in the sample produced the phoneme correctly in at least two words. Table 6.4 summarises the data. Girls and boys alike acquired all 19 syllable-initial consonants or clusters by five years, and all eight syllable-final segments by four years six months. The girls' acquisition initially proceeded more rapidly than that of the boys, but by four years each had mastered 15 syllable-initial phonemes. Unaspirated plosives and nasals were acquired before fricatives and affricates, unaspirated phonemes before their aspirated partners. The Cantonese-acquiring children's order of acquisition of phonemes is similar to that of children learning English. Like English-acquiring children, Cantonese-speaking children first acquired nasals, glides and bilabial and alveolar stops and thereafter /h/ and /k/. Aspirated plosives, affricates and voiced fricatives were acquired later.

Vowels

Ninety percent of the children in the youngest age group were using all vowels contrastively and all the children in the other age groups did the same. Only 15 children (5.6%) made two or more vowel errors; the total number of vowel errors was 67, representing only 4.5% of total errors. Although there were few errors, there seemed to be one consistent pattern. Vowels were sometimes changed to harmonise with the adjacent consonants, e.g. [kɔk] /kœk/, such harmonisation accounts for 29% of the vowel errors. The other 40 vowel errors showed no consistent error pattern.

Tones

Two children (less than 1%) in the cross-sectional study made tone errors, one four-year-old made two and a five-year-old made three, a frequency of less than in one in 3000 responses. That is, by two years of age most children had mastered tonal contrasts. To gain information concerning the acquisition of tone, four younger children were assessed longitudinally between the ages of 1;2 and 2;0 years. A tone was judged to have been acquired when it was used contrastively on at least 50% of opportunities and mastered when produced correctly on 90% of opportunities. Table 6.5 summarises their acquisition of tone. All four children showed a similar pattern of order and rate of acquisition. They all first acquired two of the three level tones (high-level and mid-level tones) followed by the high rise tone and then the three entering tones. Two of the children then acquired the low level tone before the low fall and low rise tones, whereas child C showed the opposite pattern and child D acquired these three tones simultaneously. The patterns of the children's acquired tones were confirmed to be similar to that of adults' using a *Visipitch* instrument. All children completed their acquisition of tone by 2;0 years and the consistency of the order of acquisition of the nine tones by the four children is apparent from Table 6.5.

Syllable-initial consonant errors

Most errors affected syllable-initial consonants (see Table 6.3). The errors could be classified into three patterns: assimilation, cluster reduction and systemic simplification errors. The proportion of children in each age group who made more than two errors exemplifying phonological error patterns implementing these strategies, is listed in Table 6.6. Many children in the two youngest age groups used the following strategies: assimilation, cluster reduction, and systemic simplification error patterns resulting in stopping, fronting, deaspiration and affrication. The three-year-old children used cluster reduction, stopping and deaspiration while less than 10% of the four-year-old children any one error strategy consistently.

The error patterns used by more than 10% of the sample at any age band are described briefly below.

(1) *Assimilation.* Ninety-two percent of the 51 assimilation errors were examples of a syllable initial alveolar being realised as a velar, in the presence of a syllable final velar (e.g. [k^{h}ɔŋ$_2$] /t^{h}ɔŋ$_2$/).

(2) *Cluster reduction.* The most common realization of k$^{(h)}$w was [k$^{(h)}$]. If the /k/ was fronted it was more likely to realised as a [p] than as a [t] (e.g. [pa$_1$] /kwa$_1$/). It is different from the fronting of a singleton /k/ which was usually fronted to [t], and never to [p] (e.g. [tɐj$_1$] /kɐj$_1$/). Hence in the deletion of /w/, many children took account of its

Table 6.5 Acquisition of tone

Age (months)	16	17	18	19	20	21	22	23	24
Child A	1;3	1;3	1;2;3	1;2;3	1;2;3;6;7;8;9	1;2;3;6;7;8;9	1;2;3;6;7;8;9	Complete	Complete
Child B	1;3	1;3	1;2;3	1;2;3	1;2;3;6;7;8;9	1;2;3;6;7;8;9	1;2;3;6;7;8;9	Complete	Complete
Child C	1;3	1;3	1;2;3	1;2;3	1;2;3;4;5;7;8;9	1;2;3;4;5;7;8;9	1;2;3;4;5;7;8;9	Complete	Complete
Child D	1;3	1;3	1;2;3	1;2;3;7;8;9	1;2;3;7;8;9	1;2;3;7;8;9	Complete	Complete	Complete

Tone code: 1, high level (55); 2, high rise (25); 3, mid level (33); 4, low fall (21); 5, low rise (23); 6, low level (22); 7, high entering (5); 8, mid entering (3); 9, low entering (2).

Table 6.6 Percentage of children using phonological rules affecting syllable-initial consonants in different age groups and the error patterns

Age	2;0–2;5	2;6–2;11	3;0–3;5	3;6–3;11	4;0–4;5	4;6–4;11	5;0–5;5	5;6–5;11	Most common error forms
No errors	*3.8*	*6.1*	*23.7*	*24.2*	*50*	*41.2*	*70.6*	*75*	
Structural simplification									
Assimilation[#]	38.5	21.2	7.9	6.1	–	5.9	–	–	Alveolars harmonise with SF velars
Cluster reduction	76.9	39.4	26.3	24.2	2.9	8.8	2.9	–	kʰw: [kʰ] 43% [pʰ] 34% [t] 9% [f] 8%, kw: [k] 44%, [p] 27% [t] 8% [w] 4% [f] 16%
/h/ deletion	11.5	6.1	5.3	3.0	2.9	–	–	–	
I.C.D.[†]	7.7	9.1	–	–	2.9	–	–	–	
Systemic simplification									
Stopping	61.5	36.4	15.8	15.2	5.9	8.8	2.9	2.7	Same place 88%

Continued

Table 6.6 (Continued)

Age	2;0–2;5	2;6–2;11	3;0–3;5	3;6–3;11	4;0–4;5	4;6–4;11	5;0–5;5	5;6–5;11	Most common error forms
No errors	3.8	6.1	23.7	24.2	50	41.2	70.6	75	
Fronting	46.2	24.2	10.5	9.1	8.6	2.9	2.9	2.7	$k^{(h)}$w: [p] 61% [t] 31% [f] 8%; $k^{(h)}$: [t] 97% [ts] 3%
Deaspiration	57.7	33.3	31.6	9.1	8.6	–	–	2.7	[p t k ts kw]
Affrication	42.3	18.2	7.9	6.1	8.8	2.9	2.9	2.7	[ts$^{(h)}$]
Deaffrication	3.8	18.2	5.3	3.0	–	8.8	2.9	2.7	
F.C.D.*	15.4	21.2	–	–	–	–	–	–	
Frication	7.7	3.0	5.3	–	–	–	–	–	
Aspiration	7.7	–	2.6	6.1	8.8	5.9	–	–	
Gliding	7.7	3.0	2.6	3.0	2.9	5.9	–	–	
Backing	3.8	3.0	5.3	3.0	2.9	5.9	–	–	

#Most commonly rules assimilation; *final consonant deletion; †initial consonant deletion.

place of articulation in choosing how to mark the cluster. Older children often marked the level of aspiration of the target cluster while reducing the clusters also by realising /kw/ as [f] but /k^{h}w/ as [p$^{(h)}$].
(3) /h/ deletion. Only the youngest group of children delete /h/.
(4) *Stopping.* Fricatives and affricates /f, s, ts, ts^h/ were realised as a plosive at same place of articulation and this accounted for 88% of the stopping errors. Unaspirated /t/ was mostly used by younger children in stopping both the aspirated and unaspirated affricates /ts^h, ts/. However, the aspirated continuant /ts^h/ was realised as the aspirated plosive /t^h/ 81% of occasions by children aged 2;6 to 3;5 with only 19% /t/ substitutions.
(5) *Fronting.* The velar plosives /k/ and /k^h/ were realised as /t/ by the younger children. When the children suppressed the de-aspiration process, /k^h/ was substituted by /t^h/. When /k/ and /k^h/ occurred in clusters, the fronting pattern was different (see above).
(6) *Deaspiration.* Deaspiration was a prominent process in the Cantonese-speaking children's data. This process often occurred with other processes such as stopping and fronting.
(7) *Affrication.* Thirty percent of children under the age of 3;0 affricated fricatives (e.g. [tsy] /sy/). The Cantonese-speaking children did not acquire fricatives or affricates as part of their phonemic repertoire until they were aged at least 2;6. The error pattern of affrication was not expected, and children used [ts] to mark /s/ though /ts/ was not part of their phonemic repertoire.
(8) *Deaffrication.* Affricates /ts, ts^h/ were realised as /s/ by 22% of children under age of three.

Initial consonant deletion, frication, aspiration, gliding and backing were error patterns produced by a small number of children.

Syllable-final consonants

Relatively fewer errors were made on syllable-final consonants. Thirty-seven children (13.8%) made more than two errors on syllable-final consonants, resulting in 159 errors (10.7% of total errors). Three error patterns accounted for all errors: fronting (e.g. [pen] /peŋ/), accounting for 28.9% of syllable-final errors; backing (e.g. [mɐk] /mɐt/), 34.6%; and final consonant deletion (e.g. [sa] /sam/), 36.5%. Fifteen percent of the 2;0–2;6 group and 21% of the 2;6–2;11 group deleted syllable-final consonants.

Discussion

The results from the analyses of speech samples from 268 Cantonese-speaking suggested that Cantonese-speaking children completed their acquisition of tones before vowels and syllable final consonants, which in turn are acquired before syllable-initial consonants.

Phoneme acquisition

The order of phoneme acquisition by Cantonese-speaking children supported Jackobson's (1941/1968) law of irreversible solidarity that nasals are acquired before orals, stops before fricatives and front sounds before back sounds. The last sounds acquired by Cantonese-speaking children are the fricatives, affricates and the aspirated sounds. Cantonese-speaking children's acquisition of phonemes is at a more rapid rate than that reported for English-speaking children but the order of acquisition is similar for both groups of children. These findings are in agreement with the results of case studies of children acquiring Cantonese (Tse, 1982; Tse, 1991).

Feature acquisition

The features of affrication and aspiration are acquired last. Affrication has been reported to be acquired late in a number of languages. Prather *et al.* (1975) reported that English-speaking children acquired the affricates /tʃ, dʒ/ later than other phonemes. However, in other languages, Japanese and Italian, affricates are acquired earlier than other phonemes (Yasuda, 1970, cited in Locke, 1983; Battacchi, 1964, cited in Locke, 1983b). Differences in the sequence of phoneme acquisition in different languages may suggest the influence of the ambient language on acquisition.

Error pattern

The error patterns used by Cantonese-speaking children supported universal trends but also illustrated language-specific patterns. Assimilation, stopping, and fronting are observed in other languages such as English and Italian. Other error patterns such as affrication, and deaspiration are used by Cantonese-speaking children but not English-speaking children.

Factors affecting rate and order of acquisition

Cantonese-speaking children seem to be faster in completing their acquisition of the consonant phoneme inventory than English-speaking children. Ingram (1989a) suggests that the rate and order of acquisition of consonants are determined by their functional load, where functional load is measured in terms of the number of oppositions or minimal pairs in which a consonant occurs in a child's language environment. While variation in the order of acquisition of consonants might be elegantly explained in this way, it is a less plausible explanation for rate of acquisition of a phoneme inventory in a particular language. The way of determining functional load does not include other aspects of phonology that might contribute, relatively, to the functional loading of consonants: vowels, syllable structure, stress and tone.

Vowels are important in English phonology as they are oppositional and have distinctive syllabic value. Therefore vowels carry a heavy functional load in English. English has a large number of consonant clusters and a more complex syllable structure. Stress in Cantonese is correlated with tone, higher tones receiving greater stress (Hashimoto, 1972). Tone carries a functional load in Cantonese but not in English. The concept of functional load might be useful if expanded to include not only consonant, but also consonant clusters, vowels, tones and stress. Cantonese words are mainly monosyllables and have a relatively simple syllabic structure. There are only eight vowel phonemes. Hence consonants plus tones carry a heavy functional load and, would need to be acquired early. In English, words are differentiated by vowels, syllable structure and stress as well as consonants. Hence the functional loading of English consonants seems to relatively less than that of Cantonese. It is plausible that the relative contributions of consonants, vowels, syllable structure, stress and tones affect the rate of acquisition of these elements.

Conclusions

The prediction that the pattern of phonological errors would reflect Smith's (1973) universal tendencies of assimilation, cluster reduction and systemic simplification was confirmed. Children's understanding of the structure of Cantonese phonology was reflected in the rules used. The emergence of Cantonese-speaking children's consonant phoneme inventories provides evidence that phonological acquisition follows linguistic universal tendencies but is affected by language-specific contexts. While there maybe a universal order of acquisition, the rate of acquisition may differ depending on the need to use a particular element to mark differences between words in a language. Acquisition of Cantonese consonants is faster than English consonants. This may suggest that consonants are salient for the differentiation between words in Cantonese phonology.

Phonological ability and classification of Cantonese-speaking children with phonological disorders

So and Dodd (1994) studied 17 monolingual Cantonese-speaking children aged between 3;6 to 6;4 who were consecutively referred for assessment of disordered speech.

The aims of the study were to answer the following questions:

(1) What are the speech characteristics of Cantonese-speaking children with speech disorders?
(2) Can the phonologically-disordered children be classified into subgroups according to their speech performance?
    - articulation disorder (e.g. lisp),
    - delayed phonological development,

- consistent use of one or more unusual rules,
- inconsistent errors.

(3) What are the differences in the speech of Cantonese-speaking children with phonological disorders and those with normal development?

Method

Subjects

Seventeen children, 13 boys and four girls, aged between 3;6 and 6;4 years were recruited as subjects. They were referred to the Phonology Clinic, Department of Speech and Hearing Sciences, University of Hong Kong during one academic semester. All children attended kindergarten for five days a week. The range of parental occupations included business executives, skilled and unskilled labourers, office clerks, a teacher and a missionary. Cantonese was the children's primary language, although some English might be in daily use in some families (e.g. communicating with the Filipino maid).

In order to exclude any other factors that might affect the children's phonological development other than phonological disorder, the following criteria were used:

(1) normal hearing,
(2) normal intelligence,
(3) no abnormalities in oral structure,
(4) normal language ability.

Table 6.7 provides a summary of the subjects' characteristics and includes, as an indication of severity, the percentages of 121 consonants, 67 vowels and 38 tones spoken in error during the Cantonese Segmental Phonology Test (So, 1992). The table also lists the classification of subgroup of phonological disorder to which each child was assigned.

Procedure

Children were assessed in a sound-proof suite by a speech therapist and a final year student clinician. A parent of each child was always present. The first 10 minutes were spent establishing rapport with the children through free play. Once the children had explored the environment and were happy to cooperate, the Cantonese Segmental Phonology Test (So, 1992) was administered. After completion of the test, an oromotor examination was done and parents were interviewed to obtain case history information. All sessions were both audio- and video-taped.

Analyses

The sessions were transcribed within two days. A phoneme was judged be part of the child's phonetic repertoire if it was used correctly

Table 6.7 Speech disordered subjects' information, percentage error and diagnosis*

Subject	Age	Sex	Oral structure and function	Any additional problems	% error Tones	% error Vowels	% error Consonants	Diagnosis
N.F.	5;10	M	Tongue thrust		0	0	3.3	Articulation
K.Y.H.	5;0	F	Short velum	Hypernasality	0	0	16.5	Articulation
S.F.	3;6	M			0	0	20.7	Delay
K.P.	3;7	M			0	0	20.7	Delay
C.M.	4;6	M			0	0	5.8	Delay
K.L.	4;11	M			0	0	36.4	Delay
C.S.	5;1	M			0	0	24.0	Delay
K.Y.	5;2	M			0	0	16.5	Delay
F.W.	5;3	M			0	0	21.5	Delay
C.W.	5;4	F			0	0	31.4	Delay
J.M.	4;1	M		Language	0	10.4	28.9	Articulation and consistent P.D.
Y.Y.	4;6	M			0	1	19.8	Consistent P.D.
Y.W.	4;8	M			0	0	17.4	Consistent P.D.
Y.L	5;11	F			0	0	18.2	Articulation and consistent P.D.
O.L.	5;11	F		Voice	0	17.9	34.7	Consistent P.D.
T.C.	4;7	M		Language	3	0	20.7	Inconsistent P.D.
M.Y.	6;4	M			0	4	38.0	Inconsistent P.D.

*Also appeared in So and Dodd (1994).
P.D. = phonological disorder.

at least twice, and an error pattern was considered to be used if there were at least two occurrences of the error in different lexical items and no counter examples. Audiotapes of the Cantonese Segmental Phonology Test (So, 1992), administered in the initial assessment session, were re-transcribed by the speech therapist to check for reliability with the initial transcription. Four tapes were re-transcribed and point to point reliability was high: 98.5%. The children's patterns of errors were compared with those of the 268 two- to six-year-old children whose phonological acquisition was described in the previous section. The 17 speech disordered children were categorized into four subgroups according to their error patterns.

Results

There were four groups of children (see Table 6.7). Two children had articulation difficulties and eight children showed delayed phonological pattern. Five children consistently used at least one unusual phonological rule and two of these children also distorted /l/ and /or /s/. The other two children made inconsistent errors. Each case is briefly outlined below. Table 6.8 provides a summary of the processes and rules used by the delayed and phonologically disordered children.

Articulation

N.F.   Due to tongue thrust, this 5;10-year-old boy distorted /s, ts, ts^h/. His phoneme repertoire, tones and range of syllable structures were complete.

K.Y.H. This girl's articulation was characterised by hypernasality and exaggerated aspiration of aspirated sounds which is a result of incomplete closure of the soft palate with the oropharyngeal wall. She had a short velum. Apart from the absence of the syllable-initial /f/, all syllable-final consonants, tones and syllable structures were used correctly.

Delay

Phonemes in bold exist as part of the child's *phonetic* repertoire (i.e. were used as a substitute for other sounds or could be imitated in isolation, although not all sounds were elicited in isolation in the sessions for all children and thus the extent of the children's phonetic repertoires may be underestimated).

S.F.   (3;6 male)
- Missing phonemes were: /p^h, **t^h, k^h**, **f**, s, **ts^h**, h, k^{h}w/.
- Four delayed error patterns
    (a) stopping, e.g. [paj] /faj/, [tai] /sai/,
    (b) deaspiration, e.g. [piŋ] /p^{h}iŋ/,
    (c) /h/ deletion, e.g. [aj] /haj/,

Table 6.8 The processes and rules used by children classified as delayed and consistent disordered

Subjects:	Delayed								Disordered				
	S.F.	K.P.	C.M.	K.L.	C.S.	K.Y.	F.W.	C.W.	J.M.	Y.Y.	Y.W.	Y.L.	O.L.
Assimilation					*	*							
Cluster reduction		*		*	*	*		*					
Stopping	*		*	*	*	*	*	*					
Fronting	*	*	*	*	*	*		*					*
Deaspiration	*	*			*		*	*				*	
Affrication	*					*							
/h/ deletion	*	*				*							
Deaffrication													
F.C.D.#	*	*		*						*			*
F.G.D.‡	*			*					*	*			*
Frication										*			
I.C.D.†											*		
Aspiration													
Gliding									*			*	
Vowel rule	*								*		*		*
Backing	*										*	*	*

#Final consonant deletion; †initial consonant deletion; ‡final glide deletion (modified from So & Dodd, 1994).

(d) affrication, e.g. [tsœj] /sœj/, [tsow] /tow/.

K.P. (3;7 male)
- Missing phonemes were: /pʰ, tʰ, **kʰ**, f, s, ts, tsʰ, **h**, kʰw/.
- Four delayed error patterns
    (a) stopping, e.g. [paj] /faj/, [tai] /sai/,
    (b) deaspiration, e.g. [pi] /pʰiŋ/,
    (c) /h/deletion, e.g. [aj] /haj/,
    (d) final consonant deletion, e.g. [pa] /pan/, [tɔ] /tʰɔŋ/.

C.M. (4;6 male)
- Missing phoneme was: /s/.
- Two delayed error patterns
    (a) stopping, e.g. [tɐj] /sɐj/,
    (b) deaspiration, e.g. [piŋ] /pʰiŋ/.

K.L. (3;7 male)
- Missing phonemes were: /**k**, kʰ, kʰw/.
- Four delayed error patterns
    (a) cluster reduction, e.g. [paj] /faj/, [tai] /sai/,
    (b) fronting, e.g. [tɐi] /kɐi/, [bwa] /kwa/, [pʰɐ] /kʰwɐn/,
    (c) final consonant deletion, e.g. [ha] /ham/, [wu] /wun/, [pe] /peŋ/,
    (d) final glide deletion, e.g. [fa] /faj/, [tsi] /tsiw/, [ma] /maw/.

C.S. (5;1 male)
- Missing phonemes were: /**tʰ, k**, kʰ, f, s, **ts**, tsʰ, kw, kʰw/.
- Five delayed error patterns
    (a) assimilation,
    (b) cluster reduction, e.g. [pʰɐn] /kʰwɐn/,
    (c) stopping, e.g. [tɐj] /sɐj/,
    (d) fronting, e.g. [tɐj] /kɐj/,
    (e) deaspiration, e.g. [piŋ] /pʰiŋ/.

K.Y. (5;2 male)
- Missing phonemes were: /f, **s**, kw, kʰw/
- Six delayed error patterns
    (a) assimilation, e.g. [kɐk] /kɐt/,
    (b) cluster reduction (optional), e.g. [pʰɐn] /kʰwɐn/,
    (c) stopping, e.g. [tœj] /sœj/,
    (d) fronting, e.g. [pɐj] /kɐj/,
    (e) affrication (optional), e.g. [tsʰœj] /sœj/,
    (f) /h/deletion, e.g. [a]/ha/.

F.W. (5;3 male)
- Missing phonemes were: /**pʰ, tʰ, kʰ**, f, s, ts, tsʰ, kʰw/.
- Two delayed error patterns
    (a) stopping, e.g. [paj] /faj/, [tuk] /tsuk/, [tœj] /sœj/,
    (b) deaspiration, e.g. [piŋ] /pʰiŋ/.

C.W. (5;4 female)
- Missing phonemes were: /pʰ, tʰ, kʰ, f, s, ts, tsʰ, kw, kʰw/.
- Four delayed error patterns
  (a) cluster reduction, e.g. [wa] /kwa/,
  (b) stopping, e.g. [tœj] /sœj/,
  (c) fronting, e.g. [tɐj] /kɐj/,
  (d) deaspiration, e.g. [piŋ] /pʰiŋ/.

Phonological disorder: Consistent errors
J.M. (4;1, male)
- Missing phoneme was syllable final alveolar nasal /-n/.
- Three unusual error patterns
  (a) final glide deletion, e.g. [pa] /paj/, [hi] /hœj/,
  (b) backing, e.g. [fɐŋ] /fɐn/,
  (c) vowel errors, confusion between two vowels, /ɐ, e/ e.g. [mɐj] / mej/, [tʰej] /tʰɐj/.

Y.Y. (4;6 male)
- Missing phonemes were, /tʰ, kʰ, tsʰ/,
- Three unusual error patterns
  (a) frication, e.g. [hœ] /sœj/,
  (b) syllable-final nasals are deleted, e.g. [wu] /wun/,
  (c) Syllable-final glides are deleted, e.g. [ha] /haj/, [pu] /puj/.

Y.W. (4;8 male)
- Missing phonemes were: syllable-initial, /s, f, ts, tsʰ/.
- Two unusual error patterns
  (a) syllable-initial fricatives (except /h/) and affricates delete, e.g. [aj] /faj/, [i] /tsi/,
  (b) syllable-final /n/ is velarised, e.g. [paŋ] /pan/.

Y.L. (5;11 female)
- Missing phonemes were: syllable-initial /pʰ, tʰ, kʰ, tsʰ, kʰw/.
- Three unusual error patterns
  (a) deaspiration, e.g. [piŋ] /pʰiŋ/, [kɐm] /kʰɐm/,
  (b) backing, alveolar plosives become velar, e.g. [kow] /tow/, [kɐj] /tʰɐj/,
  (c) gliding, syllable-initial /l, n/ are realised as /j/, e.g. [jaj] /laj/, [jɐw] /nɐw/.

O.L. (5;11 female)
- Missing phonemes: syllable-initial /k, kʰ, kw, kʰw/, and syllable-final consonants: /p, t, m, ŋ w, j/. Two vowels were also missing: /ɐ, œ/.
- Five error patterns
  (a) fronting, e.g. [tœk] /kœk/, [pʰwa] /kʰwɐn/,
  (b) syllable-final nasals deletion, e.g. [wu] /wun/,

(c) backing, syllable-final /p, t/ are realised as /k/, e.g. [mɐk] / mɐt/, [ak] /ap/,
(d) syllable-final glide deletion, e.g. [tsi] /tsiw/, [pu] /puj/,
(e) vowel substitutions, e.g. /ɐ/ → [a]; /œ/ → [ɔ].

O.L. had a phonotactic constraint that specified that /k/ could not be used in the initial syllable position but was used as the only syllable-final consonant. Such a syllable constraint is atypical of normal development.

Phonological disorder: Inconsistent
T.C. (4;7 male)
- Missing phonemes were /**s, tʰ, n**/.
- Most errors affected alveolar consonants /s, tʰ, n/ and are summarised below
  (a) /t/ → [j], or delete, e.g. /tin/ was realised as [jin] and [in],
  (b) /tʰ/ → [h], or delete, e.g. /tʰɔŋ/ was realised as [hɔŋ] and [ɔŋ],
  (c) /s/ → [h], [t], or delete, e.g. /sœj/ was realised on different occasions as [hœj], [tœj] and [œj],
  (d) /l/ → [j], delete or correct, e.g. /lej/ was pronounced as [jej], [ej] but also as [lej],
  (e) /n/ → [l], or delete, e.g. [lɐw] /nɐw/, [ɐw] /nɐw/.

There were also some other odd substitutions e.g. /j/ → [m]; /m/ → [n], f → [m] and inconsistent initial consonant deletions of /k, j/.

M.Y. (6;6 male)
- Missing syllable-initial consonants: /**pʰ, t, tʰ, k, kʰ, l, s, ts, tsʰ, kʰw**/ and syllable-final consonants /**p, t, m**/.
- The characteristics of M.Y.'s phonology were
  (a) initial consonants deletion,
  (b) syllable-final consonants e.g. [ak] /ap/, [mɐk] /mɐt/,
  (c) all consonants are deaspirated,
  (d) clusters were reduced inconsistently: e.g. [wɔɐŋ] /kʰwɐn/; /kʰw/ → [f], e.g. [fɐŋ] /kʰwɐn/; /kʰw/ → [kw], e.g. [kwɐŋ] /kʰwɐn/; e.g. [ɐŋ] /kʰwɐn/. There were also inconsistent vowel errors, e.g. /œ/ → [u], /e/ → [ɐ], /a/ → [e]; and consonant substitutions, e.g. /p/ → [f]; /pʰ/ → [f]; /j/ → [h]; /w/ → [m], /k/ → [m].

M.Y.'s phonology is not a straightforward inconsistency case. This may be due to the fact that he deletes many syllable-initial consonants and marks all syllable-final consonants as /k/. When a child starts receiving therapy and breaks the syllable constraints, inconsistency may become more apparent. For example, Woodyatt and Dodd (1995) reported a child who produced all syllables as [hV] when phonological contrast therapy successfully suppressed the syllable constraint, a variety of phonemes were inconsistently used to mark word initial consonants.

Discussion

Four subgroups of speech disorder were identified in a group of children. The errors could be classified as articulation disorder, delay, consistent use of unusual (non-developmental) rules and inconsistent errors. Articulation disorders can be found in the acquisition of all languages. Two of the Cantonese-speaking children had pure articulation difficulties of organic origin. An additional two children, who used unusual error patterns also had difficulty articulating /s/ and /l/. The two disorders can occur together (Elbert, 1992), although it is important to distinguish between articulation and phonological disorder because treatment approaches for the two disorders differ markedly (Fey, 1992).

Eight of the Cantonese-speaking children exhibited delayed phonological development. Some straightforward cases of cluster reduction indicated a phonological system that was typical of a specific younger age group, e.g. C.S., a five-year-old boy, was behaving, phonologically, like a typical three-year-old. Some other children used error pattern that occur in early development and in later development. This provided examples of chronological mismatches (Grunwell, 1985). K.L.'s treatment of syllable-final consonants is an example of a chronological mismatch. None of the delayed children exhibited syllable structure constraints or were identified as having delayed acquisition of expressive or receptive language. They did not make a significant number of vowel or tone errors. Their phonological delay was restricted to the consonant system.

Delayed phonological development has been found in children acquiring other languages. For example, Yavaş and Lamprecht (1988) reported that two of the four phonologically disordered Portuguese-speaking children showed a delayed pattern of acquisition while Bortolini and Leonard's (1991) group of nine phonologically disordered Italian-speaking children used developmental error patterns. Some of the Cantonese-speaking speech disordered children used unusual phonological error patterns. Such an error may arise from an impaired understanding of the nature of the phonological system being acquired (Vasanta & Dodd, 1991). Phonologically disordered children may not be able to make use of the phonetic regularities of the language to govern their output (Leonard et al., 1989).

Two of the phonologically disordered children made many vowel errors. Many words in Cantonese consist of CV syllables, so vowel errors are associated with unintelligibility. There are few reports in the literature of vowel difficulties in children. It is surprising, then, that two out of five Cantonese-speaking phonologically disordered children made a high percentage (more than 10%) of vowel errors. It may be that the Cantonese vowel system is more vulnerable to disorder than the English.

In contrast, the entire data set revealed only one tonal error. Tones carry a heavy functional load in Cantonese, e.g. /ji$_1$/ aunty, /ji$_2$/ chair, /ji$_3$/ meaning, /ji$_4$/ move, /ji$_5$/ ear, /ji$_6$/ two, where each subscript number denotes a different tone. And, in line with the present results, clinicians working in Hong Kong anecdotally report tone disorders to be very rare.

The two children classified as inconsistent each had distinctive patterns of errors. T.C.'s pattern of inconsistency was mainly limited to alveolar consonants, and his range of errors was also limited to deletion of /h, t, j/. These sounds were allophones for T.C. whose error pattern might reflect his impaired ability to assemble phonological plans for words that contrast alveolar consonants.

M.Y.'s pattern of errors might be attributed to a similar deficit. He deleted a wide range of syllable-initial consonants and used /k/ to mark all syllable-final consonants except glides. This might suggest the use of a syllable strategy to overcome an impaired ability to assemble contrastive phonological plans for words (Dodd et al., 1989). Bradford (1990) argues an alternative account of inconsistent errors that, although the ability to assemble phonological blueprints for words is intact, these plans fail because of the speaker's inability to plan the sequences of fine motor movements for speech production. Both accounts of the deficit underlying inconsistent errors seem plausible. Without further and more incisive research the nature of the deficit or deficits that might underlie inconsistent speech errors will remain elusive.

Conclusion

The 17 cases of Cantonese-speaking speech-disordered children reported here could be categorised into the same four groups reported for English-speaking speech-disordered children (Dodd, 1993): articulation disorder, delayed phonological development, consistent use of unusual phonological rules and inconsistent errors. The speech characteristics of these four groups of children differed from that of normally developing children and also from each other. The different patterns of surface speech errors arguably relate to a range of deficits at different levels of the speech processing chain. Consequently the more important question for clinical research is which specific remediation approach is most successful for each subgroup of phonological disorder and not whether one remediation approach is better than another for phonologically disordered children in general (Gierut, 1990).

Notes

1. Some phonologists view the labialised velar clusters /k^{h}w, kw/ as labialised velar stops /k^h, k/.
2. Some phonologists stated that there were 11 vowels /i, y, ɪ, e, œ, ə, a, ɐ, ɔ, u, ʊ/ and 11 diphthongs /ai, ɐi, au, ɐu, ei, əy, ɔi, ui, iu, ou, eu/ in the Cantonese vowel system.

Chapter 7
Phonological Development of Maltese-Speaking Children

H. GRECH

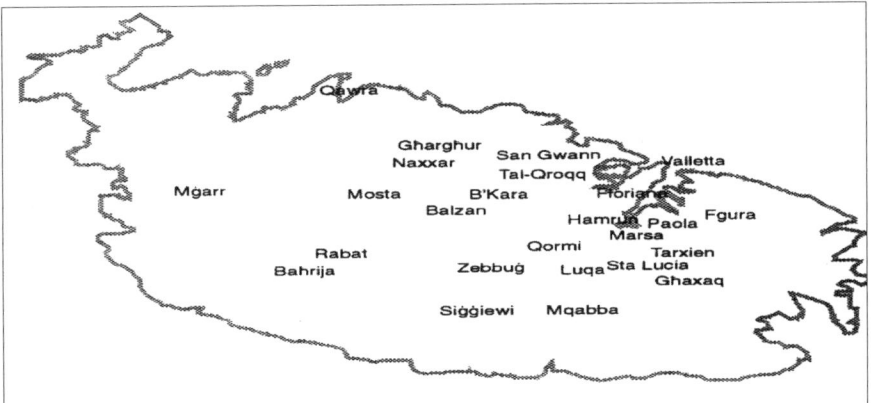

Figure 7.1 Geographical distribution of the sample

Introduction

Maltese is the vernacular of most people living on the Maltese Islands, situated in the middle of the Mediterranean Sea. Maltese is a derivative of Arabic introduced to the Maltese Islands sometime between AD 870 and 1090. Maltese has developed independently ever since the end of the Arab occupation of the Maltese Islands in 1090 AD. It is spoken by one third of a million people living on the islands. However, it is claimed that there are more Maltese emigrants, living mainly in Australia and the United States of America, than there are Maltese living in Malta and Gozo (unavailable data, National Statistics Office, 2003a). Some of these emigrants (especially the first generation members of families, who are now senior citizens) still speak Maltese with their families outside their home countries.

Before the Maltese Islands became a Republic in 1978, they were controlled by various colonies including the Phoenicians, Romans, Normans, Knights of St John and finally the British. All these left an impact on the spoken language of the Maltese. The Maltese grammar is

Semitic amalgamated with influences from other languages. The vocabulary contains English, French and Italian influence. This progressive meshing of other languages on to the original Arabic dialect has made it a unique, independent and a separate language.

Sociolinguistics of Maltese

Until 1800, standard literary Italian and the indigenous vernacular were Malta's two languages. From 1814 the British colonists in Malta commanded the diffusion of the English language among the Maltese inhabitants and the adoption of every means of substituting English for the Italian language. Despite the modest revival of Italian in recent years, it is now considered and studied as a 'foreign' language through the medium of English. Maltese was often considered as a utility rather than a real medium of modern culture (Hull, 1993). Today English still carries prestige in Malta. Borg (1980) refers to the Maltese English used which is really utterances containing both Maltese and English words/phrases, i.e. code-switching. He claims that the amount of mixing of the two languages depends on the linguistic abilities, social context, sex and social background of the individual. The supremacy of English in the schools, in the past decades, reflects on the fact that nowadays many Maltese still find it easier to write English than Maltese. Apart from local newspapers, most educated people still prefer reading English books to the relatively few available in Maltese. Malta is experiencing linguistic change primarily resulting from inter-ethnic marriages, the more positive attitude of the Maltese towards their indigenous language, the increasing incidence of bilingualism and multilingualism amongst the local population, the official status of Maltese as one of the languages of the European Union and the push by local education authorities, politicians and parents towards multilingualism claiming it beneficial for employment prospects and for intercultural mixing. Figure 7.2 highlights published data following the National Census (Malta Central Office of Statistics, 1995) and the Lingua Survey

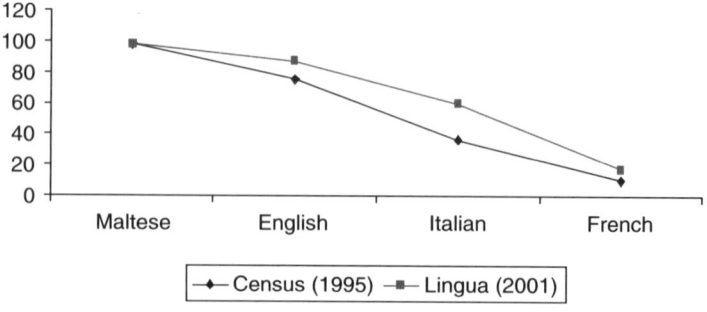

Figure 7.2 Languages known by the Maltese (% of sample population)

(Sciriha & Vassallo, 2001) related to the main languages used by the Maltese. The National Minimal Curriculum (Ministry of Education, 1999) endorses bilingualism as the basis of the educational system. Most children are taught a third language in schools. Sciriha (1999) reports that more than 80% of children attending Church or Independent schools and 10% of those in state schools are taught a fourth language. What we have today, is children who from a very early age use Maltese with English words amalgamated and meshed into Maltese child language.

The Phonetics of Maltese

Azzopardi's (1981) analysis of sound patterns is based on a stricter phonetic approach than previous studies had taken in deciding which phonemes are Maltese. She introduces the sound system of Maltese in terms of minimal contrast including minimal pairs (relatively few in Maltese) plus consonantal and vocalic duration differences. Table 7.1 and Figures 7.3 and 7.4 include the derived consonants, monophthongs and diphthongs of Maltese following Azzopardi's research project which she later updated in Borg and Azzopardi-Alexander (1997). She claims that her system of phonemes does not take into account any morphological, lexical or syntactic considerations. The sound system of Maltese that Azzopardi derives includes 22 consonantal phonemes[1] (three of which are affricates), 11 monophthongs and seven diphthongs.

The Phonetic Description of Groups

The consonantal phonemes

Table 7.1 below summarises the place and manner of articulation of each phoneme.

Oral stops (plosives)

Voiceless plosives /p/, /t/ and /k/ are generally aspirated in all contexts. Aspiration is not contrastive in Maltese. Oral stops are always audibly released in Maltese irrespective of their position in the word. This also applies when they occur in clusters. The consonants /p/ and /b/ are produced as labial oral stops. /t/ and /d/ are considered as flat apical advanced alveolar stops. /k/ and /g/ have their main stricture occurring just forward of the post palatal region though it usually extends as far back as the velar region. The glottal stop in Maltese is produced with complete closure of the glottis and is always audibly released same as other voiceless oral stops even when it occurs in clusters.

The nasals

Consonant /m/ is a labial nasal in Maltese. /n/ is a flat apical advanced alveolar nasal. The nasals almost always lose their characteristic place of articulation. Assimilation occurs when they precede the stops or /f/ and /v/.

Table 7.1 The 22 Maltese consonant phonemes organised by their articulatory features

	Bilabial	Labiodental	Alveolar	Postalveolar	Palatal	Velar	Glottal
Plosive	p b		t d			k g	ʔ
Nasal	m		n				
Fricative		f v	s z	ʃ			h
Affricate			ts	tʃ dʒ			
Approximant/ tap/trill	w		r		j		
Lateral approximant			l				

Note: Phonetic transcription as in the IPA alphabet (revised to 1989).

The fricatives

/f/ and /v/ are labiodental fricatives and are often articulated with the lower lip introverted. The stricture for the realisations of /s/ and /z/ occurs just at the end of the alveolar ridge with the tongue being grooved. /ʃ/ is released in the post-alveolar region. Azzopardi (1981) reports that many Maltese speakers have a consistent secondary articulation of labialisation with /ʃ/. The fricative /h/ varies in place of stricture. It can be post-palatal, velar, glottal or pharyngeal. It is voiced if it precedes a voiced consonant except in case of /m, n, l, r, w, j/ which do not participate in the voicing harmony.

The affricates

The three Maltese affricates, namely, /ts/, /tʃ/ and /dʒ/ are recognised by Azzopardi as unified segments. /tʃ/ and /dʒ/ are cupped lamino-pastalveolar affricates while /ts/ and /dʒ/ are cupped apical alveolar affricates. The affricate /dʒ/ very rarely occurs fully voiced. [dz] could be considered as a separate phoneme from /ts/ since it is not restricted to a phonetic context requiring a voiced obstruent. [dz] occurs very infrequently in Maltese and when it does so it usually occurs in words which are not part of the lexicon of young children. Hence, it did not merit its status as a phoneme. In this text [dz] is considered as an allophone of /ts/ in the context of adult gloss or when this is used by the children as a match to the adult version.

The approximants

The stricture for /w/ realisations is one of open approximation at the lips and velum. /j/ is released as open approximation in the palatal or less commonly in the pre-palatal region. /j/ and /w/ are always released as voiced. /l/ is released at the end of the alveolar ridge as with /s/ and /z/. The air flow could be bilateral, right sided or left sided. Hence /l/ is the lateral approximant in Maltese. The allophones of /r/ are usually slightly retroflexed when produced and can have a secondary articulation of labialisation. The allophones could be apico post-alveolar (or retracted alveolar) approximants or taps and occasionally trills. Some speakers use [ɾ] and [r] respectively in the same contexts and some use [ɾ], [ɻ] and [r] as free variants.[2]

Maltese vowels

Azzopardi (1981) distinguishes quantitatively as well as qualitatively (through formant structure) between the 11 monophthongs which can all exist as stressed vowels. She reports relative distances between cardinal vowels and the Maltese vowels as indicated in Figure 7.3. Vowels are longest in monosyllables. Their duration depends on the number of syllables in the word. Long vowels never occur in unstressed syllables.

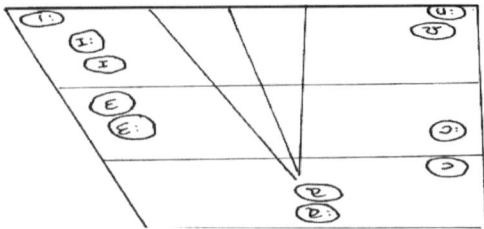

Figure 7.3 The 11 Maltese monophthongs organised according to relative distance between cardinal vowels. *Source*: Adapted from Azzopardi (1981); Maltese phonemic transcription as in Borg and Azzopardi-Alexander (1997). The relative distances are only approximations as variation exists between speakers

The diphthongs

The diphthongs have been less controversial in the past regarding their symbolisation. Figure 7.4 below indicates the auditory quality that again is relative to the cardinal vowel system. The arrows indicate the direction of movement where they start from any of the four vowel places /ɪ, ɛ, ɐ, ɔ/ and moving on to the /ɪ/ or /ʊ/ place. Azzopardi considers Maltese diphthongs as a combination of vowels plus consonant. She states that the greatest degree of closeness of this combination is heard when the second element comprising the diphthong functions both as syllable final and syllable initial of the preceding and following syllable respectively, e.g. /hlɛuːɐ/. Since this work concentrates mainly on discussing data of the development of consonantal segments in Maltese speaking children, a broader description of vowels and diphthongs will not be given in this text.

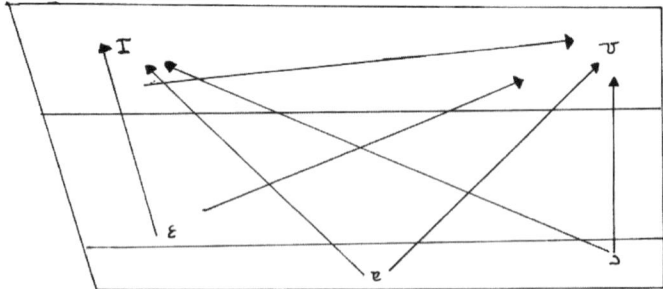

Figure 7.4 The seven Maltese diphthongs with reference to the cardinal vowel chart. *Source*: Adapted from Azzopardi (1981). The relative distances are only approximations as variation exists between speakers

Maltese phonological processes/rules

Katamba (1989) discusses the attempt to make a distinction between phonological processes and rules. He reports that a case has been made in the literature for restricting phonology to processes with a genuine phonetic basis and reserving for the morphological component of the grammar any rules regulating alternations that are determined by non-phonetic factors. A broad description of Maltese natural processes and morphophonemic rules (as defined by Katamba), is given below. Some rules, which are syllable dependent, are described with the syllabic structure of Maltese later on in the text.

Maltese natural processes

(1) There is no opposition between voiced and voiceless obstruents in word-final position. Only voiceless obstruents occur word-finally. One exception to this rule occurs when the following word in the utterance has a voiced obstruent word-initially and the two words are not separated by a pause.

(2) Gemination occurs when two identical consonants are adjacent to each other. It occurs when a particular segmental articulation is prolonged to cover what would otherwise be two distinct segments. No geminated consonant occurs word initially or syllable initially in Maltese since this would be preceded with a short epenthetic vowel /ɪ/. Geminated consonants have dual syllable memberships (except word finally) even when the first operates syllabically.

(3) Voicing assimilation occurs when pairs of voiced and voiceless sounds are brought together as a result of grammatical process or juxtaposition of words (usually regressive), e.g.

/rɐbɐt/ → /rɐptɐ/   'he tied'   'tie/knot'

(4) Complete assimilation where the modified segment takes on the complete bundle of distinctive features proper to its neighbour also occurs in Maltese. Such is the case with the definite article /l/ or /il-/, as in the case of Arabic. The article assimilates in words whose syllable initial word initial phoneme is any of the following phonemes: /t, d, n, s, z, ʃ, ts, tʃ, r, l/. Phonemes affected are termed 'sunny consonants'; e.g.

/ɪt: ɪ:ʔɐ/ → 'the window';   /ɪts:i:u:/ → 'the uncle'

(5) Sibilant assimilation is displayed in two ways in Maltese. One occurs by the juxtaposition of /ʃɪ/ meaning 'what' with words beginning with /s/ and /z/; e.g.

/ʃsɛrɐʔ/   becomes   /s:ɛrɐʔ/ → 'what did he steal'

The other kind of assimilation occurs when there is co-occurrence of the discontinuous morpheme /ma......ʃ/ (indicating 'negative') with the verb form ending in /s/ or /t/; e.g.

/mɐbɐbɐsʃ/ becomes /mɐbɐbɐʃ/ → 'he did not tamper with'

(6) Diphthong alternation occurs in keeping with the general phonological constraint that Maltese vowels do not cluster. Thus, the morpheme /u/ meaning 'and' alternates depending on the presence and absence of vowels in adjacent positions; e.g.

/mɐrɐ u: rɐːdʒɛl/ becomes /mɐrɐuːrɐːdʒɛl/ → 'a woman and a man'

Similarly, in the third person singular and plural of verb forms in the imperative; e.g.

/uːɐ ɪmuːr/ becomes /uːɐɪmuːr/ → 'he goes'.

In both examples the two adjacent vowels become a diphthong (/ɐʊ/, /ɐɪ/ respectively).

(7) Metathesis is common in Maltese also where two contiguous phonemes exchange position to conform with certain phonological rules or preferences attested in the language; e.g. some Maltese speakers reverse the positions of the first and second radical as in the pronunciation of certain verb forms and say, e.g.

/kpɛɪt/ → 'I cried' rather than /pkɛɪt/.

Metathesis is restricted to /l/, /r/ or word forms with labial and a velar (or glottal stop).

Maltese morphophonemic rules

(1) Stress shift and loss of segmental length: In Maltese stress tends to co-occur with vocalic length. Thus any stress shift concomitant with grammatical processes such as pluralisation, negativisation, etc., is often accompanied by loss or displacement of vocal length; e.g.

/biːp/ → 'door'   /bɪbiːn/ → 'doors'

Changes in consonantal length too can be phonologically conditioned, as when some final geminated consonants suffer reduction when followed in close transition by a sequence beginning with a consonant, e.g.

/kɛmː/ → 'how much'
/kɛmtɐːk/ → 'how much did he give you?'

(2) Replacement of vowels in unstressed position: Stress shift can sometimes also be accompanied by qualitative vowel changes in Maltese; e.g.

/kˈiːseh/ → 'cold' (singular)   /kɛshˈiːn/ → 'cold' (plural)

(3) Epenthesis in Maltese occurs in the case of the imperfective of trilateral or quadrilateral verbs, the plural of which often displays tri-consonantal clusters. Maltese phonotactics favours clusters of the shapes obstruent-obstruent-obstruent, resonant-resonant-resonant, resonant-obstruent-resonant, resonant-resonant-obstruent. Clusters conforming to these permissible phoneme sequences do not display epenthesis. Obstruent-resonant-obstruent clusters however, are not tolerated and thus feature an epenthetic vowel intervening between C1 and C2. e.g.

/nɪtɪlfʊ/ → 'we lose'   *but*   /nɪtlɛf/ → 'I lose'

(4) Dissimilation occurs very rarely in Maltese (Borg, 1975) and gives one example of such occurrence where it can be observed in the replacement of /n/ by /l/; e.g.

/nɔfsɪnɐːr/ → 'midday'   which is often realised as   /lɔfsɪnɐːr/

The Syllabic Structure of Maltese

A description of the syllable in Maltese is necessary in an investigation on child phonology. It helps the reader to understand how the sound system of children differs from the adult's. The syllable in Maltese can have the following structure in the case of monosyllabic words:

(C) (C) (C) V (C) (C)

Syllable division has preferences in that there is a tendency for one syllable division from another as indicated below. If consonants occur intervocalically the preferred pattern for occurrence is syllable initially of the second syllable, i.e. V-CV. When two intervocalic consonants or geminated consonants occur there is a preference for these to split up as consonant sequences to allow a closed syllable to precede a consonant released syllable (Azzopardi, 1981: 74). The order of preference for division is: C-C (always in geminated; preferable position with two intervocalic consonants, rather than V-CCV or VCC-V).

With a three consonant sequence intervocalically, the tendency is for the following order of preference:

C-CC
CC-C
but never
-CCC or CCC-

If the medial consonant is /m/ or /w/ the latter may constitute a separate syllable or CC-C option is used in analysis, e.g. /wɛrw-rʊ/ or /wɛr-w-rʊ/. As a rule CC-C is opted for when C2 and C3 cannot occur as syllable initial clusters but are possible as final clusters.

Assimilation of voicing, place of articulation and lip movement are not restrained by syllable division. The syllable nucleus in a Maltese syllable almost always consists of a vowel. The nasals /m/, /n/, lateral /l/ and /r/ may be syllabic when they occur word initially. Vowel length and stress are not in any way clues to syllable division (Azzopardi, 1981).

Syllable based phonological rules

(1) All consonants can occur singly in syllable initial word initial position. If they are intervocalic they usually occur as syllable initial of the second syllable of the two syllables involved. Single consonants usually function as final consonants of long vowels. They could be geminated.

(2) Although CC combinations occur as clusters word initially and word finally (see Tables 7.2 and 7.3 below), they are dismissed from qualifying as clusters within a multi-syllabic word because they are bound by syllabic division. In the circumstances they become consonantal sequences. There are only few restrictions for CC sequence combinations across syllabic boundaries (see Table 7.4 below).

(3) ccc clusters are not very common in Maltese and they do not occur word finally. There are no ccc medial clusters according to Azzopardi's definition since the tendency is to split up all word-medial consonant sequences as, c-cc or cc-c. In ccc initial clusters when a choice is given the speaker chooses the simpler structure with the introduction of the epenthetic vowel /ɪ/ when it is possible to separate the initial ccc cluster in two syllables, e.g.

/ʃɪ/ + /flɪːʃkɛn/   rather than /ʃflɪːʃkɛn/.

CCC sequences within the word are possible usually with C1 and C3 being the same and C2 being a stop. e.g. /ɪtɛptpʊ/ → 'flashing'. Syllabic division would be VC-VC-CCV. There are some distributional restrictions as to which consonants can occur in this position, e.g. no occurrence as /ʃmʃ/ but /ʃɪmʃ/ is possible as in /mɛʃɪmʃʊ/ → 'chewing

(4) Obstruents (plosives, fricatives and affricates) in a cluster are either all voiced or all voiceless depending on the last obstruent in the group. This rule does not apply to /l, m, n, r/. /w, j, h, ʔ/ are not affected by other consonants in a cluster or sequence. In addition, only voiceless obstruents occur before /ʔ/ and /h/. /h/ is often voiced when it precedes a voiced obstruent.

Table 7.2 CC (clusters) in Maltese: syllable initial

	p	t	k	s	f	ʃ	tʃ	ts	b	d	g	v	z	dʒ	ʔ	h	m	n	l	r	w	j
p	-	pt	pk	ps	pf	pʃ	ptʃ	pts							pʔ	ph		pn	pl	pr	pw	pj
t	tp	-	tk	.	tf	.	.	.							tʔ	th	tm	tn	tl	tr	tw	tj
k	kp	kt	-	ks	kf	kʃ	ktʃ	kts								kh	km	kn	kl	kr	kw	kj
s	sp	st	sk	-	sf	sʃ									sʔ	sh	sm	sn	sl	sr	sw	sj
f	fp	ft	fk	fs	-	.	ftʃ	fts							fʔ	fh	fm	fn	fl	fr	fw	fj
ʃ	ʃp	ʃt	ʃk	ʃs	ʃf	-	ʃtʃ	ʃts	ʃb					ʃdʒ	ʃʔ	ʃh	ʃm	ʃn	ʃl	ʃr	ʃw	ʃj
tʃ	tʃp	tʃt	tʃk		Tʃf	.	-									tʃh	tʃm	tʃn	tʃl	tʃr	tʃw	tʃj
ts			tsk		tsf			-											tsl			
b									-	bd	bg	bv	bz	b dʒ			bm	bn	bl	br	bw	bj
d									db	-	dg	dv					dm	dn	dl	dr	dw	dj
g								gdz	gb	gd	-	gv	gz				gm	gn	gl	gr	gw	gj
v									vb	vd	vg	-	vz	vdʒ					vl	vr	vw	vj
z									zb	zd	zg	zv	-	zdʒ			zm	zn	zl	zr	zw	zj
dʒ									dʒb	dʒd	dʒg			-			dʒm	dʒn	dʒl	dʒr	dʒw	dʒj
ʔ	ʔp	ʔt		ʔs	ʔf	ʔʃ			ʔb	ʔd		ʔv	ʔz		-	ʔh	ʔm	ʔn	ʔl	ʔr	ʔw	ʔj
h		ht	hk	hs	hf	hʃ			hb	hd			hz	hdʒ	hʔ	-	hm	hn	hl	hr	hw	hj

(Adapted from Azzopardi, 1981.)

Table 7.3 CC (clusters) in Maltese: syllable final

	p	t	k	s	f	ʃ	tʃ	ts	b	d	g	V	z	dʒ	ʔ	h	m	n	l	r	w	j
p	-	pt				pʃ										ph						-
t	-	-																				
k		kt	-			kʃ																
s		st	sk	-		sʃ									sʔ							
f		ft			-	fʃ																
ʃ		ʃt	ʃk			-																
tʃ		tʃt					-															
ʔ		ʔt				ʔʃ									-							
h						hʃ									hʔ	-						
m	mp	mt				mʃ										mh	-					
n		nt	nk				ntʃ											-				
l	lp	lt	lk		lf	lʃ		lts							lʔ	lh	lm		-			
r	rp	rt	rk	rs		rʃ									rʔ	rh	rm			-		
w		wt	wk													wh	wm	wn	wl		-	
j	jp	jt	jk													jh		jn	jl	jr		-

(Adapted from Azzopardi, 1981.)

Table 7.4 Possible cc sequences between syllables in Maltese (representing syllable final and syllable initial phoneme respectively)

	p	t	k	s	f	ʃ	tʃ	ts	b	d	g	v	z	dʒ	ʔ	h	m	n	l	r	w	j
p	-	pt	pk	ps		pʃ	ptʃ								pʔ	ph	.	pn	pl	pr		pj
t	tp	-	tk		tf										tʔ	th	tm	tn	tl	tr	tw	tj
k	kp	kt	-	ks	kf	kʃ	ktʃ									kh	km	kn	kl	kr	kw	kj
s	sp	st	sk	-	sf										sʔ	sh	sm	sn	sl	sr	sw	sj
f		ft	fk	fs	-	fʃ	ftʃ								fʔ	fh	fm	fn	fl	fr	fw	fj
ʃ	ʃp	ʃt	ʃk		ʃf	-									ʃʔ	ʃh	ʃm	ʃn	ʃl	ʃr	ʃw	ʃj
tʃ	tʃp	tʃt	tʃk	tʃs	tʃf		-									tʃh	tʃm		tʃl	tʃr		
ts								-									tsm	tsn				tsj
b									-	bd			bz	bdʒ				bn	bl	br		bj
d									db	-							dm	dn	dl	dr	dw	dj
g									gb	gd	-	gv	gz				gm	gn	gl	gr	gw	
v										vd	vg	-	vz	vdʒ			vm	vn	vl	vr		vj
z									zb	zd	zg	zv	-	zdʒ			zm	zn	zl	zr	zw	zj

Continued

Table 7.4 (Continued)

	p	t	k	s	f	ʃ	tʃ	ts	b	d	g	v	z	dʒ	ʔ	h	m	n	l	r	w	j
dʒ									dʒb	dʒd			dʒz	-			dʒm	dʒn	dʒl	dʒr	dʒw	dʒj
ʔ	ʔp	ʔt		ʔs	ʔf	ʔʃ	ʔtʃ		ʔb	ʔd			ʔz		-	ʔh	ʔm	ʔn	ʔl	ʔr	ʔw	ʔj
h		ht	hk	hs	hf	hʃ			hb	hd			hz	hdʒ	hʔ	-	hm	hn	hl	hr	hw	hj
m	mp	mt	mk	ms	mf	mʃ	mtʃ	mts	mb	md	mg	mv	mz	m dʒ	mʔ	mh	-	mn	ml	mr	mw	mj
n	np	nt	nk	ns	nf	nʃ	ntʃ	nt	nb	nd	ng	nv	nz	n dʒ	nʔ	nh	nm	-	nl	nr	nw	nj
l	lp	lt	lk	ls	lf	lʃ	ltʃ	lts	lb	ld		lv	lz	l dʒ	lʔ	lh	lm	ln	-		lw	lj
r	rp	rt	rk	rs	rf	rʃ	rtʃ	rts	rb	rd	rg	rv	rz	r dʒ	rʔ	rh	rm	rn	rl	-	rw	rj
w		wt	wk	ws	wf	wʃ	wtʃ		w	wd	wg		wz	w dʒ	wʔ	wh	wm	wn	wl	wr	-	
j	jp	jt	jk	js	jf	jʃ	jtʃ		jb	jd			jz		jʔ	jh	jm	jn	jl	jr	jw	-

(Adapted from Azzopardi, 1981.)

Suprasegmental Phenomena in Maltese

Aquilina (1959) and Azzopardi (1981) agree that the stressed syllable plays the dominant role and is given the rhythmic prominence in Maltese. Borg (1973) gives a more detailed account and reports that Maltese stress is related to segmental length and it is predictable and therefore non-phonemic. Azzopardi implies that Maltese is stress-timed similar to the rhythm in English. All long vowels are stressed but that not all vowels are long. Aquilina claims that there can only be one stress in the same Maltese word. He also claims that in Maltese the stress falls on the penultimate or on the last syllable in multi-syllabic words. In Maltese, intonation amalgamates with stress. When word stress interacts with intonation, one of the words in a sentence has a syllable which stands out above the rest. Variation in pitch is only functional at sentence level in Maltese. Tone is not relevant at word or syllabic/segmental level. Borg (1988) states that Maltese can have the same sentence structure carrying different meanings, all dependent on intonation varieties.

The Orthographic System

The Maltese orthographic system was officially devised in the 1920s. Though spoken Maltese is Semitic in orgin yet its orthography employs Roman letters. It is a relatively transparent orthography, except for two 'silent consonants' namely, the <għ> and <h>. The Maltese alphabet consists of 30 letters of which 24 are of a consonantal nature, whilst six are vowels. These are: a, b, ċ, d, e, f, ġ. g, għ, ħ, h, i, j, k, l, m, n, o, p, q, r, s, t, u, v, w, x, z and ż. In his dictionary, Aquilina (1987) adapts the 'phonetic' orthographic principle for loan-words including those from English and other languages. This claim is to date controversial.

Review of Previous Studies

Studies on phonological acquisition of the Maltese population are very limited. A small scale study investigating the development of Maltese consonants and some consonant clusters in four-year-old children was carried out by Azzopardi in 1997. This involved a cross-sectional study of 10 children acquiring Maltese who were following a normal developmental pattern. The phonetic inventories of all the children in Azzopardi's study included all the Maltese adult phonemes and some additional ones. Results indicated that the four-year-old informants were exhibiting few developmental processes. The processes exhibited by some of the informants in Azzopardi's study included fronting of /ʃ/ (three subjects); compensatory vowel lengthening (two subjects); gliding (one subject); lateralisation of /r/ (one subject); devoicing in syllable initial position (one subject); and consonant deletion in syllable final position (two subjects). These results indicate that by four years of age the Maltese informants were approximating adult phonology. Azzopardi concluded that the phonological characteristics exhibited by the Maltese four-year-old informants were similar to the universal trends.

This study has several methodological and analytic limitations. It was conducted on a relatively small sample and trends of the 'normal' developmental pattern cannot therefore be concluded from this study. The speech sample was only elicited via picture naming. Ideally a spontaneous speech sample plus the picture naming task would have been a more valid procedure to collect the necessary data. Transcription reliability was not measured. The analysis of the speech samples was restricted to the phone and phoneme inventories of each child and a description of the developmental processes exhibited by the children. The phoneme inventory did not include phonemes in syllable final within the word position (SFWW). The patterns observed may have highlighted other phonemes and/or developmental processes if consonants were analysed in SFWW position also. The criteria for identifying phones and developmental phonological processes were discussed whereas, the criterion for phoneme inclusion was not included. Mastery of phonemes was also not discussed in Azzopardi's study.

Another small scale cross-sectional study was carried out by Frendo in 2002. This study looked at aspects of the phonological system of three Maltese-speaking three-year-old twin sets and compared them with three individually matched Maltese-speaking three-year-old singletons. The selected subjects had been selected to ensure that they were following a normal developmental (including language) pattern. They also had normal hearing acuity, no significant medical conditions, no anatomical, physiological, oro-facial difficulties or neurological deficits and had no apparent emotional difficulties that could have reflected negatively on their speech development. Data were collected via a picture naming task that represented Maltese phonemes in different syllabic positions. Inter- and intra-transcriber reliability was calculated. The result indicated 92% and 96% inter- and intra-rater agreement, respectively. A modified version of *PACS* was used for analysis. Each speech sample was analysed to highlight the phonetic inventory, the system of contrastive phones in syllable initial and syllable final position, the mastered phonemes, the phonotactic potential and the structural and systemic phonological processes used by the subject. The criteria adopted by Grech (1998) to identify these aspects of phonology were applied in this twins' study. The analysis indicated similarities between the phonological systems of the twin sets and the singleton control subjects. Results compared well with the available trends of phonological acquisition of three-year-old Maltese speaking children (Grech, 1998). The criteria for selecting the twin sets were very strict and may not represent 'typical' twin sets who often exhibit developmental difficulties, particularly reflecting on speech development (McMahon & Dodd, 1995). The children's overall developmental profile was based on parental rather than professional assessment and analysis. The speech sample was collected using a picture naming task and any spontaneous utterances were not included for analysis. This may not have reflected the true picture of the children's functional communication skills.

The Main Study on Phonological Development of Normal Maltese Speaking Children

The first and only major contribution in connection with trends of development of phonology of the Maltese speaking child is that carried out by Grech (1998). This was an exploratory longitudinal study of the phonological development of 21 normally developing Maltese speaking children. The reader is referred to Grech (1998: 138–43) for justification for opting for a longitudinal study. The data were also analysed cross-sectionally to look into the possibility of generalising data at one point in time (specific developmental stage).

Data from the Maltese children were collected over a period of 18 months. It was decided that 'lexical phonological organisation' would be avoided in this project. Hence, data was first collected at 2;0 years of age to ensure that basic phonemic organisation was developed. The period between 2;0 and 3;6 years of age was chosen specifically to include the 'crucial' years for phonological change to occur. It was expected as from other research findings (e.g. Grunwell, 1985; Ingram, 1989b) that changes in a child's phonology would become less apparent after three years of age. The fourth recording period provided the researcher with the possibility of observing further changes which occur after three years of age. In this longitudinal language sampling, each child was visited at home at five different stages, for a reasonable length of time not exceeding 45 minutes, with the purpose of collecting a reasonable language sample.

A pilot study was carried before the main study was conducted. Eleven subjects were selected coming from stable families who use non-dialectal Maltese and who are monolingual speakers. The ages ranged between 1;1 and 4;10. All children were following a normal general developmental pattern. The recording equipment was identical to the one used in the main study. Material used included, free conversation, elicited conversation through toys, books and picture naming. The original plans in connection with the methodology for the main study were amended following identification of certain pitfalls in the pilot study.

The sample size

Since the researcher's concerns in the main study were both to gather knowledge of the process of phonological acquisition and the establishment of age norms, this created controversy regarding sample size since the former information is best gained through the study of a few children whereas the information to establish age norms must be obtained on data from many children. Considering the size of the Maltese population, the number of yearly births which equates with around 5000 and the number of monthly births which goes down to about 400 the minimum sampling number to obtain generalisable information is 30–40 (Butler, 1985). In view of the questions put forward in this project and considering practical issues, it was decided that data would be collected from 30–40 children.

The gender, sibling position and multiple-birth considerations

Some studies affirm that gender and sibling position affect speech and language development. Evidence to the contrary also exists. Since this investigation dealt with collecting data from a large sample of children, gender and sibling position were not controlled; nor were multiple birth children ruled out, so that variation of the 'norm' could be picked up.

Sample selection

This ongoing study was initiated by drawing a full random sample from the birth records of the only general hospital in Malta. Because phonological changes occur so rapidly in the early years, the variation in birth date of the chosen subjects was required to vary by no more than a month. To cover this specific population birth and to double check, birth lists were also obtained from the Public Registry. The implications of working with an absolute random sample include that data would have results from all possible socio-economic groups who are randomly geographically distributed. Figure 7.1 indicates geographical distribution of the sample.

The exclusion of subjects mentioned below was done to endorse the aim of studying the normal population. Because the study was primarily concerned with normal children in ordinary family situations, only those children who passed the following criteria were selected from the original list of 405 children:

(1) Apgar scores at birth greater than 3 (McCormick, 1992);
(2) child not admitted to special care baby unit neonatally;
(3) child not born with congenital abnormalities;
(4) child not illegitimate and both parents living together at birth; the public register indicates if father is unknown or if mother is a single parent or if the child is illegitimate; the number of illegitimate

children is not high in Malta; thus they could be eliminated without affecting the sample size required;
(5) both parents spoke fluent Maltese (to eliminate variability in linguistic input. This was considered important as it would have otherwise skewed the data provided, and more foreign words than is normally expected, would have been included).

After elimination of these children, the list was reduced to 394 children. A number random distribution chart was then consulted to draw the random sample of forty subjects from these presumably 'normal' children. Parents of the selected children were visited at home prior to the commencement of data collection. They each completed a questionnaire with the help of the researcher which indicated whether their child was following a normal developmental pattern, whether they were healthy and whether the input language was Maltese. During the same session the respective children went through a language screening test administered. This gave a broad view of the verbal comprehension and expression abilities. Prior to data collection the selected children were also screened for cognitive and hearing abilities. Children failing these screening measures were eliminated from the main study. Consequently, data proceeded to be collected from 33 children for the first recording session following a drop out after the screening during the initial interview. Thirty children completed all recording sessions. Descriptive analysis was carried out on 21 children since transcript size was only acceptable for 23 children for all the recording sessions. Furthermore, one child had to be eliminated because there were more English than Maltese words in her transcript. One child's transcript was eliminated from analysis since her recordings were not consistent with other subjects' recordings.

Data collection

Types of material used for data collection

Spontaneous speech sampling was considered for data collection in this project. An elicited picture naming test was also included to provide the consistency required. Since sessions were to be spaced by five to six months intervals, the 'learning effect' of exposing the same material to the children was minimised. Moreover, such a picture test was also meant to maintain inter-subject consistency since all children were exposed to the same test.

A *picture naming test* which was constructed specifically to suit the needs of this study. It included an adult consonantal phonemic inventory. Each consonant was represented in a mono-, di- and multi-syllabic word each in picture form. A few words with syllable initial word initial consonant clusters were also included on a separate form. Consonant clusters chosen were the most commonly used as were picked up from the samples recorded in the pilot study. The reader is referred to Grech (1998: 186–88) for details of criteria applied in constructing the picture naming test. Modelling picture naming was still impossible to avoid in the case of early sessions when the children were less than or at age 2;5 years, as they did not have a vast vocabulary at the time. It was thought that the application of delayed imitation would minimise such a difficulty. Such a procedure was adopted by Weiner (1979).

Spontaneous speech sampling, elicited using toys and play material with mother and/or siblings, was planned to take approximately 10–15 minutes per session. Consonant phonemes and cluster combinations, through picture naming, in all word positions were the primary target for analysis. Although as mentioned above, spontaneous speech sampling would not provide the consistency among subjects that the picture naming test would, yet, it was crucial to include it as part of the data to be collected. Stemberger (1988) reports that multi-word utterances present a new challenge to children who are coming out from their one word utterances. More than one word would have to be encoded at the same time and joined together to form the multi-word utterance. Stemberger argues that this is likely to create some difficulty with the result that 'between word processes' occur in child phonology which mismatch with the respective adult multi-word utterances.

Transcript size

To date no universal convention is applied for transcript size. Grunwell (1985) and Crary (1983) commented on the sample size of the picture naming test and spontaneous speech sampling, respectively. Grunwell agrees that a minimum of 100 different words should be used while she comments on a preference for at least 200–250 words. Crary's study on the influence of sample size indicated that samples of 50 words provided descriptive information similar to samples of 100 words. The pilot study carried out in conjunction with this research project indicated that a word sample of less than 100 might not include enough opportunities for all adult representations to occur with the expected frequency. On the other hand, it was difficult to collect a relatively large speech sample from the younger age groups. A specific criterion was devised for sample size for this project (Grech & Hesketh, 1996). The authors recommend that transcripts should be accepted for analysis if they contain a minimum of 50 spontaneous/elicited single word utterances and a few multiple word utterances in case of children who are 2;0+ years old. In view of Crary's (1983) findings and considering data obtained from the pilot study this seems to be valid and justified.

Recording the data

Reliable audio-recording for phonetic transcription was essential in this project. The sessions were video-recorded also. Information about situational context, direction of the child's attention, gestures and accompanying vocalisations could be provided via video-recordings. The children were audio- and video-recorded in free play with their mothers in their homes as well as during the administration of the picture and non-word naming tests. This system was also adopted by Vihman et al. (1986) where detailed phonetic transcripts could then be prepared from the audiotapes with the video-tape as a back up. Lip to microphone distance was maintained at 15–30 cm. This was made possible by using a wireless microphone with a small transmitter (Connevans, Type CRM-T200) attached to the child's pocket or trousers and the receiver (Connevans, Type CRM-R200) connected directly to the audio-cassette. The frequency response of the radio microphone equipment used was 90 Hz–5.5 KHz. The microphone (BT 1754 Electret) used was AGC controlled. The audio-cassette (Nokia recorder type, SL 837 AV stereo) is a stereo-recorder with a built in condenser microphone (mono) and built in slide signal generator, a two channel sound mixer plus tone control availability. The video-camera (Panasonic NV-MS4E) was also supplied with a 'gun' microphone. The signal to noise ratio was more than 47 dB. These methods yielded excellent quality tapes in which as reported by Shriberg et al. (1984), consonant allophone features such as aspiration were clearly audible and vowels were not distorted.

Transcription

Most of the phonetic transcription was done in situ. This was completed and matched with the audio-tape and video-tape recordings when it was reviewed as early as possible following each session as was recommended in Grunwell (1985). The International Phonetic Alphabet (IPA) has been used for language analysis by various researchers e.g. Boysson-Bardies and Vihman (1991), Dobrich and Scarborough (1992), Vihman et al. (1986). Duckworth et al. (1990) reported on the extensions to the IPA that have been recommended for the narrow transcription of disordered speech. The issue of how to transcribe children's speech is not discussed clearly and comprehensively in the literature. Crystal (1985) remarks on the objectives behind transcription. He emphasises that a good transcription should give the reader a comprehensive reproduction to be able to 'hear' the speech sample that is being transcribed. Creaghead et al. (1989) recommend close phonetic transcription (i.e. including diacritics) when transcribing child speech. They emphasise that this would give a clearer picture of the generalisations in the child's system as the child may use phones which are not included in the adult phonology of the language in question. Grunwell (1985) also recommends the use of the IPA (both segments and diacritics) and narrow transcription as much as the knowledge of the transcriber can take. Since her PACS procedures do not take vowels into consideration she recommends that vowels are recorded phonemically. Ball and Kent (1997) stress the importance of recording phonetic detail as this may reveal more information about the child's system. On the other hand it is important to transcribe significant rather than the fine details of the articulatory set of movements. In view of such perspectives, a set of conventions were constructed and applied in transcription (Grech & Hesketh, 1996).

Reliability and validity

The investigator went through all the manual analysis for each child twice. This approach was also applied for the group results which were collated on respective tables and figures. Differences recorded between the original results and the reviewed ones were minimal implying, that the investigator was consistent in her ratings. The possibility of investigator bias needed to be eliminated. Hence, inter-transcriber reliability was calculated by applying Boysson-Bardies and Vihman's (1991) comprehensive approach, whereby agreement was sought for consonantal place and manner features; consonantal count in pre- and post-vocalic position; and vocalisation length in syllables. A sample of the recordings was also transcribed by a Maltese phonetician. The transcription reliability between the phonetician and the researcher ranged from 91.2–100%. This is comparable to findings obtained from similar studies. Validity was evaluated and confirmed by associating the statement of the question with the description adopted and results obtained. For example, in order to consider PACS as a valid descriptive tool for Maltese child phonology, modifications had to be made. Otherwise, PACS would have lost its validity since it would not have catered for the Maltese child's pronunciations.

Scoring criteria

Criteria for process occurrence

Reynolds (1986) states that unless empirical criteria are applied, children's 'errors' could reflect free variation within child's system, a transcription error, an idiosyncratic production or they could be an example of a phonological process. Adaptations of Dinnsen *et al.*'s (1979) qualitative criteria were applied in this study. Hence, a process was said to occur if criteria (a) and (b) below were both met:

(a) The 'phone/s' affected by the process would react similarly in the same position for different words, for example: stopping of /ʃ/ as in

[tɪtɐ]   for /ʃɪtɐ/   → 'rain'
[tɐdɪnɐ] for /ʃɐdɪnɐ/ → 'monkey'
[tɛmt]   for /ʃɛmʃ/   → 'sun'

(b) If different adult phonemes in the same place or manner category of articulation reacted similarly as 'mismatches', say, fronting of alveolar consonants, these sounds would be said to be affected by a process irrespective of whether the specific sound is part of the child's phonetic/phonemic inventory. Examples are:

[θɪdʒ:ʊ] for /s ɪdʒ:ʊ/ → 'chair'
[θi:ɐ]   for /tsi:ɐ/   → 'aunt'

Though /ts/ may not yet be in the child's phonetic inventory, yet, the above examples would indicate process occurrence as other alveolars (which are part of the child's phonetic system, such as /s/ above) react similarly.

Criteria for phonetic inventory

Ingram (1986a) discusses the issue regarding the determination of the child's phonetic inventory. Ingram proposes that a criterion of frequency be applied to the child's sounds, such as a quantitative measurement to decide when a sound becomes part of child's inventory. The criterion of frequency (Ingram, 1981) is based on the arbitrary assumption that any sound used by the child should at least occur once in any random selection of 25 phonetic forms or lexical tokens (lexical tokens: an adult word used by the child; phonetic form: a distinct phonetic shape independent of lexical token). The calculation is as follows:

$$\frac{(\text{number of lexical token} + \text{phonetic forms})}{2} \div 25$$

The answer is rounded up to the nearest whole number. This criterion of frequency was applied in this investigation. This way sounds which occurred marginally could be excluded from the phonetic inventory and a clearer picture of the child's sound system at one point in time could be easily established.

Criteria for the phonemic inventory

The set of criteria used for considering a sound to be a phoneme were:

(1) the sound had to be used frequently. Ingram's quantitative criterion for phonetic inventory (mentioned above) is applied first. Any identified marginal phones were not considered as possible phonemes.
(2) The sound occurred in minimal or near minimal pairs.

(3) It assigned a specific contrast from analysing the child's substitution patterns.

Criterion for mastery of phoneme

A distinction had to be made with regards to the frequency of matched phonemes of the child with those of the adult. Once a child starts using phonemes contrastively as adults, he may take some time until he does this consistently. The criterion adopted to mark the consistency of usage was that suggested by Stoel-Gammon and Stone (1991). This criterion requires a phoneme to be produced correctly in at least half the word positions tested, so that it is classified as 'customarily' produced. It is said to be 'mastered' if produced correctly in all positions. Customary usage implies development but not mastery of phonemes.

Analytic framework

All the data collected during the recorded sessions were organised and analysed for each child and each recording session so that charts related to phoneme and cluster realisations, phonetic inventories and phone distribution, systems of contrastive phones, syllabic structure (phonotactic possibilities) and phonological process (structural and systemic) were compiled. This analytic framework was originally used by Grunwell (1985) in *Phonological Assessment of Child Speech (PACS)*. Grunwell's charts were modified for Maltese with kind authorisation. Tables and figures were organised for the group for each recording session. These were then summarised to give the developmental profile for the group. The above analysis was to be the source from which the phonetic, phonemic and phonotactic components with regards to the Maltese phonological acquisition were drawn out. Elbert (1992) suggests that for children to be able to use the phonological system of a language for communication optimally, they need to be able to master all the above mentioned components. Nonlinear analysis for speech samples was applied for selected processes. Some of the processes which were described nonlinearly are not mentioned in *PACS*. These were chosen specifically as it was felt that they merited more attention. Due to the vastness of data and processes exhibited, this study had to limit the number of processes addressed in nonlinear terms.

Results

Tables 7.5–7.10 provide a summary of the key stages for phone/phoneme inventories the developmental processes and canonical syllabic structures used across ages. Other patterns of the developmental profile were highlighted in the main study though not included in the tables below. For a more comprehensive description of the developmental profile the reader is referred to Grech (1998).

Discussion

This study was mainly concerned with looking at possible trends that could help a clinician with diagnosing a phonological impairment. Hence, inter- and intra-language commonalities were highlighted. It does not deny the presence of individual variation. In fact, it was also observed that children may choose their own idiosyncratic path for some aspects or at some stage during their progress towards phonological maturity. For example, subject 21 showed a relatively advanced phonetic/phonological development, compared to the other subjects; yet, she rarely used the voiced bilabial plosive and used a nasalised version of it at 3;6.

Developing sound classes

The *nasals* [m, n] were used commonly very early. No other nasals were used by any of the subjects at any stage. This reflects stability of these

Table 7.5 Phone inventories for the Maltese speaking subjects (used by 75% or more of the children)

Age	Nasal	Plosive	Fricative	Affricate	Approximant
2;0	m	p b		h	w
	n	t d			l
		k			j
		ʔ			
2;5	m	p b	f		w
	n	t d	s		l
		k	ʃ		r
		ʔ	h		j
3;0	m	p b	f v		w
	n	t d	s	tʃ	l
		k g			r
		ʔ	h		j
3;6	m	p b	f v		w
	n	t d	s z	tʃ	l
		k g	ʃ	dʒ	r
		ʔ	h		j

Table 7.6a Adult phonemes used by the Maltese children to convey the same contrast at syllable initial position (used by 75% or more of the children; most of the phonemes were produced with variation)

Age	Nasal	Plosive	Fricative	Affricate	Approximant
2;0	m	p b			1
	n	t d			
		ʔ			
2;5	m	p b	f v		w
	n	t d	s		l
		k g			r
		ʔ	ʃ		j
			h		
3;0	m	p b	f v		
	n	t d	s z	tʃ	l
		k g	ʃ		r
		ʔ	h		j
3;6	m	p b	f v	ts	w
	n	t d	s z	tʃ	l
		k g	ʃ	dʒ	r
		ʔ	h		j

Note: /w/ is not represented as a phoneme at age 3;0 but is observed at age 2;5. This is because some children did not have the opportunity for its occurrence and not because it had disappeared as a phoneme since the earlier recording stage. Although this phoneme inventory seems to follow a progressive hierarchy, yet some discrepancy may occur because of not having enough opportunities for realisation.

phones but not necessarily stabilisation as phonemes. To some extent this ties in with Locke's theory and other Universalists' view that children show more or less a similar sequence of acquisition. The adult *plosives* were all used consistently by most of the children since age 2;0. This includes glottal stop which was used by most children throughout the 18 months. The 'non-adult' plosives produced were used less often and by fewer children. This could mark early phonological maturity for plosives.

The number of different *fricatives* produced by the children is more than the number of different fricative phonemes produced by the native adult speakers at any stage recorded. This outnumbering increased progressively; it must be related to free variation with most of the

Table 7.6b Adult phonemes used by the Maltese children to convey the same contrast at Syllable final position (used by 75% or more of the children; most of the phonemes were produced with variation)

Age	Nasal	Plosive	Fricative	Affricate	Approximant
2;0					w
	n				
2;5	m	p	f		w
	n	t	s		l
		k	ʃ		r
					j
3;0	m	p			
	n	t	s		l
		k			r
					j
3;6	m	p b	f	ts	w
	n	t	s	tʃ	l
		k	ʃ		r
		ʔ	h		j

Note: /f/, /ʃ/ and /w/ are not represented as a phoneme at age 3;0 but are observed at age 2;5. This is because some children did not have the opportunity for its occurrence and not because it had disappeared as a phoneme since the earlier recording stage. Although this phoneme inventory seems to follow a progressive hierarchy, yet some discrepancy may occur because of not having enough opportunities for realisation.

fricatives being allophones of the other. Edwards (1979) reports data from six English-learning children indicating that correct production of fricatives fluctuated with various types of substitutions. This could mark cross-linguistic similarities in the acquisition of fricatives. [h] was used by most children in the early recording stages and later on was seen in all the phonetic inventories. This is in line with Sloat *et al.*'s (1978) expectations for [h] to be one of the earliest fricatives to develop universally. For each recording period, there were always more children using voiceless fricatives than their voiced counterparts. However, in general there were relatively more voiced fricatives recorded as marginal phones than their voiceless counterparts throughout the recording stages. Apart from possible developmental reasons this could have resulted from the voiced fricatives having had less opportunity for occurrence in children's transcripts and/or because they are less frequent in the native adult system.

Table 7.7 Mastered contrastive phones for the Maltese speaking subjects

Age	Nasal	Plosive	Fricative	Affricate	Approximant
2;0	m	ʔ	f		w
			v		j
2;5	m	p ʔ	v		w
3;0		b	f v		w
		d	h		j
		ʔ			
3;6	m	p b	f v		w
		t	h		j
		k g			
		ʔ			

Note:
(1) Mastered phonemes are those used without variation or misarticulation by 70% or more of the subjects who had the opportunity.
(2) Phonemes that have not been mastered at age 3;6 include /n, d, s, z, ʃ, l, r, ts, tʃ, dʒ/.
(3) /f, j/ are not highlighted at 2;5 though they seem to have been mastered at age 2;0; /m, p/ are not highlighted at 3;0 though they seem to have been mastered at age 2;5; /d/ is not highlighted at 3;6 though it seems to have been mastered at age 3;0. See Discussion for an explanation of this 'apparent regression'.

Table 7.8 Percentage of children making use of structural processes

Process description	Age 2;0	Age 2;5	Age 3;0	Age 3;6
Weak syllable deletion	85.7	80.95	85.7	61.9
Syllable final consonant deletion (single segments)	100	90.5	95.2	90.5
Syllable final consonant deletion (cluster reduction)	52.4	71.4	85.7	61.9
Consonant harmony	80.95	57.1	42.85	19.0
Reduplication	100	76.2	95.2	66.7
Syllable initial consonant deletion (single segments)	80.95	85.7	80.9	47.6
Syllable initial consonant deletion (cluster reduction)	80.95	95.2	80.9	71.4
Compensatory vowel lengthening	52.4	76.2	71.4	38.1
Gemination of consonant in sequence	80.95	57.1	66.7	52.4
Other structural processes	52.4	66.7	61.9	33.3

Table 7.9 Percentage of children making use of systemic processes

Process description	Age 2;0	Age 2;5	Age 3;0	Age 3;6
Fronting	95.2	100	100	90.5
Stopping	100	95.2	90.5	57.1
Gliding	57.2	47.6	61.9	66.7
Lateralisation of /r/	42.8	66.7	80.9	57.1
Delinking of affricates	95.2	95.2	85.7	80.95
Devoicing	47.6	28.5	42.9	38.1
Other systemic processes	95.2	90.5	76.1	66.7

The Maltese children used a variety of *affricates*, particularly the alveolar affricate. Affricates present as a single segment with two mutually exclusive properties – a complex underlying configuration. Although the children used various affricates, the trend was to use the adult ones

Table 7.10 Canonical structures of the children

Syllabic structures	Canonical structures		Percentage of children
Monosyllables	Age 2;0	CV	66.6
		CVC	23.8
	Age 2;5	CVC	95.2
	Age 3;0	CVC	100
	Age 3;6	CVC	100
Disyllabic	Age 2;0	CV,CV	61.9
		V,CV	19.05
		CVC,CV	14.29
	Age 2;5	CVC,CV	33.3
		CV,CV	28.5
		V,CV	23.8
	Age 3;0	CV,CV	28.57
		CVC,CVC	23.8
	Age 3;6	CVC,CVC	38.1
		CV,CVC	23.8
		CVC,CV	9.52

Note: C = non-syllabic segment; V = syllabic segment.

more often as the children grew older. It is likely that the Maltese recognise the three adult affricates very early; most of them start using a variety of them relatively early and gradually reduce the degree of free variation until the target affricates are stabilised. This assumption infers that phonemic acquisition could be ahead of 'phonetic stability' for affricates. Two of the three 'adult' affricates (i.e. /tʃ, dʒ/) were used by more than half the group at 2;5 years of age and by 75% or more of the subjects when they were three and a half years old. Studies concerning age norms for English consonant sounds report affricates as among the later acquired consonants; for example, Prather *et al.* (1975) mention that the said affricates are not acquired before 3;8 years of age; Templin (1957) reports age of acquisition for /tʃ, dʒ/ as being 4;6 and 7;0, respectively. Although such studies need to be interpreted with caution, yet the general tendency is perhaps for Maltese children to produce affricates relatively early. Such an assumption supports the notion of the influence of language exposure on the development of child 'speech'. Among the data collected in this project, affricates were scarcer than corresponding plosives and fricatives. Perhaps the element of articulatory maturity for the surfacing of 'complex' segments such as affricates plays a role in sequence of acquisition. This is in support of the view of the influence of neuro-motor articulatory development on cognitive-linguistic aspects of speech development.

Amongst the *approximants*, [r] was used unexpectedly early. This is reputed to develop late as a phoneme for other languages such as English (Grunwell, 1985). The articulatory competence seemed to be established by most Maltese subjects. This could be a language-specific phenomenon if it proves to be contrastive at this age. The velar approximant was only apparent in a few of the children's inventories (again stressing language-specificity). This could prove to be a free variant for /r/. Other approximants used, were those included in the adult inventory. Most children produced these early. This is in accordance with the language specific expectations model (i.e. that of early linguistic processing).

Dinnsen *et al.* (1990) adopted a hierarchical framework for the development of phones (for phonologically delayed children) which focused on feature distinctions as the units of analysis as opposed to the more conventional 'phones'. They claimed that this approach to studying phonetic contrasts compares better across different language speaking children's inventories. These were later found to hold also for normally developing systems (Dinnsen, 1992). This approach was adopted to look at the development of Maltese phones in more detail (see Table 7.11 below). It led to the conclusion that such natural phenomena of phonetics apply for Maltese. One discrepancy between Dinnsen *et al.*'s model and the data obtained in this study is the establishment of

Table 7.11 Implicational hierarchy of phonetic features

Dinnsen et al.'s (1990) levels	Maltese age equivalent (for 75% or more subjects)
Level A [syllabic] [consonant] [sonorant] [coronal]	2;0 (includes nasals, glides and stop phones)
Level B [voice]	2;0 (including voiced and voiceless stops; all dimensions at level A are valid)
Level C [continuant] [delayed release]	2;5 3;0 (fricatives and/or affricates includes all dimensions at levels A & B)
Level D [nasal][1]	2;0 (incorporates a liquid phone [r] or [l]; all features of Levels A–C are valid)
Level E [strident][2] [lateral]	2;5 (laterality difference among liquids)

Notes:
1. The feature [nasal] was introduced at this level as a non-redundant feature to distinguish the nasal consonants from the liquid consonants. Up till level C this was not necessary since the nasals were the only sonarant consonants and therefore nasality was predictable.
2. Stridency difference amongst fricatives in <50% of subjects.

the [delayed release]. This feature occurs before the liquid phone distinction in Dinnsen et al.'s model. The latter not only developed earlier for Maltese, but even the laterality distinction among liquids was marked as an earlier feature than the [delayed release] distinction.

In conclusion, the Maltese findings so far are indicating a clear effect of the influence of neuro-motor-articulatory development (e.g. affricates taking longer to surface); universal patterns for certain class sounds to develop earlier (e.g. nasals, plosives surfacing earlier and in more children than other class sounds); and language specific trends (e.g. laterality distinction developing relatively early).

Developing consonantal clusters

More consonantal clusters were produced at syllable initial position than in final position for all recording stages. The explanation for such behaviour could be three fold; one being that clusters develop earlier in this position; a second reason could be related to the fact that consonantal clusters occur more often in speech in initial syllable position; while a third reason could be because the picture naming tasks were included for syllable initial clusters but not for syllable final position. A marked increase in cluster production was observed between each recording stage and the following session. This is due to phonetic stability, expansion of vocabulary, increase in complexity of utterances, progress in morphophonemic development, and possibly disappearance of the cluster reduction process. One major implication of these findings is that from 3;0 years onwards almost all the children are able to use consonantal clusters of some type. This indicates a certain degree of articulatory maturity. The phonotactics of the input language which includes so many possible cluster combinations is bound to have an influence on the respective children's productions.

The development of the contrastive system

Children's early speech production is typified by limited inventories and having one phone signifying more than one contrast of the adult system (e.g. Dinnsen, 1996). Such mismatches were observed in the Maltese speaking children. The Maltese children's developing contrastive system reflected degrees of *stabilisation*, where variants were progressively reduced to a phoneme. Variants in this study refer to *potential phonetic progress* where two phonetically similar phones may be competing for phoneme establishment; or *contextual variation* with different phone use across word positions; or *variety of use across time* with phones appearing and disappearing occasionally; or *free variation* when two or more different phones are used separately in different occasions in the same place in structure to signal the same contrast. These are distinguished from the potential phonetic progress type as they would only affect sounds which are established adult phonemes.

Nasals and plosives were among the sound classes to stabilise first as phonemes. This can be clearly seen in Table 7.7. The phonemic inventories were progressively *expanding* also. This is clearly noticeable in Tables 7.6a and 7.6b. More phonemes were incorporated in more syllabic positions as the children grew older. A geometric framework based on feature distinction for phoneme acquisition of the Maltese informants is given below. This is comparable to the similar model constructed for the development of consonantal phones, illustrated above.

One factor which must be noted is the apparent regression between recordings for some phonemic feature distinctions. For example the [dorsal] place feature within glides (/w, j/ distinction) seems to be acquired at age 2;5; but /w/ disappears phonemically at 3;0. Various explanations may be possible such as the fact that some children did not have enough opportunities for phoneme occurrence at particular

Table 7.12 Implicational hierarchy of phonemic features* (common phonemic distinctions acquired by the Maltese subjects) (adapted from Gierut *et al.* 1994)

Gierut et al.'s typology	Maltese typology	Basic feature distinctions	Maltese age equivalent (for >75% of subjects)
Type I:			
nasals	nasals /m,n/	[syllabic]	2;0
stops	stops /p,b,t,d,ʔ/	[consonant]	
glides	glide /w/	[sonorant]	
	liquid /l/	[voice]	
		[labial]	
		[coronal]	
Type II:			
nasals	nasals /m,n/	the above +	2;5
stops	?	[continuant]	
glides	glides /w,j/	[dorsal]	
fricatives	liquids /l,r/	[distributed]	
	fricatives /**f,v,s**, ʃ, **h**/	[anterior]	
Type III A:			
nasals	nasals /m,n/	the above +	3;0
stops	stops /p,b,t,d,k,g,ʔ/	[delayed release]	
glides	glide /j/		
fricatives	liquids /l,r/		
affricates	fricatives /f,v,s,z,ʃ,h/		
	affricate /tʃ/		
Type III B:			
nasals			
stops			
glides			
fricatives			
liquids			
Type IV:			
nasals	nasals /m,n/	as at age 3;0	3;6
stops	stops /p,b,t,d,k,g,ʔ/		

Continued

Table 7.12 (*Continued*)

Gierut et al.'s typology	Maltese typology	Basic feature distinctions	Maltese age equivalent (for >75% of subjects)
glides	glides /w,j/		
fricatives	liquids /l,r/		
affricates	fricatives /f,v,s,z,ʃ,h/		
liquids	affricates /ts, tʃ, dʒ/		

Note: Most of the phonemic distinctions were produced with variation indicating incomplete mastery.

stages of recording; the vocabulary became wider and more phonotactically complex as the children grew older. Therefore the larger the frequency of occurrence of a particular phoneme the greater was the chance for it to mismatch especially if syllabic complexity within words increased; in the younger children avoidance strategies may have been employed for some phonemes and therefore the 'more mastered phonemes' were more frequent in the earlier stage; as the children grew older other features started to surface with a lot of variability. Such variability involved previously acquired phonemes. This gave the impression of regression in the previously acquired phonemes; e.g. as /s/ started to surface, this was in free variation with /t/; hence the latter phoneme re-appeared in free variation.

A comparison of the phonetic and phonemic development of the Maltese subjects indicates that similarity exists in the hierarchical expectations and in types of sound classes expected at different stages of development. However, when analysis goes beyond basic class contrasts into within-class distinctions associated with place and voice in particular, there does not seem to be a one-to-one correspondence. One such example occurs at Level B whereby all voiced and voiceless stops were established phonetically by 2;0; but mastery of these phones as phonemes was not yet established. This is in line with universal expectations as children introduce sounds which are at first not used as contrastive phones in the same way as adults. Later these begin to conform to the adult system.

The development of syllabic structures

Table 7.10 highlights the change in canonical syllabic structures of children as they grew older. Since there exist a wide range of syllabic structures, the data were summarised depending on syllabic size.

Multi-syllabic words other than disyllabic ones are not tabulated due to the limited space allowed for this chapter. However, the discussion below refers to more comprehensive data sheets that are available for each session per child.

A more complex structure seems to become common among the children as they grew older. Data analysis indicated a high degree of matching of monosyllables with the adult form even at age 2;0. An average of 88% monosyllabic matches was produced at this age. With regards to disyllabic matches, this averaged to 76.4% for this age group, whereas production of multisyllabic words was matched for structure 35% of the time. The trend for matches increased progressively, so that by age 3;6, matches for monosyllabic words were 94.4%; disyllabic words: 95%; multisyllabic words: 89.4%. This implies that most children mastered their phonotactics by the time they reached 3;6 years of age, irrespective of whether these include multisyllabic words or words with syllabic complexity. This is an interesting finding especially when it is compared with results obtained for the same subjects regarding their phone/phoneme systems. Data indicates that for the Maltese subjects syllabic structure development precedes segmental development. Maltese can have monosyllabic words as complex as C_3VC_2 and words can frequently have up to five syllables. Perhaps this high proportion of structural matching with the adult system could be the influence of the structure of the language in question.

Contrastive consonantal cluster matches

Lleo and Prinz (1996) report on the reduction of clusters in young children's speech resulting in the production of a single consonantal segment. The segment which the child uses to represent the cluster is not necessarily identical 'to one of the target segments'. It may constitute a natural class with one of the segments constituting the cluster. Such a phenomenon was observed with some of the Maltese children but as they grew older there seemed to be more variability reflecting potential phonetic progress, e.g. /sn/ → [θn]. A possible explanation to this is that the process of 'cluster reduction' is typical of early phonological development. Clusters are then mismatched in a different way as phonology matures so that this is taken over by potential phonetic progression. This phenomenon was particularly common amongst clusters containing fricatives, affricates and liquids which tend to develop later as singletons.

Developmental patterns for specific processes

This section reports what is specific to the Maltese children's phonological behaviour. It also compares the informants' behaviour with that of children acquiring other languages.

Weak syllable deletion – 61.9% of the informants were still applying this process at age 3;6. Grunwell (1987) does not expect this process to disappear before 3;6–4;0. The results for the Maltese subjects are consistent with the expected English patterns for this process.

Syllable final consonant deletion for singletons was common for all children at age two. This is apparently a 'natural' process as the child uses his/her basic syllable structure (i.e. CV – the open syllable) and consequently the final consonant is omitted from the syllable. This process was produced by fewer children five months later, so that 90.5% of the children produced it. At age 3;0 this process seems to be used by more children than in the earlier session. However, this could be explained in terms of phonotactic development whereby multisyllabic word usage seemed to have increased significantly at this stage with the consequence that the string of syllable sequences reverted to the open syllable style. By the time they reached age 3;6 their phonotactics had matured so that fewer subjects applied this process.

Cluster reduction in syllable final position – By age 3;0 most children were using this process so that the percentage went up to 85.7%. There is a noticeable decrease in cluster reduction at age 3;6. Perhaps this is the stage when children were starting to master their consonantal clusters at syllable final position; or perhaps certain morphological progress is established at this stage. The overall impression is that clusters surface early for Maltese probably due to the influence of the structure of the language; however, this has a less positive effect on phonological progression; perhaps because of the numerous cluster combinations and the morphophonemic complexity, stability and mastery takes a relatively longer time to be completed.

Consonant harmony is characterised by having *all* consonants in a word 'harmonised' so that they share similar phonetic characteristics (Grunwell, 1985). Grunwell (1987) reports that it usually affects the place of articulation. However, it has been noticed among the Maltese subjects that this process could affect the harmonisation by manner and voice also. The use of this process phased out gradually so that only 19% of the children used it at 3;6 years of age.

Reduplication in this study refers to the term used in Grunwell (1985) where it is defined as repetition of an adult target syllable (complete reduplication), or part of the syllable (partial reduplication). At age 2;5 reduplication started to disappear in some of the children so that it went down to 76.2%; at 3;0 the number of children engaging in reduplication went up again to 95.2%. This apparent regression could be related to a significant increase in multisyllabic word usage which may not have necessarily matched with the corresponding adult words. Grunwell (1987) expects this process to disappear by 2;0–2;6.

The Maltese subjects were not necessarily extending its use by a year or so. The phenomenon of gemination of consonants in sequence seemed to be the dominating factor as children grew older with regards to characterisation of partial reduplication and this may be a persevering process for Maltese.

Syllable initial consonant deletion – Initial consonant deletion is not considered as a frequent occurrence in Grunwell (1985, 1987) and Ingram (1981). Results indicate that a high proportion of the Maltese children applied syllable initial consonant deletion until age 3;6. This process includes the deletion of the syllable initial component of a consonantal sequence. As indicted in Table 7.4, cc sequences are very common within words in Maltese. Further research may need to be carried out on this phenomenon as it may be a language specific process that may yield useful information for theoretical application.

Syllable initial cluster reduction is a more universal process which the Maltese subjects applied throughout the recording period. This process was exhibited mostly at age 2;5; from this age until 3;6 there was a gradual disappearance so that at the last recorded stage the percentage of children exhibiting this process went down to 71.4%. Syllable initial cluster reduction may be accountable for lack of morphological maturity. Pluralisation may involve introduction of syllable initial consonant cluster.

Compensatory vowel lengthening – Vowel length is phonemically meaningful for Maltese. Hence, the investigator hypothesised that this was being used meaningfully by Maltese speaking children to perform contrasts between consonantal segments that were not yet established in their phoneme inventories. This postulation ties up with Waterson's theory that prosodic development precedes segmental development. A possible explanation to this was that the subjects were aware of the underlying consonantal segment contrastiveness and because of restrictions in their own 'production system' they applied the more established prosodic contrast.

Gemination of consonant in sequence – This process also merited a separate heading in view of its frequency of occurrence and the possible underlying explanation for its application. It was observed that the Maltese speaking children were mismatching 'abutting consonants' (consonantal sequences) in a consistent manner. Frequently, they were lengthening one constituent of the consonantal sequence while deleting the other. A possible explanation reflects similar phenomena to compensatory vowel lengthening. These two processes support early linguistic processing, since they seem to be tied in with over-generalisation of some phonological aspects of the native adult system.

Other 'structural' processes – This term was used in this project to include processes which were not common among all the children, or which were used less frequently (even though commonly) by the group. For further details the reader is referred to Grech (1998).

Fronting is a very common process among the Maltese subjects. Nearly all the children used this process during all the recorded sessions throughout the 18-month period. However, the high degree of application of this process could be related to the broad definition that it was given in this study. Besides, there are more Maltese phonemes than English ones that could be susceptible to this developmental process (e.g. /ts/). This is a relatively late developing affricate and as a result fronting persevered even up till 3;6.

Stopping – This process seems to disappear earlier than fronting in Maltese speakers. Grunwell (1987) reports that stopping begins to disappear for most fricatives and affricates by 2;6–3;0 even though complete mastery is gradual. Chiat (1989) reported her findings where fricatives were not stopped word finally or medially between strong and weak syllables. There is some analogy with the Maltese findings, in that there was less stopping at syllable final position compared to the other syllabic position for all recording stages.

Gliding is not applied by most Maltese children at age 2;0. It may be recalled that [r] was already being used by about half the group at age 2;0 and [l] was applied by most children as a phone at that age. Thus, it seems that /r/ and /l/ started off relatively early as phones/phonemes. Therefore, the 'gliding' process was perhaps required less because children could use the 'lateralisation' of /r/ as an alternative process.

Lateralisation of /r/ is not highlighted as one of the main children's processes in many protocols. Lateralisation of /r/ was used by almost half the group at age 2;0. This score increased progressively though. A significant decrease in number of children applying this process was noticed at age 3;6, so that it only persevered in about half the group. Perhaps at this stage some of the children may have already mastered /r/. This finding puts a lot of weighting on specific linguistic processing. It is reported in Gan *et al.* (1996), that in Hebrew the substitution for gliding would involve /j, l/. Hebrew is a Semitic language and /w/ is not a phoneme of the respective language adult language. More comparative research on languages sharing such phonological similarities needs to be carried out.

Delinking of affricates – Ingram (1981) includes this phenomenon as a substitution process while Hodson (1986) considers it with miscellaneous phonological processes. Delinking of affricates was a relatively common phenomenon observed in the Maltese subjects. The fact that three affricates are included in the phoneme inventory of the adult Maltese system may be a contributing factor. This is linked with the relatively long process which is associated with the development and mastery of affricates as phones and phonemes.

Devoicing was a phenomenon observed among the Maltese children in positions where it is not normally exhibited by the native adult speakers, that is, syllable initial position and syllable final within the word positions. The researcher postulates that the young Maltese speakers neutralise the adult phonological rule of devoicing by applying it to other positions. Devoicing was applied by about half the group at age 2;0. There do not seem to be significant changes in the number of children exhibiting devoicing at the different stages of recording. The fact that the same children who produced the process initially seemed to have persevered in its use could imply that devoicing may be predictable for some children at later stages. However, this possibility would need to be supported by further research.

Other systemic processes – These processes were grouped together due to their infrequency of occurrence among the group; or because they represented realisations by specific subjects; or else because very few (one to three) occurrences occurred in the children who applied the specific process rendering it difficult to be 'accepted' as a process. Further details are cited in Grech (1998).

The Influence of Sub-components of the Maltese Language on Findings

The findings will be discussed below in terms of how they are influenced by the development of other sub-components of the language. This ties in with applying findings to the context of assessment and diagnosis of the phonologically impaired. It also merges with specific issues that may need to be addressed in the remediation of Maltese children with phonological deficit. The influence of other sub-components of language, particularly the *impact of lexical and morphological acquisition* is evident in the Maltese findings. Maltese words can be composed of a series of morphemes; for example, possession, the feminine and some plural forms may be expressed through a suffix. Hence, lexical expansion may be indicated by an increase in the number of morphemes attached to or merged in a word. Consequently, syllabic complexity and the number of syllables in the word increases as more morphemes are included in the word. Therefore, progress in lexical and morphological development puts demands on Maltese child phonology. Some examples related to this issue are expressed below.

For example, the early use of consonantal clusters ties in with morphosyntactic advancement. In some cases, pluralisation in Maltese is signified by the substitution of a syllable initial consonantal cluster for a singleton; e.g. /tɪflɐ/ → /tfɐːl/ 'child' (feminine) → 'children'.

The fact that more syllable initial clusters were recorded when the children were older could have been influenced by the advancement of such aspects morphological development. Similarly, in Maltese, verb forms are derived from the same verb base. More clusters were produced in syllable initial position for all recording stages. This could be due to the fact that some verb forms signifying past tense (which may involve the introduction of syllable final clusters in a word, as in the example below) may take longer to develop, than other morpho-syntactic aspects, such as pluralisation, e.g. /ımːuːr/ → /mɔrt/ 'I go' → 'I went'.

Ingram (1989b) explains that phonological disorders are usually characterised by a discrepancy between lexical development and phonological progress. How can this be considered in the Maltese context when the respective distinction may not be so clear cut? An apparent delay in syntactic/lexical/morphological development may be consequent to slow development in phonology and vice versa. This also has an impact on intervention strategies. Influences of the *phonotactics* of Maltese are noticeable. Clusters surfaced early, so that by 3;0 most children were producing some. However, their stability in respect of contrastivity and matching to the adult system seemed to take a relatively long time for mastery (possibly even longer than for learners of other languages). Implications could be that the complex phonotactics of the language in question have an influence on phonological stability/mastery.

Phonological Systems of Maltese-Speaking Children with Speech Disorders

To date, there are no publications related to studies of speech disorders in Maltese-speaking children. However, clinical records of the developmental profiles of such children are available. This section will describe aspects of the phonological systems of two Maltese children who exhibit atypical patterns.

A.B. is an 8;6-year-old boy born with a bilateral cleft lip and palate. The boy was also diagnosed as having congenital heart defects and mild pulmonary stenosis. He has gone through 10 surgical procedures in connection with his congenital defects. A.B. was also diagnosed with attention deficit and hyperactivity disorder. He speaks Maltese and English fluently though his speech is unintelligible to unfamiliar people. There are no concerns about his verbal comprehension and expression skills; he has basic writing skills although he cannot read yet. A.B. produced all the adult phones except for /ts/ in his spontaneous utterances as phonemes. [k, g, w] were produced marginally. There were not enough representations of /w/ in the speech sample. However, there were many opportunities for the occurrence of /k/ and /g/ and yet these were often uttered as [ʔ]. The boy produced most of the phonemes with a lot of variation. Analysis indicated the use of processes such as cluster reduction, gemination of consonants in sequence and glottalisation. There were other potential developmental processes used. The criterion for process inclusion was strict and hence these could not be considered as 'processes'. However, other than 'glottalisation' none of these processes are atypical of a normally-developing Maltese speaking child. A.B.'s speech is highlighted by cleft-type characteristics (Sell, Harding & Grunwell, 1994) and his phonology is relatively delayed. However, glottal substitution occurred not only for voiceless plosives as is usually the case with cleft palate speakers (Sell et al., 1994) but also for fricatives, affricates and one voiced plosive /g/. This characteristic could be language specific (resulting from the influence of the glottal stop as a Maltese adult phoneme).

G.M. is a 5;4-year-old Maltese-speaking child who was referred for speech therapy by his mother earlier on following her concern about his speech and language development. Assessment by different professionals indicated no concern other than communication difficulties. Assessment by a speech-language pathologist indicated difficulties at syntactic, morphological and phonological level. His speech difficulties are not related to an organic problem. His phone inventory included all the adult phonemes though some were marginal (probably due to the limited size of the speech sample). His system of contrastive phones was similar to that of the Maltese adult though marked with variation indicating instability of phonemes. The child exhibited no oral dyspraxia; DDK rate was less than the expected mean. His speech errors were relatively consistent for mono- and disyllabic words though phonotactics became inconsistent with polysyllabic words. Some vowel errors were also observed. Various potential developmental processes were noted. These did not meet the strict quantitative criteria, devised by McReynolds and Elbert (1981) for process inclusion. However, while some behaviour was typical relative to the phonology of the Maltese speaking 3;6–4;0-year-old, yet some atypical patterns were noted. This included the substitution of a fricative by an affricate (affrication) and the substitution of a stop by a fricative. This 'atypical' behaviour could be considered as language specific possibly related to the relatively large number of affricates and fricatives in the adult phonological system.

Speech-Language therapy service in the Maltese Islands

Speech therapy in Malta and Gozo is relatively young and is expanding gradually. Fifty full-time practitioners are currently providing the speech therapy service. In the 1980s the Maltese who benefited from the local speech therapy service were limited in number, mainly because of the scarcity of staff and lack of awareness of the service. The increase in the number of recruited personnel brought about an expansion in the type and number of caseloads managed by speech-language pathologists.

The service has also opened up for client groups such as adults with mental handicap and those encountering specific difficulties with understanding and/or producing written language, as well as other forms of non-vocal communication. Individuals with drinking, eating and swallowing difficulties also form a significant proportion of the speech-language pathologist's caseload today. Nowadays, the service is offered in a range of settings that includes community-based clinics (health centres), acute hospitals (in-patients and out-patients), institutional settings, rehabilitation centres, day centres, school settings (special and mainstream) and the clients' homes. Therapy may take various forms, such as individual or group therapy, direct or indirect intervention and may include early intervention, rehabilitation, counselling, consultations and participation through a multidisciplinary team. Local education in logopedics has developed to address needs and culture of the Maltese population. The University of Malta took up the education and training of SLPs in 1991, with the help of expatriate colleagues from Ireland, United Kingdom and the United States. The undergraduate training course is a four-year full-time programme leading to the award of B.Sc. (Hons) in Communication Therapy. Eligibility to register and practise as a speech-language pathologist in Malta is subject to having this qualification or its equivalence. Strategies such as sending students on overseas placements, inviting overseas experts to run courses for students and in clinical teaching for practitioners, engagement in European staff/student exchange programmes and the establishment of a teaching and research clinic within the University of Malta have been adopted to provide optimal training.

Conclusion

The data reported in this chapter are bound to make a substantial contribution in local clinical settings. The identified stages of phonological development are applicable for assessment purposes in speech therapy and allied professional settings. The conventions applied in the main study for transcribing child phonology, in particular addressing the local bilingual situation, may help in the standardisation of assessment procedures which have not yet been done with universal agreement. The data helps with differential diagnosis of delayed, uneven and deviant development. Such a developmental profile would have clinical implications for the planning of treatment strategies.

The main study also contributed to a larger body of work. A cross-linguistic examination of data revealed analogous phonological acquisition trends especially in the early sampling ages, in spite of language structure and cultural differences. This research study places some weighting on the importance of sound exposure in relation to phonological development. For example, the glottal stop was one of the children's earliest developing contrastive phones in this study. This could be related to the rate of exposure of this sound. The data obtained does not rule out the applicability of the natural/biological theory. For example, the Maltese affricates /ts, /tʃ/, /dʒ/ took a relatively long time to stabilise and by the last recording stage they had not been mastered as phonemes by most of the subjects. These are complex phones to articulate; such complexity of utterance may have been influential in shifting /ts, /tʃ/, /dʒ/ acquisition to the later developmental stage. Perhaps they are more complex to articulate than some consonantal clusters. In fact, most of the children matched most of the clusters they produced with corresponding adult ones by age 3;6. Findings in the main project gave support to existing models on phonological acquisition. For example, Waterson (1987) and Fee's (1995) proposition that some sounds may not be able to surface in early child speech as a result of the segmental tier not mapping with the prosodic level, have been given more weighting by the Maltese children's behaviour in terms of compensatory prosodic lengthening.

Notes

1. [dz] is not usually given full phonemic status (see description of affricates below for details).
2. In this text this adult phoneme is represented symbolically as /r/ and referred as a liquid approximant. The children's respective production is transcribed as [r] unless it deviates from adult allophonic variation.

Appendix: Chronology of developmental processes (Maltese)

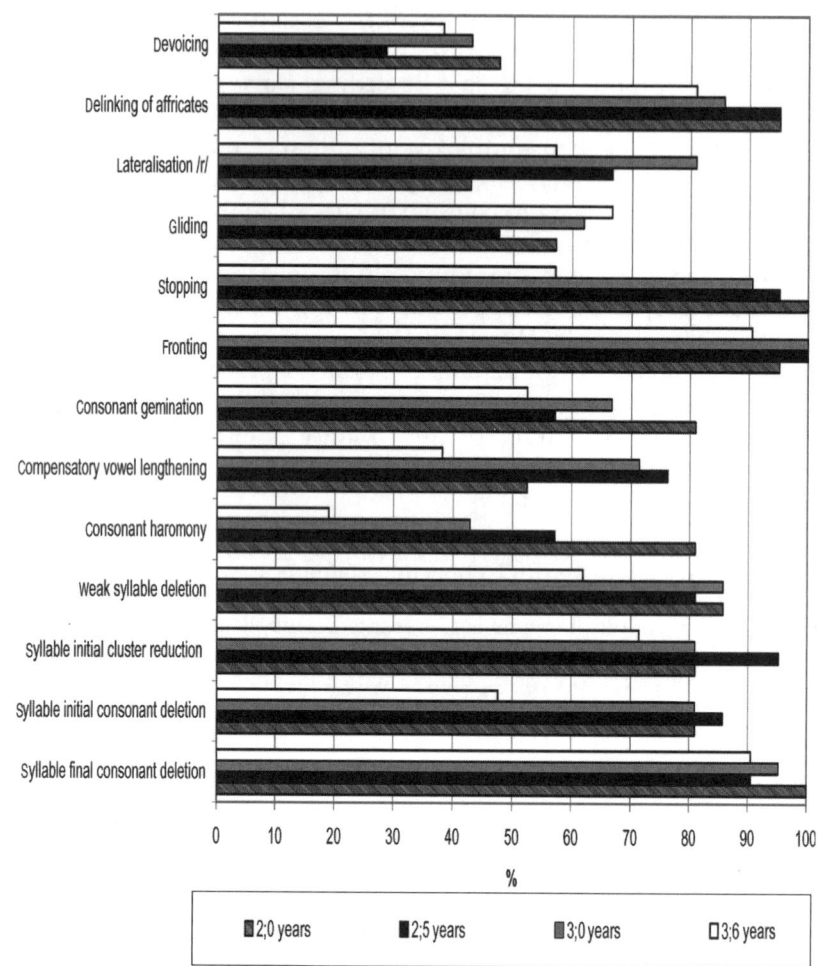

Chapter 8
Syllabic Constraints in the Phonological Errors of Children with Pre-lingual Hearing Loss: A Perspective from Telugu

D. VASANTA

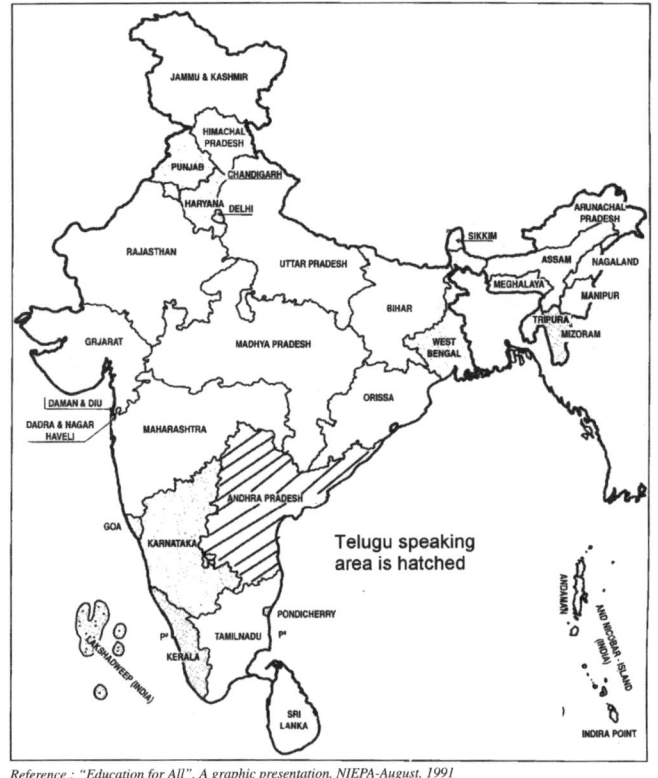

Reference: "Education for All", A graphic presentation, NIEPA-August, 1991

Figure 8.1

Introduction

Telugu belongs to the Dravidian language family. With more than 60 million people speaking this language, Telugu constitutes the largest of all the Dravidian languages. Since 1966, Telugu has been the official language of the state of Andhra Pradesh which was formed in 1956 from the Telugu speaking districts of the former presidency of Madras along with nine Telangana regions under the Nizam's dominions (Campbell, 1995). Hyderabad, the capital of Andhra Pradesh belongs to the Telangana region (see Figure 8.1).

There are four major dialects in Telugu: *Northern* – spoken in the nine Telangana districts; *Southern* – the four inland districts of Rayalasima together with Nellore and Prakasam districts; *Eastern* – Vishakhapatnam and Srikakulam districts close to the Oriya speaking area; *Central* – Midcoastal districts of East and West Godavari, Krishna and Guntur. According to Krishnamurti and Gwynn (1985), the central variety is considered as the 'standard' variety of Telugu in that it is this variety that is used in the radio, TV, textbooks, newspapers and creative writing. Both the researcher (this writer) and the hearing impaired children discussed in this study spoke the Central dialect of Telugu the phonological structure of which is described below. For other details about the distinctive features and allophones of various phonemes of Telugu, the reader is referred to Bhaskara Rao (1982), Kostic *et al.* (1977), Nagamma Reddy (1987), Prabhavathi Devi (1990), Prakasam (1978), Ramarao (1969) and Sastry (1972).

Consonants and Consonant Clusters

The Central dialect of Telugu has as many as 43 segmental phonemes of which 33 are consonants, and 10 vowels in addition to two diphthongs and aspirated consonants as shown in Tables 8.1 and 8.2.

In the standard dialect, a distinction is maintained between alveolar and alveo-palatal affricates and fricatives. Phonemes /t/ and /d/ are realised as dentals in Telugu. Phoneme /w/ is a voiced labial frictionless continuant. When it precedes front vowels, it tends to become [v], i.e. voiced labiodental fricative. [f] is a borrowed sound from English and Urdu, and is therefore not counted as part of the phonemic system of Telugu. There are as many nasal allophones as there are stops. All the stops have their aspirated counterparts, whereas only alveopalatal affricates are aspirated. However, it should be noted that aspiration is not a distinctive feature in the native vocabulary with the exception of perhaps one or two words. It occurs mainly in Tatsamas, i.e. unassimilated loan words from Sanskrit which are often abstract words (e.g. *bhayam* 'fear'; *abhivriddhi* 'progress'; *subham* 'good' etc.) which cannot be

Table 8.1 Telugu consonants

			Bilabial	Labio-dental	Dental	Alveolar	Alveo-palatal	Palato-alveolar	Retroflex	Velar	Glottal
Stop	Vl.	Unasp.	p		t̪				ʈ	k	
		Asp.	pʰ		t̪ʰ				ʈʰ	kʰ	
	Vd.	Unasp.	b		d̪				ɖ	g	
		Asp.	bʰ		d̪ʰ				ɖʰ	gʰ	
Affricate	Vl.	Unasp.				ts	c				
		Asp.					cʰ				
	Vd.	Unasp.				dz	ɟ				
		Asp.					ɟʰ				
Fricative				f		s	ś	ʃ			h
Nasal			m			n			ɳ		
Lateral						l			ɭ		
Trill						r					
Semi-vowel			w				j				

Note: Vl.: voiceless; Vd.: voiced; Asp.: aspirated; Unasp.: unaspirated.

Table 8.2 Telugu vowels and diphthongs

	Front	*Central*	*Back*
Close	i:		u:
	i		u
Half close	e:		o:
	e		o
Half open	(æ:)		
Open		a	
		a:	
Diphthongs		ai	au

picturized and as such are of little use in clinical contexts. The alveolar and alveo-palatal distinctions among affricates and fricatives are also confined to very limited vocabulary with restricted frequency of occurrence. For these reasons, a two way rather than a three-way distinction among affricates and fricatives is maintained in this study. Thus, out of the phoneme inventory for the central dialect of Telugu, only 21 different consonants, five vowels both short and long versions were utilized in designing assessment tools for the present study. The 21 different consonant phonemes allowed for contrast of the features: nasality, voicing, continuancy and place. There are minimal pairs for each of these features in both word initial and word medial positions.

Consonant clusters occur primarily in word medial position in Telugu. In the initial position they occur in loan words and typically take the form stop +y, w, r, l clusters. The clusters operating on the native vocabulary are primarily geminates (kk, cc, tt, pp, gg, etc.); nasal + homorganic stops (nt, nd, nk, ng; mp, mb, etc.); stops or affricates combining with /y/, /r/, /l/ and /w/. In all the clusters, fricatives can be followed by a plosive, but not vice versa. The trill /r/ can occur after any major consonant types other than an affricate. Semivowels do not occur before voiced aspirated stops. Similarly nasals do not occur after breathy voiced stops. Fricatives also do not occur after aspirated consonants and affricates. Three consonant clusters occur word medially in Telugu. The permitted combinations are fricative + plosive + trill; nasal + obstruent + liquid /semivowel; trill + obstruent + trill/semivowel.

Vowels

The 10 vowel phonemes in Telugu (/i, e, a, u, o/ plus their long counterparts) occur in all three positions of a word, although not with the same frequency. Vowel length is phonemic in Telugu in that just the length of the vowel alone distinguishes the meaning (e.g. *nela* 'month' – *neːla* 'floor'; *nadi* 'river' – *naːdi* 'mine'; *kona* 'end' – *koːna* 'forest'). Vowel /æ/ is always long and is not counted as an independent phoneme as it does not occur in the other dialects. The high and mid-back vowels are rounded, all the rest are unrounded. Phonetically, front vowels are preceded by a homorganic onglide [y] when they constitute an initial syllable (as in *yiːḍu* 'marriageable age'; *yeːru* 'river'); and back vowels in the same environment are preceded by [w] as in *wuːru* 'village' and *woːḍa* 'ship'.

It is a common observation that open vowels (e.g. /a/, /aː/) are longer than their corresponding close vowels (e.g. /i/, /u/) and that the diphthongs are about the same duration as the long vowels. Vowel duration is subject to a number of contextual effects. For instance, vowels preceding voiced consonants are longer than those preceding voiceless consonants; a vowel occurring after an aspirated consonant is longer than that occurring after an unaspirated consonant; a vowel in word final position is longer than the same vowel in other word positions; a vowel in the first syllable of a disyllabic word is longer than the same vowel in a trisyllabic word; a vowel in a stressed syllable is longer than that in an unstressed syllable; both vowel and consonant duration can be used effectively to achieve emphasis.

It can be seen from the above discussion that the most (functionally) important vowel contrasts are: vowel duration; vowel height, vowel place and vowel versus diphthong. Perception of vowel as well as consonant length is crucial in that it signals phonological contrastiveness as evident in the examples given in Table 8.3.

Phoneme Frequencies

Based on 96,882 printed Telugu syllables drawn from a random sampling of modern fiction, newspapers and scientific literature, Kostic *et al.* (1977) offered the following phoneme frequencies: Vowels constituted 47.21% compared to consonants which occurred at 52.79%. The frequency of central unrounded vowels (a, aː) is reported to be more than the combined frequencies of the front unrounded and back rounded vowels. The mid-vowels (e, eː, o, oː) are less frequent than the high vowels and long vowels less frequent than the corresponding short ones. Among the consonants, in terms of place of articulation, coronals (dentals, alveolar and retroflex) were very frequent (29.63%) followed by palato-velars (12.15%) and then labials (10.78%). In terms of manner, stops had the highest frequency of occurrence (23.79%); followed by nasals (10.06), liquids (9.63), semivowels (5.63%) and fricatives (3.45). The frequency of aspirated stops and fricatives was very low suggesting their foreign

Table 8.3 Examples of Telugu words showing contrastiveness in vowel and consonant length

VCCV/CVCCV	VVCV/CVVCV	VNCV/CVNCV	VVCV/CVVCV
aḍḍu obstruction	a:ḍu to play	kanḍa meat	ka:ḍa stem
uppu salt	u:pu to swing	unḍa ball	u:ḍa prop root
oḍḍu bank	o:ḍu defeat	panṭa crop	pa:ṭa song
ekku to climb	e:ku cotton spindle	enḍu to dry	e:ḍu seven
wippu to open	wi:pu back	wampu bend	wa:pu swelling
guḍḍu egg	gu:ḍu nest	gunḍu bald head	gu:ḍu nest
pakku boil	pa:ku to crawl	pongu to boil over	po:gu earring
callu to sprinkle	ca:lu enough	cempa cheek	ce:pa fish
burra head	bu:ra balloon	maamsam meat	ma:sam month
gitta calf	gi:ta line	ninḍaa full	ni:ḍa shade

Note: Notice that the vowel preceding a germinate consonant is always short, whereas, a consonant cluster can be preceded by a long vowel (as in maamsan 'meat').

origin. In the unaspirated series, voiceless stops were more frequent relative to voiced ones.

Syllable Structures

Some of the published facts pertaining to Telugu syllable structure are described only to provide a background against which the results of this study can be discussed. The examples of the canonical syllable structures in Telugu are: VCV (e.g. *ala* 'wave'); VVCV *uuru* 'village'; VCCV *atta* 'aunt'; CVCV (e.g. *kala* 'dream'); CVC1C1V (e.g. *ceyyi* 'hand'); CVVCV (e.g. *kaalu* 'leg'); CVVCVC (e.g. *kaaram* 'chilly powder'); CVC1C2V (e.g. *waarta* 'news'); CVNC1C2VC (e.g. *gunḍram* 'round'); CVCVCV (*goḍugu* 'umbrella'); CVVCVCV (e.g. *naalugu* 'four'); CVCVCVCV (e.g. *tiragali* 'grinding stone').

Although very little published information is available on the frequency of occurrence of different syllable structures, going by native speaker intuitions, it appears that disyllables of the type CVCCV, CVVCV and CVCV are more common than the others. One of the characteristic features of Telugu is that there are more open syllables than closed syllables. The first syllable of every word receives the primary stress. In disyllabic words like *ga:li* 'wind', the second syllable is unstressed. However, the second syllable of a disyllabic word receives secondary stress if the coda of the first syllable and onset of the second syllable contain similar consonants as in words, *akka* 'sister' or *patti* 'cotton' etc. Sastry (1994) provides a detailed description of the stress rules governing both native and borrowed vocabularies in Telugu.

Typically Developing Children

Acquisition of segments and syllables

One of the exhaustive accounts of acquisition of Telugu in normal children is that of Nirmala (1981a), who studied four children in the age range 1;6–3;0 years over a period of next six months. For each child, speech samples were collected in six different sessions (separated by one month interval) of one to one and half hour duration each. The data were later transcribed by the experimenter herself who is a professionally trained linguist. The results revealed that even the youngest child of 1;6 years old was able to produce and contrast all the major vowel phonemes except [æ] which anyway is not treated as a separate phoneme in the language. Among the consonants, nasals appeared first, followed by stops, laterals, affricates, fricatives and trills/flaps in that order. Voiceless phonemes were acquired earlier than voiced ones. Contrasts among the voiceless stops and nasals were established before those among voiced stops affricates and semivowels. Aspirated phonemes were acquired by 3;5 at which point the distinction between retroflex versus non-retroflex sounds was still emerging. Glottal fricative /h/ had no substitutes and it was deleted in the speech of all four children until the age of 3;5 years. There were many substitutions among medial consonant clusters produced by 2;6–3;5-year-olds. These involved dentals for alveolars and retroflex consonants; affricates for fricatives; laterals for trills. Geminate and homorganic clusters were acquired earlier than the others. There were many instances of two consonant culsters being rendered as geminates in the first session, but by the last session (six months later) two of the four children learned to differentiate them into clusters. Most of the substitutions affected words longer than three syllables but rarely two syllable words. Discussing her acquisitional data pertaining to consonant clusters, Nirmala (1981b) stated that three major phonological processes seem to govern consonant cluster acquisition, *viz.*, deletion, substitution and assimilation. She posited the following hierarchy: (1) total deletion of the cluster, (2) reduction + substitution, (3) substitution + assimilation, (4) substitution of one or both the consonants, and (5) adult like clusters.

To summarise the salient points of this section, in Telugu, the frequency of central unrounded vowels (/a/, /ai/) is more than the combined frequency of front unrounded and back rounded vowels. Mid vowels are less frequent than high vowels, and long vowels less frequent than short vowels. Among consonants, coronals (dentals, alveolars and retroflex) are more frequent than palato-velars and labials. In terms of manner of articulation, stops and nasals are more frequent than liquids and fricatives. Medial consonant clusters, especially geminates, are more common among native Telugu words compared to initial clusters which are confined primarily to loan words. The acquisition data reveals that all the vowel contrasts are mastered before the consonantal contrasts. Contrasts among nasal and voiceless stops are acquired before those involving voiced stops, affricates and semivowels. The contrast between retroflex and non-retroflex is still emerging around the age of 3;5 years. Telugu words typically end in an open syllable. Two syllable words are more common than three or tetrasyllabic words. In child language, syllable reduction is observed mainly with respect to three syllable words. There is a tendency for consonant clusters to be realised as geminates and for C1 and C2 in words to harmonise according for place. Sonority constraints are not always respected in developing phonologies of Telugu children. However, the concept of sonority is discussed in greater detail in the next section in order to explain its relevance in understanding disordered phonological systems.

Sonority

Theoretical aspects

There is a general agreement among researchers that a syllable can be divided into two primary parts: an initial consonant or a consonant cluster called the *onset*, and the vowel together with the following consonants called the *rime*. The vocalic portion of the rime (including diphthongised vowels) is referred to as the *nucleus* or peak, and the consonant(s) in the rime constitute the *coda*. Thus, in the monosyllabic English word 'feet', /f/ is the onset, and /it/ the rime; in the word, 'feast', the rime is /ist/. In both these words, /i/ is the nucleus; /t/ and /st/ are the codas respectively. English word, 'fee' represents a syllable without a coda.

Every language has co-occurrence restrictions specifying legal/illegal onsets and rimes. It was observed that while many languages permit onsets, few require codas and no language prohibits onsets. The 'best' syllable (one that enhances production and perception) is the one that is made up of single consonant (onset) and a vowel (nucleus) with no coda, that is, a syllable with CV structure. Syllables with complex onsets (CCV) or those with a coda (CVC) or those which lack an onset (V) are all considered to add a degree of complexity to the basic CV template. For a review of distributional evidence for the distinction between onsets and rimes, see Selkirk (1982). According to Clements and Keyser (1983), syllables can be ranked according to complexity (from simple to complex) as follows:

(1) CV
(2) V, CCV, CVC
(3) VC, CCVC
(4) VCC

Since optimal syllables are those which should enhance production and perception, it was predicted that simple syllables should occur more often in the languages of the world than complex syllables. This turned out to be true. For instance, frequency counts of syllable types (based on dictionary entries as well as predicted through computational models) for a diverse group of 10 different languages have shown that CV syllables outnumber any other type of syllable structures (Joanisse, 1999). Cross-linguistic studies dealing with syllable structures revealed that there exist implicational universals such that if a language allows a template of a given complexity, it should also allow the simpler template (see Greenberg, 1978).

Vennemann (1988) argued that a hierarchy of CV syllable templates is inadequate to capture all the linguistic facts, and that syllables should be ranked not only based on their structural properties (whether they have onsets, if so, whether those onsets are simple or complex, etc.), but also according to the nature of the segments contained in the syllable (for instance, whether the onset consonant is an obstruent or a sonorant). The reason for this argument is that different classes of speech sounds are known to differ from one another along a property called, *sonority* or perceived loudness. Two factors determine the sonority of a sound; one, the degree of jaw opening or stricture, and two, its propensity for voicing. Thus, it was noted that stops, affricates and fricatives (obstruents) with greater degree of stricture are less sonorous than liquids and nasals. Within each category, voiced ones have greater sonority than their voiceless counterparts.

Drawing on the sonority theory which dates back to late 19th century, Clements (1990) among several others, proposed a sonority hierarchy (SH) that puts Obstruents (O), that is, stops, fricatives and affricates at the bottom end of the hierarchy and Nasals (N), Liquids (L), Glides (G), and Vowels (V) in that order towards the most sonorous end of the scale:

Stops < Fricatives < Nasals < Liquids < Glides < Vowels
[t, d]   [s, f]   [m, n]   [l, r]   [y, w]   [a, i]

It should be noted that the ONLGV scale is fundamentally determined by the degree of vocal tract constriction for production of that class of speech sounds. Other researchers have specified the sonority values of different sounds such that one can calculate sonority distance between adjacent sounds within or across syllables (see Hogg & McCully, 1987, for elaboration of this point).

Phonologists also noted that the optimal syllables prefer a sonority contour that includes a sharp rise in sonority from initial consonant (onset) to the vowel (nucleus) and a minimal or no sonority descent from nucleus to the coda resulting in peaks and troughs as in CVCV syllables. This principle seems to have been based on the observation that obstruents (with low sonority) tend to occur mostly in the onset position, whereas liquids and glides (relatively high sonority) predominantly occur in the coda position in the languages of the world. Further, there is no language that permits obstruent codas and prohibits sonorant codas suggesting that sonorants are more natural codas than obstruents. In other words, liquids cohere with a vowel to a greater degree than obstruents. The perceptual implication of this distributional evidence is that the transition from high sonority nucleus (vowel/diphthong) to liquid codas may be perceptually less salient than the transition from obstruent onsets to the nucleus.

Some of the behavioural evidence reviewed by Treiman (1989) showed that the division of the rime (into nucleus and coda) depends upon the nature of the consonant that follows the vowel. That is, there is a differential affinity between the vowel and the post-vocalic consonant(s) in the coda such that, liquids for instance, are more closely tied to the vowel than nasals and that obstruents have the weakest vowel–consonant bond; that rimes made up of vowels followed by obstruents are easier to segment into phonemes than rimes made up of vowel plus relatively high sonority consonants like liquids.

Sonority and developing phonologies

Data from developing phonologies also demonstrated that syllables with CV structure where the C is a stop (which is maximally distant from the vowel in terms of sonority) is preferred during the initial stages over other syllables of same structure such as [ra] or [wa]. That is, stop plus vowel combinations are acquired earlier than liquid plus vowel or glide plus vowel combinations. The sonority theory also predicts that initial consonant clusters will reduce to whichever consonant that creates a maximal sonority rise (see Ohala, 1995 for a detailed discussion based on English). Sonority has been shown to play a role in the phoneme awareness abilities of four and six-year-old English-speaking children in tasks involving phoneme segmentation (Yavaş & Gogate, 1999). Sonority hierarchies have permitted prediction of speech error types in individuals with language disorders (see Christman, 1992 for English; Romani & Calabrese, 1998 for Italian data on aphasics).

It has been shown that languages differ not only with respect to the types of onsets and codas but also with regard to the prosodic profiles of the syllables. That is, factors such as stress and durational units like mora have been shown to influence performance in sound blending and segmentation tasks in Japanese (Kubozono, 1996). In other words, prosodic information interacts with the orthoghic units and influences the preferred pattern of segmentation. Otake *et al.* (1993) also noted with regard to French, English and Japanese that the language's rhythm determines the segmentation unit. Much of this research has shown that the way listeners accomplish speech segmentation is influenced by the way their native language organises its rhythm and whether or not this information is encoded in the orthography. This point is corroborated in several other cross-linguistic investigations (see Cutler *et al.*, 2001, 2003; Derwing & Yoon, 1999; Lisker & Krishnamurti, 1991; Sailaja, 2000).

Goswami *et al.* (1998) argued that the level of phonology that is represented in the orthography varies considerably across different languages. In a language such as Serbo-Croatian, the orthography is transparent (shallow) in that there is a more or less one-to-one relationship between letters and phonemes. In English on the other hand, such a relation is absent making the orthography rather deep. The level of child's phonological knowledge at any given point interacts with his/her orthographic representations in the processing of words (Goswami, 1999a, b). In other words, reading development is basically an interactive process by which phonological knowledge is interlinked with orthographic representations.

Telugu Orthography

Telugu as well as the other Dravidian languages make use of orthographies which are termed syllabic alphabets. Syllabic alphabets basically consist of two kinds of graphemes: vowels (Vs) and consonants (Cs) with an inherent neutral vowel transliterated as [*a*]. V graphemes come in two different forms: independent form in word initial (syllabic) vowels and conjunct forms to be combined with a C + [a] letter with the conjunct V superseding the inherent V. In addition, there are some auxiliary devices such as the V muting *virama* and *visarga* to indicate nasalisation. A written symbol that denotes a speech syllable as is the case in all syllabic alphabet systems is called graphic syllable or syllabogram, the basic unit of such writing systems. Complex syllables are often represented synthetically by combining two or more syllabograms. Not all languages with syllabaries or syllabic alphabet type of writing systems analyse spoken and written utterances the same way. In other words, the unit of speech analysis and the unit of written representation differ from one another (Coulmas, 1999).

Telugu has as many as 56 graphemes and allographs: 16 graphemes corresponding to the vowels; 22 to the stop consonants; five to the nasals; one to the alveolar flap; two to the two laterals; three to the voiceless fricatives; two to the frictionless continuants; one to the glottal fricative; one representing the visarga (nasal before the consonants) and a few others to represent complex syllables. It was pointed out that the system is more complex with 12 graphemes for the primary vowels which would generate 12 × 22 or 264 CV sequences; 22 × 22 or 484 consonant plus consonant combinations, although only 140 of the latter actually occur in the language. All in all, more than 400 printed characters (12 + 264 +140) are needed to represent the various speech sounds and sound combinations in Telugu language (see Krishnamurti & Gwynn, 1985). Charts displaying the primary and secondary graphic symbols of Telugu consonants and vowels are given in Tables 8.4 and 8.5.

In complex words involving clusters, the ordering of the secondary form of vowel and consonant graphemes is not dictated by the way the word is articulated. For instance, in a word like *kurci*: 'chair', the vowel marker associated with the long vowel /i:/ is attached to /r/ and not /c/ eventhough the latter follows /r/ in pronunciation. Similarly, words containing anuswara [o] indicating a nasal before an obstruent take on

Table 8.4 Combinations of consonant and vowel

		k	c	T	t	p	g	j	D	d	b	N	n	m	y	r	l	w	ś	S	s	h	L	
అ	్	క	చ	ట	త	ప	గ	జ	డ	ద	బ	ణ	న	మ	య	ర	ల	వ	శ	ష	స	హ	ళ	a
ఆ	ా	కా	చా	టా	తా	పా	గా	జా	డా	దా	బా	ణా	నా	మా	యా	రా	లా	వా	శా	షా	సా	హా	ళా	aa
ఇ	ి	కి		టి		పి							ని		యి		లి							i
ఈ	ీ	కీ							డీ								లీ							ii
ఉ	ు	కు				పు		జు	డు									వు	షు		హు	శు	u
ఊ	ూ	కూ		తూ		పూ		జూ										బూ						uu
ఎ	ె	కె	చె												యె	రె								e
ఏ	ే	కే												మే		లే								ee
ఐ	ై	కై																						ai
ఒ	ొ	కొ		టొ	పొ									మొ	యొ				షొ	సొ	హొ			o
ఓ	ో	కో		టో	పో									మో	యో				షో	సో	హో			oo
ఔ	ౌ	కౌ			పౌ									మౌ	యౌ				షౌ	సౌ	హౌ			au

Table 8.5 Combinations of consonant and consonant

	k	c	T	t	p	g	j	D	d	b	N	n	m	y	r	i	w	ś	S	s	h	L
k	క్క	క్చ	క్ట	క్త	క్ప							క్న	క్మ	క్య					క్ష	క్స		
c	చ్చ																					
T	ట్క		ట్ట									ట్న		ట్య	ట్ర	ట్ల						
t				త్త																		
p				ప్త	ప్ప							ప్న	ప్మ	ప్య	ప్ర	ప్ల				ప్స		
g						గ్గ						గ్న	గ్మ	గ్య	గ్ర	గ్ల						
j							జ్జ							జ్య		జ్ల						
D								డ్డ						డ్య	డ్ర	డ్ల						
d									ద్ద			ద్న	ద్మ	ద్య	ద్ర	ద్ల						
b										బ్బ		బ్న		బ్య	బ్ర	బ్ల						
N											ణ్ణ											
n		ంచ	ంత	న్ప	ంగ	ంజ		ంద				న్న	న్మ	న్య	న్ర	న్ల				న్స		
m				ంప									మ్మ									
y														య్య								
r	ర్క	ర్చ	ర్ట	ర్త	ర్ప	ర్గ	ర్జ	ర్డ	ర్ద	ర్బ	ర్ణ	ర్న	ర్మ	ర్య		ర్ర	ర్ల			ర్స	ర్హ	
l	ల్క	ల్చ	ల్ట	ల్త	ల్ప	ల్గ		ల్డ		ల్బ		ల్ణ	ల్మ	ల్య		ల్ల				ల్స	ల్హ	
w														వ్య	వ్ర		వ్వ					
ś														శ్య	శ్ర	శ్ర		శ్శ				
S			ష్ట									ష్ణ		ష్య					ష్ష			
s	స్క	స్చ		స్త	స్ప							స్న	స్మ	స్య	స్ర	స్ర				స్స		
h												హ్న	హ్మ	హ్య	హ్ర	హ్ర					హ్హ	
L														ళ్య		ళ్ర						ళ్ళ

different values depending on the preceding consonant and yet such phonological information is not encoded by the orthography. This means, children have to make use of their orthographic knowledge as well as phonological awareness skills in learning to read and spell Telugu words (see Vasanta, 2004 for details).

Syllabic Alphabets and Phonological Awareness

Studies of speech segmentation abilities of illiterate and biliterate Telugu and English-speaking adults (Sailaja, 1997, 1998) have shown that illiterates had considerable difficulty segmenting spoken words into syllables and that orthography strongly affects analysis of a spoken word in the literate population. The preferred syllable division by the literate subjects, however, violates the sonority sequencing principle which states that from the syllable peak (vowel) onwards there must be a decline in sonority. The violation of this principle is evident in VCV syllables getting divided as V-CV; VCCV as V-CCV and VNCV as VN-CV in their production. In a later study Sailaja (1999) argued that the reason for this is that Telugu does not permit consonants in word final position (no coda principle) except for [m]. When asked to indicate their preferred syllable division among three alternatives provided by the experimenter (the participants had to judge which division sounded right as opposed to segmenting the spoken word themselves) biliterate adults showed a preference for splitting consonants across syllables and thus accepting a coda (e.g. *bhak-ti* 'devotion' was preferred over *bha-kti*). However, when there is a homorganic nasal and obstruent cluster in words, they preferred VN-C over V-NCV and VNC-V option probably because Telugu orthography has that rule (i.e. the preferred division for gampa 'basket' is gam.pa and not gamp.a or ga.mpa). Commenting on the results of her studies, Sailaja stated that in Telugu, the influence of orthography over phonology is so strong that sometimes certain phonological principles of the language are violated in experiments dealing with speech segmentation.

Vasanta (2003) presented evidence on how phonological awareness interacts with the orthographic knowledge in tasks involving segmentation of Telugu words in normal hearing children from 4th and 6th grade. The target words (20 meaningful and 20 nonsense words of two syllable lengths each word having a cluster) were divided into two lists: List A had all the words/nonwords in which the first syllable had obstruents in the coda whereas list B words/nonwords had sonorants in the codas of the first syllables. Going by sonority considerations, List A words/nonwords had less optimal first syllables than list B words/nonwords. However, Telugu orthographic conventions dictate that the first syllabogram of the cluster be written in its primary form, whereas, the second syllabogram appears in its secondary form. In other words, in both the lists, it is easier to isolate the first segment of the cluster than the second one (which does not carry the vowel marker) based on orthographic knowledge. If sonority considerations alone play a role in segmentation, there should not be any difference in the percent correct performance in segmenting the two components of the syllable and identifying the vocalic element. However, if orthographic knowledge acts as a variable, then children should recover the first component of the cluster better irrespective of its sonority status. The children were asked to write, next to each target word, the two orthographic syllables constituting the cluster; the vowel shared by the two consonants in the syllable; delete one of the syllables in the cluster and make up a new meaningful word (e.g. for the target word *padyam* 'poem', the expected correct response was, [d], [y], [a], *padam* 'word'). The results revealed developmental trends in the ability to do this segmentation task. While both the groups of children scored better in isolating the first component of the cluster, the younger children exhibited considerable difficulty in isolating the second component of the cluster especially in list B items. Younger children also made more errors in identifying the vowels and making up new words. Together the results suggested that in the processing of visually presented words, both phonological and orthographic considerations play a role and that for Telugu, the minimal functional unit of reading need not be a syllable. Children from both the groups were able to segment phoneme sized units even though the orthography is primarily syllabically coded.

In the course of spoken language acquisition, hearing infants encounter unsegmented audiovisual signals and not the phonological categories discussed thus far. How do they then learn to segment the input signals? How does awareness about words, syllables and phonemes develop? Considerable research evidence shows that children's attentional, perceptual/cognitive abilities, and literacy training enables them to acquire and use the various phonological categories relevant to their language. Beckman and Edwards (2000) argued that the acquisition of the phonological categories in hearing infants is influenced by the pattern frequency in the lexicon of the ambient language and that we need age-appropriate models of how the lexicon influences a child's interaction with the ambient language.

In the case of hearing impaired children, the issue (acquisition and use of phonological categories) gets more complicated, because their phonological representations are influenced by their limited auditory and lip-reading capacities as well as their reliance on written language. A considerable number of orally trained hearing impaired children (who have little or no exposure or training in sign language) use speech as their primary mode of communication. Two decades ago, Kent (1983: 26) argued that speech has to be recognized as a motor skill, but also as a mode of language expression. A child who cannot articulate speech sounds of a language being leaned (as many hearing impaired children do), will, necessarily, develop a phonology that is different in important ways from the adult model (Fey, 1992). The sub-category called developmental phonological disorders proposed by Shriberg and Kwiatkowski (1982) describes (a) children who may have deficits such as hearing impairment, mental retardation or emotional disturbances and (b) children who may have minimal or no involvement other than speech errors, essentially children with functional disorders.

Much of the published information on the manifestation of phonological disorders (in monolingual or bilingual children) is confined to category (b) children mentioned in Shriberg and Kwiatkowski's definition. Hearing impaired children learning a phonological system must acquire the phonetic component (how different sounds are articulated) the phonemic component (how sounds contrast to distinguish meanings) and phonotactic component (how to use sound sequences appropriately in different positions and contexts). An understanding of how these three components are functioning in a given child is essential for planning treatment. The purpose of this paper is to present and discuss results of an earlier study (Vasanta, 1994) which throws light on the nature of syllabic constraints that operate in the speech of orally trained Telugu-speaking hearing impaired children and, to discuss some of the implications of the results.

Before going into the details of the study, it is necessary to comment briefly on the speech-language clinical service situation in the context of India.

The Term 'Phonological Disorder' in Relation to Indian Languages

The term, phonological disorder itself does not have the same currency in our context as it does in relation to English. I offer the following reasons to justify my statement:

First, the training of speech-language therapists does not include a course such as structure of an Indian language. The one or two courses in linguistics offered as part of the graduate programmes make use of books that deal with English or languages other than those spoken in India. Second, speech-language therapists are not employed in schools nor do they work in University-based centres. It is not possible to offer clients comprehensive speech-language assessment in the hospitals or private clinics. Third, there is little, if any published information on the acquisitional aspects of linguistic structures, and language processing abilities in relation to Indian languages. Fourth, computerised corpora are not available on the statistics of phonological structures in the spoken language of children. There is no readily accessible information about orthographic neighbourhood size and other such psycholinguistic variables in relation to Indian languages. Fifth, standardised assessment techniques are also not available in relation to Indian languages. Finally, there is a great demand for learning English right from the elementary grades and therefore, it is becoming increasingly difficult to find participants who are monolingual in Telugu. Phonological assessment becomes all the more difficult when one has to deal with bilingual/ biliterate populations. Thus, 'phonological disorder' is not a routine clinical entity in our context, in that, clinicians are not diagnosing children as having phonological disorder and therefore are not making use of phonologically based intervention approaches. The use of this term is primarily confined to teaching centres, conference papers and research publications.

The Study

The data to be discussed in this chapter comes from three prelingually hearing impaired Telugu children who had little or no exposure to sign language. In India, most of the children with congenital hearing impairment, especially when it is not profound, are admitted into regular schools and often into schools where the medium of instruction is

Telugu. The oral language input to these children both at home and in school is primarily Telugu. The three children of the study are monolingual Telugu speakers, although they are exposed to some common English words borrowed and used in day-to-day conversations (words such as bulb, brush, spoon, bucket, blade etc.). Going by Shriberg and Kwiatkowski's (1982) classification system, I consider these three children to have developmental phonological disorder. I will discuss the nature of the phonological errors noted in their speech and writing with a focus on syllable level errors.

Traditional approaches to phonological analysis based on phonetic transcription and listing of phonological processes will not reveal the differences in the phonological knowledge of subgroups of hearing impaired children at the qualitative level. Some of the errors might be confined to the temporal domain – errors in the realisation of syllable internal rhythmic structures. Such errors often go unrecognised in process-based analysis which focuses more on consonantal articulation with total exclusion of vowel and suprasegmental aspects (see Butcher, 1989).

The Sample

I had studied, in detail, the phonological systems of six Telugu speaking deaf children. Of these, only three children's data has been analysed and presented here. These three children had prelingual hearing loss which was detected even before the age of two years. They started wearing hearing aids from the age of four years, and were admitted to regular schools. Each of them also received speech-language therapy on an individual basis for an average period of two years before they started going to regular school. None of these children had any middle-ear infections, as ascertained by tympanogram and impedence tests. The background information is summarised in Table 8.6.

Phonological Assessment

The children named 100 colour pictures of familiar objects, fruits, body parts, vehicles, etc. The recorded responses were transcribed and ana-

Table 8.6 Subject information

Subject	Age (years)	Sex	Grade	No. of siblings	PTA HL in dB	Lip reading scores
L.S.	10.8	F	V	One	91.25	80.9
S.D.	10.9	F	VI	One	76.87	79.3
K.A.	13.6	F	VII	One	94.37	83.58

lysed for phonetic competence. Instrumental analysis was done to examine production of vowel length and consonant germination. The phonetic inventories did not show up any major problems or deviations compared to normal hearing children. The phonemic inventories revealed that there were hardly any vowel contrast errors and consonants were produced more accurately in the medial position than in the initial position. Phonological contrastivity was tested in this study using a specially designed test described below.

Telugu Test of Phonological Contrastiveness (TTPC)

This test, developed specifically for the purposes of this study (Vasanta, 1994) is capable of evaluating production and/or perception of six different phonemic contrasts in Telugu, *viz.*, vowel place, vowel height, vowel duration, consonant voicing, consonant place, and consonant manner. As evident in the phonological description given earlier in this chapter, in Telugu, consonants, for the most part occur in word initial and word medial positions and not in word final position. Therefore, all the three consonant feature contrasts (voicing, place and manner) have two components; word initial contrast and word medial contrast. Thus for instance, consonant voicing contrast in alveolar stops is evaluated in word initial position using Telugu minimal pairs such as *tummu* 'sneez' – *dummu* 'dust' and the same contrast in the medial position is evaluated using a minimal pair such as *baatu* 'duck' – *baadu* 'to beat'. This test made up of 100 minimal pairs evaluates the following phonemic contrasts:

Vowel place (front-back): 10 items;
Vowel height (high-low): 10 items;
Vowel duration (short-long): 10 items;
Vowel vs. diphthong: 10 items;
Consonant voicing: 10 items;
Consonant place: 20 items;
Consonant manner: 30 items

Based on the well established information on the relationship between feature perception and deafness (Boothroyd, 1984; Vasanta, 1986), it may be predicted that children whose average hearing loss of 90 dB or more will be able to perceive almost all the vowel contrasts, voice contrasts and some of the place contrasts, whereas, those with hearing loss less than 90 dB may be able to perceive all the vowel contrasts, the place contrasts and some of the voice and manner contrasts as well. However, whether they can maintain these contrasts in their production to generate differences in meaning is something that needs to be tested empirically. This test provides an opportunity to do so. A binary scoring method was used to assign a score of one for the presence of a given contrast as judged by the two trained linguists (who transcribed the tape recorded data independently) and zero for absence of the contrast.

To check whether the child understood the meaning of each word in each minimal pair and has the linguistic potential to use it to fill an incomplete sentence, each of the 100 minimal pairs was placed next to an incomplete sentence. Completion of 25 of the total 100 sentences required the child to make a morpho-phonemic alternation, for instance by adding a plural marker. Binary scoring of right and wrong was used for the presence or absence of a given contrast. Child's ability to produce morphophonemic alternations was assessed separately.

To facilitate easy reading, and at the same time maintain print size and quality, all the word and sentence stimuli in this test were processed on a computer. The results based on this test provided information on phonemic inventories of the subjects of this study.

Reading and spelling tests

Each child was asked to 'read thirsty crow' story in a quiet room. The recorded samples were analysed for errors besides obtaining intelligibility ratings from 12 experienced and 12 inexperienced listeners. Data was also collected regarding direct spelling of words and nonwords and spelling via lipreading of words.

All the traditional segment based analyses (e.g. phonetic and phonemic inventories, phonological contrastiveness, reading and spelling test, phonological processes, etc.) revealed some differences among the three children. While they were able to use the most simple rule of plural formation, viz., addition of suffix [–lu] to the noun stems, none of them had adequate knowledge of morphophonemic alternations in words. The rest of the results are shown in Table 8.7.

The acoustic analysis (formant frequencies of vowels, vowel duration rations, consonant closure durations, etc.), and the results of reading

Table 8.7 Results of phonological contrastivity, word comprehension, and speech intelligibility of the three hearing impaired subjects

Subject	Vowel contrastivity reading minimal pairs	Consonant contrastivity reading minimal pairs	Word comprehension in sentence completion	Intelligibility score (%)	
				EL $n = 12$	IL $n = 12$
L.S.	82.5	48.88	82	57	33
S.D.	92.5	63.88	72	70	67
K.A.	92.5	39.44	79	65	52

Note: EL = experienced listeners; IL = inexperienced listeners.

Table 8.8 Syllable structures in oral reading

Subject	VCV/VCVC CVCV/CVVCV (82)	VCCV $CVC_1C_1V(C)$ (76)	CVC_1C_2V $CVVC_1C_2V$ (24)
S.D.	104	58	20
L.S.	92	84	4
K.A.	80	95	6

and spelling tasks revealed that S.D. who had better hearing ability seems to possess phonological knowledge that is somewhat different from that of L.S. and K.A. For instance, an examination of the syllable structure produced by S.D. during oral reading (disyllabic words alone are discussed here since none of the children had difficulty producing CVCVCV structures) revealed that she had difficulty with words containing geminate consonants with $CVC_1.C_1V$ syllable structure (e.g. pakka 'bed') which became CVVCV structures (pa:ka). L.S. and K.A. on the other hand had difficulty with CVNCV structures (e.g. sanci 'bag'). These results are displayed in Table 8.8.

Basically, S.D. demonstrated a tendency to change two syllabic words with geminates into two open syllables without codas (this tendency was also evident in developing phonology); whereas both L.S. and K.A. had considerable difficulty in producing two syllable words with clusters which are basically homorganic nasal and stop clusters. In their speech, they became geminates after the nasal got deleted (refer to my earlier analysis of cluster to geminate transformations in developing phonology of Telugu). With a view to understand the constraints that reduced geminates and clusters in disyllabic Telugu words in the speech of the hearing impaired children, I have classified these errors into onset errors and coda errors and displayed the results in Tables 8.9 and 8.10.

On the whole, the children made very few errors in the onsets of disyllabic words they red aloud. In contrast, the total percentage of errors in the codas at the syllabic boundaries of words containing geminates and

Table 8.9 Errors noted in the syllable onsets during oral reading

Subject	OV (47)	NV (16)	LV (3)	GV (4)	Total (70)
S.D.	1	1	–	–	2
L.S.	–	6	3	–	9
K.A.	1	–	–	1	2

Syllabic Constraints in the Phonological Errors of Children

Table 8.10 Errors noted in the syllable codas during oral reading

Subject	VG (1)	VL (13)	VN (32)	VO (48)	Total (94)
S.D.	–	5	2	14	21
L.S.	–	4	25	9	38
K.A.	–	5	15	4	24

Note: OV = obstruent followed by vowel; NV = nasal followed by vowel; LV = liquid followed by vowel; GV = glide followed by vowel in Table 8.9; reverse notation applies in Table 8.10.

clusters is much higher. This finding, that a majority of errors in the oral reading of minimal pairs by prelingually hearing impaired Telugu children are confined to the coda component of syllables, is predicted by the sonority theory.

Following the sonority sequencing, and dispersion principles discussed by Clements and Keyser (1983) and Clements (1990) that 'between any member of a syllable and the syllable peak, a sonority rise or plateau must occur' the hierarchy in Table 8.11 can be proposed for disyllabic Telugu words.

Based on this hierarchy, we can predict that optimal syllables have the shape OV, NV in onsets and VG and VL in codas. If we go back and look at the data presented in Table 8.9 we can see that all the three children have made most of their errors on VN (vowel nasal); VO (vowel obstruent)

Table 8.11 Hierarchy of complexity for onsets and codas of Telugu syllables

	Complexity	Str. of syllable onset	Examples		
			Syllable	Word	Gloss
Onsets					
Less	1	OV	Ga	*ga.di*	Room
	2	NV	Na	*na.di*	River
	3	LV	Li	*li.pi*	Script
More	4	GV	we:	*wee.lu*	Finger
Codas					
Less	1	VG	Ey	*cey.yi*	Hand
	2	VL	Al	*al.lam*	Ginger
	3	VN	ṇḍ	*Kuṇ.ḍa*	Pot
More	4	VO	Ak	*KuK.Ka*	Dog

codas which are not optimal in terms of dispersion of sonority. It is only in the CVCV or CVVCV syllabic structures that we can expect peaks and valleys of sonority associated with minimum to maximum lowering of jaw movement repeating itself. And it is these structures that appear early in developing phonology and seem to be resistant to breakdown in the speech of hearing impaired children. This is an important feature from the point of view of visual phonology as well. Some examples (see Table 8.12) of words containing VO codas were difficult for S.D., and VN codas were more difficult than VO codas for L.S. and K.A. These findings underscore the point that sonority has some influence on the phonological patterns in the speech of these children.

It is noted that a majority of S.D.'s errors exhibited compensatory vowel lengthening caused by deletion of consonants in coda position (of the first syllable). She seemed to have had problems in controlling glottal opening and closing resulting in consonant voicing errors in addition to reduction of geminates into singletons. L.S. and K.A. on the other hand, had problems controlling the movements of the velum such that in words containing homorganic nasal plus stop clusters, nasals got omitted but the duration of the intervocalic consonants was prolonged resulting in geminates in place of clusters. One can see that all the three subjects, despite problems in realising correct articulatory movements associated with complex syllable structures, had some knowledge about temporal relationships among Telugu speech sounds, that is, knowledge about syllable rhythm (see Vasanta, 1997 for an elaboration of this point).

Table 8.12 Examples of wrongly produced syllable structures during oral reading

Subject	Target	Gloss	Response
S.D.	(1) *gaddl*	Grass	Kaadi
	(2) *rubbu*	to grind	Roopu
	(3) *boKKa*	Hole	BooKa
	(4) *mabbu*	Cloud	Maapu
L.S.	(1) *campu*	to kill	Cappu
	(2) *Konga*	Crane	KooKa
	(3) *Kundi:*	Pot	Kooti:
	(4) *panda*	unripe fruit	Pitta
K.A.	(1) *pinda*	unripe fruit	Pidda
	(2) *mandu*	Medicine	Maddu
	(3) *sanci*	Bag	Taddi
	(4) *Konga*	Crane	Kogga

Table 8.13 Examples of errors noted during spelling of Telugu words

Examples of Viseme based errors			Examples of grapheme based errors		
Subject	Response/Target	%	Subject	Response/Target	%
L.S.	kuḍukoo/goḍugu Umbrella	76.19	L.S.	uyala/uuyala Swing	23.80
S.D.	babu/paamu Snake	66.66	S.D.	daara/daaram Thread	33.33
K.A.	gaaslu/gaajulu Bangles	83.33	K.A.	gaajlu/glaasu Glass	16.66

I would like to argue that this phonological knowledge interacts with the orthographic knowledge in determining the performance of hearing impaired children in experiments involving manipulation of spoken/written language. Unless our phonological assessment batteries include tests of orthographic knowledge, we will not be able to differentiate subgroups of hearing impaired children and plan differential therapy. To illustrate this point, I would like to discuss the results of these children on reading and writing tasks.

In the oral reading of the 'thirsty crow' story, the percentage of errors made by the three children did not differ markedly (the error percentages were 35.0; 38.33 and 40.0 for L.S., S.D., and K.A., respectively). However, a detailed examination of their spelling errors revealed that while L.S. and K.A. exhibited primarily viseme-grapheme confusions, a majority of S.D.'s errors were based on the use of wrong graphemes (she appears not to draw on her lipreading skills in retrieving stored lexical representations). This is illustrated by the examples in Table 8.13.

It appears that L.S. and K.A. were trying to draw on their (viseme based) phonological knowledge to recover stored representations during spelling. Those segments and features that are not easily available through lipreading (e.g. voicing and duration) are neither stored accurately nor retrieved properly during spelling tasks by these two children. S.D. who possesses better hearing ability compared to the other two children seems to be relying on a mix of phonological and orthographic knowledge for spelling words. More details about reading and spelling data and the implications of these results for remediation are provided in Vasanta (1998, 2001).

Conclusions

The syllable based analysis of the hearing impaired children's phonological errors in speech and writing revealed that their speech was subject to the influence of orthographic awareness, lipreading and residual hearing. In addition, their phonological patterns not only resembled those of typically developing children, but also respected certain universal phonological principles. For instance, S.D. showed a preference for open syllables, providing evidence for the operation of the sonority principle. She may also have derived some phonological information through her moderately impaired auditory system given her preference for CVCV syllable structures with close open jaw patterns which are perceptually more salient than other structures. Consequently she may have drawn less on her orthographic abilities than K.A. and L.S. who had a more severe hearing loss. These two children's phonological knowledge seemed more dependent on lipreading and/or orthographic cues than that of S.D.

Implications

The results reported in this chapter have a number of important implications for assessment and treatment of phonological disorders and for future research.

Assessment

There is a need to develop phonological awareness tasks that are sensitive to the phonological and orthographic features of a given language. Such tasks need to be language specific if they are to provide an understanding of phonological disorder among subgroups of hearing impaired children. For instance, the assessment of Telugu speaking hearing impaired children necessitated use of tasks such as reading of minimal pairs varying along six different vowel and consonant features (see description of the test: TTPC). Performance on language specific tasks would provide clinical information about deficits and children's implicit and metalinguistic phonological knowledge that would allow appropriate formulation of therapeutic goals.

Treatment

Some children might produce appropriate segments in isolation, but may fail to use them correctly in clusters and multisyllabic words (Velleman, 2002). Others might produce two consonants in a row only if they belong to two different syllables but fail to do so if they form a complex onset. Purely linguistic analysis that provides phonetic and phonemic inventories, information about phonological contrastiveness and phonological processes/rules is inadequate in capturing such limitations. The most appropriate therapy goals for sub-groups of hearing impaired children whose errors go beyond isolated segments and encompass temporal relations among speech sounds may be phonotactic rather than phonetic ones. Knowledge that if two consonants of a cluster are of very different sonority (e.g. /t/-/w/), that cluster is less marked and hence learnt earlier than more marked clusters (those that are uncommon in the languages of the world and are difficult to perceive and produce) will certainly influence treatment plans and goals. It has been shown that treatment of more marked clusters will cause generalisation to less marked clusters even if the latter are not targeted in treatment (see Barlow, 2001; Gierut, 1999).

Research

Children with immature or disordered phonologies demonstrate phonotactic limitations in addition to phonetic errors. Olson and Nickerson (2001: 421) concluded that 'the syllable is a unit of linguistic organization that is abstract enough to apply to both spoken and written language'. Their study demonstrated that profoundly deaf children relied more on syllabic structure than letter frequency in the visual processing of English words. Similarly, Allman (2002) demonstrated that in tests of alphabetic knowledge, concept of word and word recognition, hard-of hearing and deaf children did as well as the hearing children. However, deaf children with poor phoneme awareness displayed spelling patterns that were markedly different from hard-of hearing children who performed similarly to their hearing peers. Allman (2002) concluded that future studies need to explore the question of how phonological information is perceived and used in reading and writing processes by deaf students. The study reported here endorses this conclusion.

Chapter 9
Phonological Development and Disorders: Colloquial Egyptian Arabic

WAFAA AMMAR and RANYA MORSI

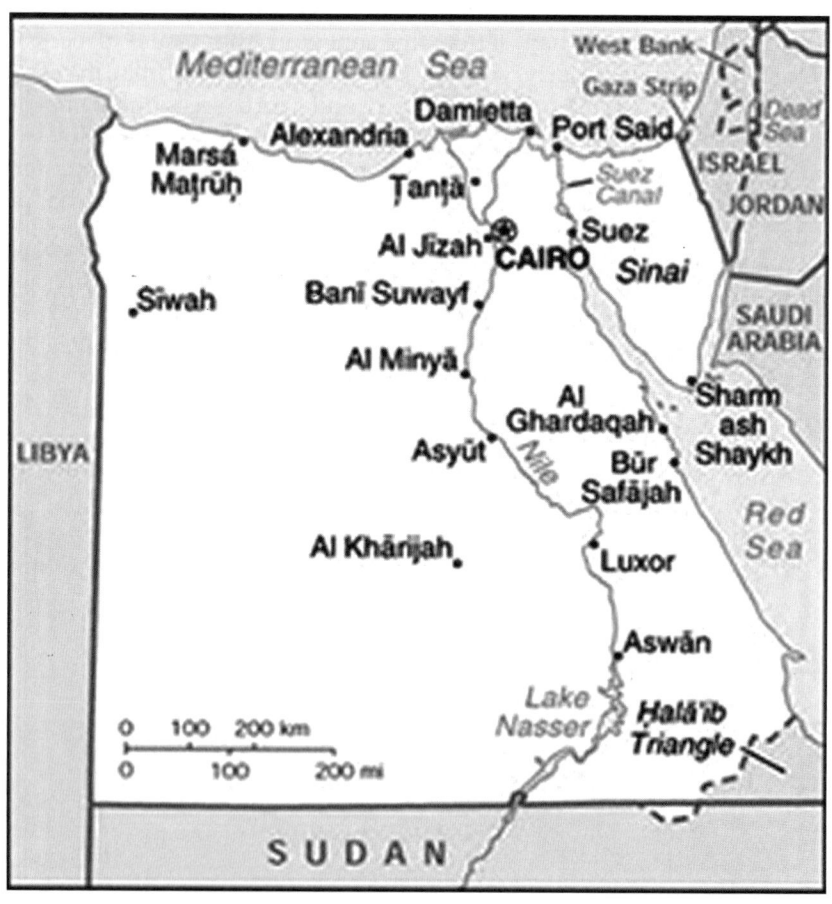

Source: http://www.nvtc.gov/Iotw/months/august/EgyptianArabic.html.

Introduction

This chapter includes an account of the main characteristics of the phonology of Egyptian Arabic, a review of previous studies of normal and disordered phonology and two recent studies. The first study is on the phonological development of normal Egyptian children between the ages of three and five years. The second is on the speech of Egyptian children with phonological disorders.

The Phonology of Egyptian Arabic

General characteristics

Colloquial Egyptian Arabic (CEA), being a dialect of Arabic, is a consonantal language. It contains 27 consonant phonemes that span the whole vocal tract from lips to glottis. Its vowel system is a simple one, containing eight vowel phonemes; with only five different qualities. Consonants are usually considered to be the cause of all vowel allophonic variations. For example, in [ʕædd] 'counted' and [ʕɑdd] 'bit', [æ] changed into [ɑ] because of the influence of the emphatic consonant [d]. The vowel allophonic variations of CEA can be accounted for by the variables of emphasisation, pharyngealisation, and tension (see Harrell, 1957). Emphasisation and pharyngealisation are caused by the spreading power of emphatic and pharyngeal consonants. Vowels are categorised as tense and lax as a function of phonemic length and stress.

Consonants play the major role in forming different syllable types in the phonology of CEA. The syllable plays an important role in both Colloquial and Classical Arabic phonology. This fact is widely recognised and any analysis of Arabic phonology must thoroughly relate to the syllable structure (Bird & Blackburn, 1990; Kay, 1987; McCarthy, 1981). The importance of the syllable can be summarised as follows:

(1) Stress is almost completely predictable in terms of syllable structure in both Classical and Colloquial Arabic (Welden, 1980).

(2) There is some evidence that intonation is predictable in terms of the syllable structure. The intonation of Arabic is 'simple'; there are few types of pitch accents and contours (Rifaat, 2003). In addition, there is a tendency for each pitch accent to be 'accented', i.e. have a peak.[1] Pitch accents are always associated with stressed syllables (Abdalla, 1960; Mitchell, 1990/1993; Rifaat, 1987, 1991, 1994, 2003).

(3) It has been noted that emphasis spread could be described in terms of syllable structure of the word (Broselow, 1976).

(4) Having recognised the importance of syllable, traditional Arab grammarians described Arabic metrics in terms of sequences of consonants and vowels, i.e. in terms of syllables.

Consonants

The consonant inventory of CEA consists of 27 phonemes (see Table 9.1). These include the primary emphatic phonemes /ṭ, ḍ, ṣ, ẓ/, which distinguish the Arabic language. The emphatic phonemes (/ṭ, ḍ, ṣ, ẓ/) physiologically differ from their non-emphatic counterparts (/t, d, s, z/) in the lip being protruded, the tongue being lowered, retracted and its front part being concave. Consequently the pharyngeal cavity is small and the oral cavity is large (see Figure 9.1).

The inventory also includes /q/ and /ʒ/ that are considered to have a low frequency of occurrence in Egyptian Arabic. The phoneme /ʒ/ is considered a marginal phoneme as all the words that include it are loan words, e.g. [gara:ʒ] 'garage', [be:ʒ] 'beige'. The phoneme /q/ occurs in few words that have persisted from classical Arabic. However, it is often substituted by /ʔ/. All consonants – except /w/ and /j/ – can occur with all vowels in all positions regardless of the subject of the frequency of occurrence of each consonant in the language (Harrell, 1957).

Vowels

There are eight vowel phonemes in CEA (see Figure 9.2). Three short vowels /a, i, u/ and five long vowels /a:, i:, e:, o:, u:/. Vowels do not occur in initial position. There are no diphthongs in CEA.

Consonant clusters

CEA permits consonant clusters only in word-final position in CVCC syllable. There are some sequences of consonants that do not occur e.g. /bf/, /fb/ (see Harrell, 1957 for more details). Voiced consonants are devoiced when followed by voiceless consonants in a cluster e.g.

Table 9.1 Consonant phonemes of CEA

	Bilabial	Labio-dental	Dental	Palatal	Velar	Uvular	Pharyn-geal	Glottal
Plosive	b		t d		k g	q		ʔ
			ṭ ḍ					
Nasal	m		n					
Trill			r					
Fricative		f	s z	ç ʒ		χ ʁ	ħ ʕ	h
			ṣ ẓ					
Semi-vowel				j	w			
Lateral			l					

Phonological Development and Disorders 207

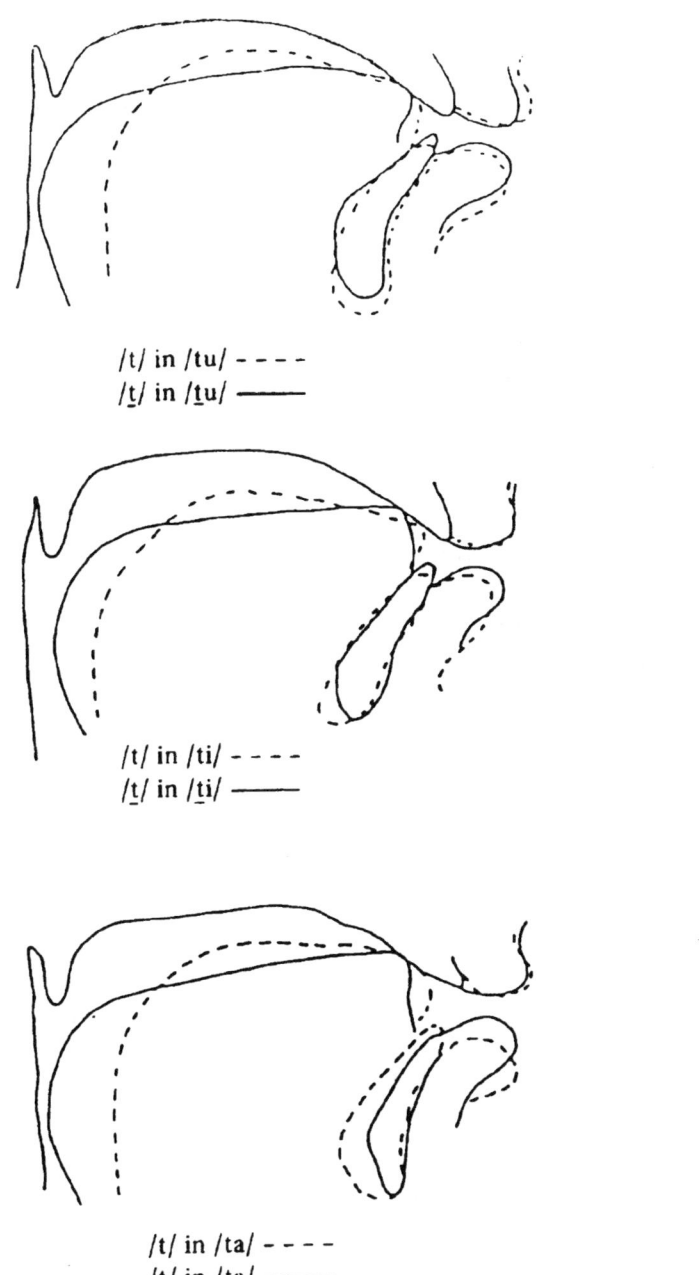

Figure 9.1 Tongue movements compared in normal versus emphatic articulation of /t/ (Al-Ani & El-Dalee, 1984: 388)

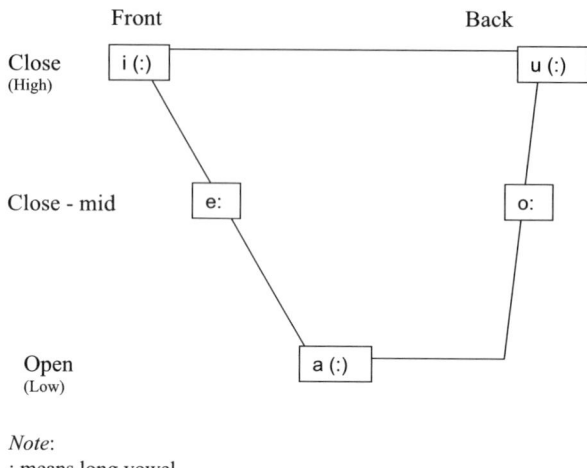

Note:
: means long vowel.
( ) means that the vowel occurs as long or short.

Figure 9.2 Vowel phonemes of CEA

/sabt/ → [sæb̥t]. When two consonants occur in medial position they are considered as abutting consonants.

Syllables

CEA has five types of syllables, two of which are short (CV and CVC) and three are long (CVV, CVVC and CVCC),[2] for examples of the five types, see Table 9.2). All types may occur as monosyllabic words. No word includes more than one heavy syllable. Concerning the positions

Table 9.2 Types of syllables in CEA

Syllable type	Length	Examples
CV	Short	ʹhæwæ ʹair'
		mæʕʹlæʔæ ʹspoon'
CVC	Short	ʹʕɑdmɑ ʹbone'
		ʹʔærnæb ʹrabbit'
CVV	Long	ʹço:kæ ʹfork'
		χıʹjɑ:rɑ ʹcucumber'
CVVC	Long	ħʊʹsɑ:n ʹhorse'
		fi:l ʹelephant'
CVCC	Long	baħr ʹsea'
		çɑʕr ʹhair'

that are allowed for each syllable, CV and CVC occur anywhere in a word, CVV occurs pre-finally, and CVVC and CVCC occur only in final position. A word may consist of one to seven syllables, although words with six and seven syllables are relatively rare.

Stress

The syllable derives a prominent status in Arabic phonology from the fact that word stress is completely predictable in terms of syllable structure of the word (Welden, 1980). There are certain rules for stress related to the syllabic structure (Gaber, 1986):

(1) Any long syllable that occurs in a word takes the primary stress. For example, [mæfæ'tiːħ] 'keys'.
(2) In any word that does not contain long syllable, the stress is pre-finally except for the following two situations:
   (a) If the second vowel in the syllabic structure CVCVCV(C) is /i/, the second syllable is stressed, for example, [çɪ'wɪlæ] 'sacs'.
   (b) If the second vowel in the syllabic structure CVCVCV(C) is /a/ or /u/, the first syllable is stressed, for example, ['ʕæg ælæ] 'bicycle'.

Previous Studies on the Typical and Atypical Acquisition of Egyptian Arabic

The study of the normal phonological acquisition of Arabic, and specifically Egyptian Arabic, has expanded in recent years. Eight studies will be reviewed.

(1) Omar (1973), in an early study, reported the order of acquisition of consonant phonemes by Egyptian children aged 1;5 to 8;0, who lived near El Menya province. Her study is concerned with the development of speech in general, so her methodology concerning the acquisition of phonemes is not well described.

(2) Ammar (1992) studied the speech of 32 Egyptian children. Sixteen children had typical development and were aged between 4;1 and 4;10. The other 16 were phonologically disordered aged between four and nine years of age. She reported their phonetic inventory, phonemic inventory and investigated 15 phonological processes that were categorized as main or secondary processes.

To determine the phonemic inventories of her four-year-old Arabic-speaking participants, Ammar (1992) followed Sander's (1972) guidelines. It was stated that there is a range for customary production of phonemes (correct responses over 50%) and a range for mastery production (correct responses over 90%). The inventory of typically developing children showed that 14 phonemes (of the 27 CEA consonants) were mastered and the other 13 were in the range of customary production. Voicing was one factor that affected the error percentages of some phonemes. The phonemic inventory of the phonologically disordered children differed considerably in terms of the percentage of phonemes in error from that of the typically developing children but the order of acquisition was almost the same.

The phonological process analysis showed that typically developing children's speech was characterised by the use of seven error patterns (/r/ deviation, sibilant fronting, devoicing, de-emphasisation, velar fronting, di- and polysyllabic word simplification and cluster simplification) but the percentage of errors was very low (less than 25%). Ten error patterns were observed in the speech of the children with phonological disorder who had high error percentages. They are di- and polysyllabic word simplification, devoicing, sibilant fronting, /r/ deviation, assimilation, velar fronting, cluster simplification, de-emphasisation, glottal replacement and final consonant deletion. Implications for the assessment and treatment of children with disordered phonology were suggested and a tentative design for an Arabic articulation test was proposed. Ammar introduced the process of de-empahasisation in the Arabic language, and relabelled some processes as '/r/ deviation' as /r/ showed several distinct patterns of deviation. In summary, the results showed that the speech of the phonologically disordered children was characterised by restrictions on the number of speech sounds used and the persistence of a considerable number of phonological processes compared to typically developing children. Some children showed deviant phenomena. Nevertheless it was concluded that phonologically disordered speech was more delayed than deviant, i.e. their speech patterns were predictable from what happens in typical development.

(3) Ammar and Rifaat (1998) studied the phonetic inventory of consonants used by three to four-year-old typically developing Egyptian Arabic-speaking children. The study included 41 children divided into two groups according to their age (using six-month age interval). The list contained 161 words and was devised to test 26 phonemes (with the exclusion of /q/) in the three different positions. The sound was considered as part of a child's inventory if it occurred more than once and as part of an age appropriate inventory if it occurred in 50% of the subjects. The results of the phonetic inventories of the two groups matched the list of consonants of adults that was drawn up by Harrell (1957). The total percentage of incorrect articulations of the younger group is higher than that of the older age group. The percentages of incorrect articulation are highest in syllable-initial position and lowest in final position for both groups. A number of phonological processes were observed in the speech of children but all registered less than 50% across children.

(4) Ammar (1999) investigated the acquisition of consonant clusters in 51 typically developing Egyptian Arabic-speaking children aged between two and four years. The children were divided into four age groups in six-month intervals. The speech material was a list that contained 100 monosyllabic words of CVCC structure. Most words were familiar to children at that age. Both quantitative and qualitative analyses were applied to this study. The former analysis was to determine correct responses and the latter to describe the different error patterns observed for the acquisition of consonant clusters. The results of the quantitative analysis showed that word final consonant clusters are acquired at an early stage compared to that of English-speaking children. Word-final consonant cluster acquisition is apparent at two years and is mastered by the age of four. There was a significant relationship between age and the acquisition of consonant clusters.

The results of the qualitative analysis showed that children used a variety of error patterns. These error patterns are: the deletion of the whole cluster, e.g. [dæʔn] 'chin' → [dæ], the deletion of one member of the cluster [ʔɪrd] 'monkey' → [ʔɪd], deletion of one member with compensatory lengthening of the vowel [kælb] 'dog' → [kæːb], deletion of one member and applying diminutization, e.g. [rʊkn] → [lʊkɪ], insertion of a vowel between two consonants (epenthesis) [bɑħr] 'sea' → [bɑħər], and finally the preservation of the entire cluster in addition to diminutisation, e.g. [çæms] → [çæmsɪ]. The results revealed that the trend of deleting one consonant of the cluster and the stability of the other was due to the degree of obstruction in the vocal tract and the age of acquiring the consonant. Plosives were the strongest consonants; fricatives came in the second stage, while trill and lateral were mostly liable to deletion. Nasals were considered to be strong but they were deleted if they occurred with certain plosives. The results also showed that although there was a general trend to delete back consonants than front ones, the manner of articulation may influence that pattern, i.e. if the front consonant was a trill or a lateral and the back consonant was a fricative, the latter was the one that was most liable to be deleted. Also, it was found that if one of the consonants of the cluster was pharyngeal, then epenthesis was more likely to happen. On the basis of the results some implications for therapy were suggested.

(5) Salem (2000) studied the syllable structure in the speech of typically developing Egyptian children aged between three and four years. It dealt with monosyllabic, disyllabic, tri-syllabic, and quadri-syllabic words and their sequences in the nominal sentences or the phrases that consist of two words. It showed the phonological processes that occur in the structure of syllables in connected speech compared with adults' speech.

(6) Morsi (2001) investigated the phonological development of CEA and designed a developmental articulation test for phonologically

disordered Egyptian Arabic-speaking children. Thirty normal Egyptian children were equally divided into three stages: 2;6–3;0 years, 3;0–4;0 years and 4;0–5;0 years. Speech data consisted of a word list of 158 nouns, to facilitate their recognition by children. It was designed to test 25 consonant phonemes (with the exclusion of /q/ and //j/ as they are considered marginal in CEA (Harrell, 1957)) and eight phonological processes (weak syllable deletion, final consonant deletion, cluster simplification, velar fronting, sibilant deviation, /r/ deviation, de-emphasisation and devoicing). Both substitution and phonological process analyses were used. Applying a 75% threshold for correct production of phonemes, the results showed that in Stage I, all consonants were acquired except /r, ḍ, ṣ, ẓ, z, ç, ʁ/. In Stage II, /ḍ, ẓ, z, ʁ/ remained un-acquired. In Stage III, only /ẓ, z/ remained un-acquired. Applying a 25% threshold for process consideration, the results showed that in Stage I, both devoicing and /r/ deviation occurred. In Stage II, devoicing occurred. By Stage III, all processes disappeared. Based on the results of typically developing children, a chart of phonological development for CEA was introduced. The results were used as the basis for designing a developmental articulation test for phonologically disordered Egyptian Arabic-speaking children, which provided the developmental norms required for the diagnosis of atypical phonological development. Also, the results guided the selection of words for the articulation test, in that those words pronounced correctly by typically developing children were included as they would allow the identification of children with disordered phonology and provide a list of keywords for therapy. In addition, the results helped in avoiding words that were often mispronounced by these typically developing children in designing the articulation test.

The test was divided into two parts. Part I is for testing 25 phonemes of CEA. They were tested in simple phonetic and phonological contexts to minimise the interference of complex structures that may influence the correct production of phonemes. They were analysed using a substitution analysis (SA). Part II assesses both structural and systemic processes (eight processes) that frequently occur in Egyptian Arabic-speaking children's speech. They were analysed using a phonological process analysis (PPA). The test was used in assessing five phonologically disordered Egyptian Arabic-speaking children. The speech data included words from both sections of the assessment of normal children, and both SA and PPA were carried out. The results indicated that the test was valid and time-efficient but still needs further testing to be reliable (for a revised version of the test, see Morsi (2003)).

(7) Ammar (2002) studied the acquisition of syllabic structure in the speech of two to three-year-old normal Arabic-speaking Egyptian children. The speech of 10 children was analysed in order to ascertain the

types of syllables they acquired and the combinations of these types in the words. Speech data were elicited through word lists, pictures and citation forms in both spontaneous and repetition modes. The results showed that 90% of the children had acquired all syllable types. Difficulties in producing syllables were manifested in CVCC syllables. As for the syllabic structure of words, the study showed that children prefer short words containing a maximum of three syllables. Quadri-syllabic words tend to be limited to one type of structure. In addition, syllabic structure is influenced by the tendency to avoid abutting consonants, thus, reducing the number of syllables or changing the types of syllables from closed to open. Closed syllables usually contain a long vowel. Prolongation of vowels seemed to be a preferred technique to facilitate articulation. In addition, the results showed that syllable structure processes always preserve the prosodic structure of the target form.

(8) Salama (2003) investigated the phonemic inventories of three to four-year-old Egyptian Arabic-speaking children in connected speech. Eight children (four boys and four girls) participated in the study. The speech data are connected speech consisting of an average of 500 words. It is elicited from children through answering questions, telling stories, singing songs, describing what they are doing while playing, and naming pictures and objects. The duration of recording, using a high quality recorder, ranged from 40 to 90 minutes. The speech data were analysed using substitution analysis. The results showed that all phonemes were produced correctly at 75% or above except for four phonemes /s̱, ẕ, ḏ, ʁ/. If the result of this study of connected speech is compared with that of single-word data collection method of Morsi (2001), it would appear that Morsi's results for the acquisition of /s̱/ and /z/ differ from those of Salama, although the difference is insignificant.

It is obvious that there are few previous studies on phonological development. Further research is needed. The following studies support the previous studies and give more comprehensive account of normal and disordered phonology in Egyptian Arabic.

Normal Phonology of Arabic-Speaking Children

Participants

Thirty-six children, aged between three and five years of age, were chosen from different nurseries representing middle socio-economic status in Alexandria. All children are typically developing with regard to intelligence, hearing and articulation. They were divided in two groups according to their age for the purpose of analysis: Group I: 10 children (five girls and five boys) aged between three and four years old, and Group II: 26 children (13 girls and 13 boys) aged between four and five years old.

Speech data

The word list consists of 228 words that included the 25 consonant phonemes (excluding /q/ and /j/) of CEA. Each consonant phoneme is tested in three word positions (initial, medial and final) and in words of different length (monosyllabic, disyllabic and polysyllabic). The words chosen are age appropriate, i.e. likely to be known by three-year-old children (see Table 9.3).

Data collection

The words are presented to children either as coloured pictures or concrete items. Speech data are elicited through picture-naming and deferred imitation tasks, depending on the children's interaction with the experimenter.

Recording

A live phonetic transcription is done during testing and all assessment sessions are tape recorded, using a high quality recorder and low noise tapes for later transcription.

Analysis

The 'relational analysis' approach is used in this study in both 'substitution analysis' and 'phonological process analysis'. In relational analysis children's realisations are compared with the corresponding adult targets (Ammar, 1992; Stoel-Gammon & Dunn, 1985).

Substitution analysis is used to determine the acquisition of each target phoneme as a whole and in the three different word positions. A phoneme acquisition is considered 'mastered' if it occurs correctly in at least 90% of responses or considered as 'customary' if it is pronounced correctly in 50–89% of responses.

Phonological process analysis reveals processes that occurred frequently in the children's speech sample. Two approaches are used to describe the children's phonological processes. The first determines the existence of a process in the speech of each child regardless of its frequency of occurrence. The second approach counts the frequency of occurrence of each process in the speech sample of each child in percentages. Both structural and systemic processes (Grunwell, 1987) are examined: di- and polysyllabic word simplification, final consonant deletion, cluster simplification, devoicing, velar fronting, de-emphasisation, sibilant deviation and /r/ deviation. The criterion for the presence of a process is 25% occurrence. Twenty-five percent is a quantitative criterion used by Bleile (1995) to show the frequency with which an error pattern occurs. In this study, this quantitative criterion is commutatively determined for the subjects. According to Bleile, below 25%, a process

Phonological Development and Disorders

Table 9.3 The word list

No.	English orthographic gloss	Arabic transcribed word	No.	English orthographic gloss	Arabic transcribed word
1	bark	hɑww	19	train sound	tuːt
2	tea	çæːj	20	basin	ħoːd̪
3	eye	ʕeːn	21	goal	goːn
4	hand	ʔiːd	22	lettuce	χɑs̪
5	bananas	moːz	23	drawer	dʊrg
6	cock	diːk	24	beans	fuːl
7	pocket	geːb	25	peaches	χoːχ
8	rat	fɑːr	26	plants	zærʕ
9	ducks	bɑt̪t̪	27	bricks	t̪uːb
10	rice	rʊz̪	28	bag	k̪iːs
11	mouth	bʊʔʔ	29	correct	s̪ɑħ
12	face	wɪç	30	monster	ʁuːl
13	day	joːm	31	clothes	lɪb̥s
14	back	d̪ɑhr	32	piaster	sæːʁ
15	egg	beːd̪	33	cheek	χædd
16	light	nuːr	34	envelope	z̪ɑrf
17	door	bæːb	35	water	ˈmɑjja
18	baa	mæːʔ	36	ball	ˈkoːrɑ

Continued

Table 9.3 (Continued)

No.	English orthographic gloss	Arabic transcribed word	No.	English orthographic gloss	Arabic transcribed word
37	watch	ˈsæːʕæ	56	drawing	ræsm
38	pen	ˈʔælæm	57	salt	mælħ
39	lion	ˈʔæsæd	58	ant	næml
40	camel	ˈgæmæl	59	pair of shoes	ˈgæzmæ
41	man	ˈrɑːgɪl	60	bear	ˈdɪbæ
42	milk	ˈlæbæn	61	bone	ˈʕɑdmɑ
43	hair	ʃɑʕr	62	carrot	ˈgɑzɑrɑ
44	ear	wɪdn	63	fish (plural)	ˈsæmæk
45	leg	rɪgl	64	cheese	ˈgɪbnæ
46	train	ʔɑtr	65	boat	ˈmærkɪb
47	monkey	ʔɪrd	66	iron	ˈmækwæ
48	food	ʔækl	67	star	ˈnɪgmæ
49	floor	ʔɑrd	68	mango	ˈmæŋgæ
50	tiger	nɪmr	69	sugar	ˈsʊkkɑr
51	comb	mɪʃt	70	cat	ˈʔʊttɑ
52	sun	ʃæms	71	bag	ˈʃɑntɑ
53	rope	ħæbl	72	sandal	ˈsɑndɑl
54	work	ʃʊʁl	73	chair	ˈkʊrsi
55	shoulder	kɪtf	74	woman	sɪtt

#	word	transcription		#	word	transcription
75	soup	ˈʃorba		96	loaf	rɪˈʁiːf
76	rabbit	ˈʔarnaeb		97	water-melon	batˈtiːχa
77	bed	sɪˈriːr		98	banana	ˈmoːzæ
78	fig	tiːn		99	proper noun	ˈnædæ
79	hair pin	ˈtoːkæ		100	proper noun	ˈraça
80	ice	tælg		101	proper noun	ˈmæhæ
81	oil	zeːt		102	elephant	fiːl
82	corn	ˈdora		103	bread	ˈʕeːç
83	cover	ˈʁaṯ a		104	sheep	χaˈruːf
84	meow (noun)	nɑww		105	horse	ħʊˈṣɑːn
85	an apple	tʊfˈfæːhæ		106	washing	ʁæˈsiːl
86	giraffe	zaˈraːfa		107	biscuits	bæsˈkoːt
87	towel	ˈfuːṯa		108	dress	fʊsˈtæːn
88	spoon	mæʕˈlæʔæ		109	key	mʊfˈtæːħ
89	fork	ˈçoːkæ		110	plate	ˈṯabaʔ
90	carrots	ˈgazaṟ		111	bell	ˈgaraṣ
91	ring	ˈχæːtɪm		112	stair	ˈsɪllɪm
92	grapes	ˈʕɪnaeb		113	pepper	ˈfɪlfɪl
93	air	ˈhæwæ		114	slippers	ˈçɪbçɪb̥
94	egg	ˈbeːḏa		115	mosque	ˈgæːmʕ
95	cane	ˈʔasab		116	officer	ˈzaːbɪṯ

Continued

Table 9.3 (Continued)

No.	English orthographic gloss	Arabic transcribed word	No.	English orthographic gloss	Arabic transcribed word
117	bus	ʔʊtuˈbiːs	137	lock	ʔɪfl
118	nose	mænæˈχiːr	138	lips	çæˈfæːjɪf
119	stove	bʊtæˈgæːz	139	flower	ˈwærdæ
120	potatoes	bɑˈtɑːtɪs	140	lighter	wælˈlæːʕæ
121	tomatoes	tɑˈmɑːtɪm	141	body	gɪsm
122	oranges	bʊrtuˈʔɑːn	142	pin	dæbˈbuːs
123	trouser	bɑntɑˈloːn	143	soap	sɑˈbuːnɑ
124	parrot	bæʁbæˈʁæːn	144	whistle	sʊfˈfɑːrɑ
125	television	tɪlfɪzˈjoːn	145	class	fɑsl
126	sock	çɑˈrɑːb	146	scissors	mɑˈʔɑs
127	lantern	fæˈnuːs	147	candles	çæmʃ
128	tongue	lɪˈsæːn	148	butter	ˈzɪbdæ
129	glass	ʔɪˈzæːz	149	trunk	zælˈluːmæ
130	water-melon	bɑtˈt iːχ	150	seeds	bɪzr
131	duck	ˈbɑttɑ	151	belt	ħɪˈzæːm
132	glass (for drinking)	kʊbˈbæːjæ	152	table	tɑrɑˈbeːzɑ
133	swing	mʊrˈgeːħæ	153	eye glasses	nɑdˈdɑːrɑ
134	lemon	læˈmuːnæ	154	girl	bɪnt
135	blood	dæm	155	sister	ʔʊχt
136	brush	ˈfʊrχæ	156	chicken	ˈfærχæ

Phonological Development and Disorders

157	mandarin	jusæˈfændi	177	carpet	sɪgˈgæːdæ
158	quilt	lɪˈħaːf	178	lollipop	mɑsˈsɑːsɑ
159	keys	mæfæˈtiːħ	179	doll	ʕaˈruːsa̱
160	cotton candy	ʁæzl	180	cucumber	χɪˈjɑːɾɑ
161	washing machine	ʁæsˈsæːlæ	181	telephone	tɪlˈfoːn
162	mule	bæʁl	182	frog	dʊfˈdɑ̱ʕa
163	flee	bærˈʁuːt	183	necklace	sɪlˈsɪlæ
164	snake	tʃˈbæːn	184	a fish	ˈsæmækæ
165	chicks	kætæˈkiːt	185	bicycle	ˈʕæɡælæ
166	aeroplanes	ṯɑjjɑˈɾɑːṯ	186	tree	ˈçɑɡɑɾɑ
167	ruler	mɑsˈṯɑɾɑ	187	jam	mɪˈɾɑbbɑ
168	fly	dibˈbæːnæ	188	French beans	faˈsʊlja
169	bones	ʕɑdm	189	strawberry	fɑˈrawla
170	white	ˈʔabjaḏ	190	umbrella	ʃæmˈsɪjjæ
171	chin	dæʔn	191	Egyptian food	tɑʕˈmɪjja
172	eye-lashes	rɪˈmuːç	192	pasta	mɑkɑˈɾoːnɑ
173	chick	kætˈkuːt	193	chocolate	çukɑˈlɑːṯɑ
174	nail	mʊsˈmaːr	194	car	ʕaɾɑˈbɪjja
175	cockroach	sʊrˈs̱ɑːr	195	tap	ħænæˈfɪjjæ
176	bird	ʕɑs̱ˈfuːɾɑ	196	molokhja	muluˈχɪjjæ

Continued

Table 9.3 (Continued)

No.	English orthographic gloss	Arabic transcribed word	No.	English orthographic gloss	Arabic transcribed word
197	blanket	bɑtˠ tɑˈnijjɑ	213	we are sitting down	bɪˈnoʕod
198	orange	bʊrtʊˈʔɑːnɑ	214	we are cutting	bɪˈnɪʔtɑʕ
199	dog	kælb	215	she dances	bɪˈtorʔʊs
200	sea	bɑħr	216	she cooks	bɪˈtʊtbʊχ
201	our God	rɑbˈbnɑ	217	he cries	bɪjˈʕɑjjɑt
202	window	ʃɪbˈbæːk	218	he hunts	bɪjɪsˈtɑːd
203	somersault	ʃɑʔlɑˈbɑːz	219	he steels	bɪˈjɪsræʔ
204	mortar	hoːn	220	he laughs	bɪˈjɪtħæk
205	gift	hɪˈdɪjjæ	221	he watches	bɪjɪtˈfɑrrɑɡ
206	proper noun	ˈnʊhæ	222	he eats	bɪˈjæːkʊl
207	alarm clock	mɪˈnæbbɪh	223	he scratches	bɪˈjʊhrʊʃ
208	hanger	ʃæmˈmæːʕæ	224	he drinks	bɪˈjɪʃrɑb
209	sign post	ˈjɑftɑ	225	he chews	bɪˈjʊmdʊʁ
210	shower	dʊʃ	226	chew (imperative)	ˈʔʊmdʊʁ
211	sleeping	ˈnæːjɪm	227	stutter	ˈtæhtɪh
212	meow (verb)	bɪtˈnɑwnɑw	228	he flew	tɑːr

is considered disappearing. From a therapeutic perspective, this percentage is the cut off for therapy.

Results and Discussion

Substitution analysis

Group I: The results of substitution analysis show that 13 phonemes /w, k, m, f, χ, ħ, ʔ, t, j, n, l, ç, h/ are in mastery production, while the remaining phonemes were in customary production (see Figure 9.3).

Group II: The results of substitution analysis show that 14 phonemes were mastered (/ʕ/ is added to the phonemes mastered by Group I) and again all the remaining phonemes are in customary production (see Figure 9.4). Comparison of the two age groups indicates a slight increase in the number of the mastered phonemes. The results also show that /w/ has the highest correct score for both groups. The results of the correct responses for the two groups show that the final position is the most difficult. The initial position and the medial positions do not differ significantly.

Phonological processes

Group I: Each child exemplifies between four and eight processes. Devoicing, de-emphasisation, cluster simplification, di- and polysyllabic simplification, /r/ deviation and sibilant deviation occur in more than 50% of the subjects. Velar fronting and final consonant deletion occur in 20% of the subjects. However, the processes occur with very low percentages

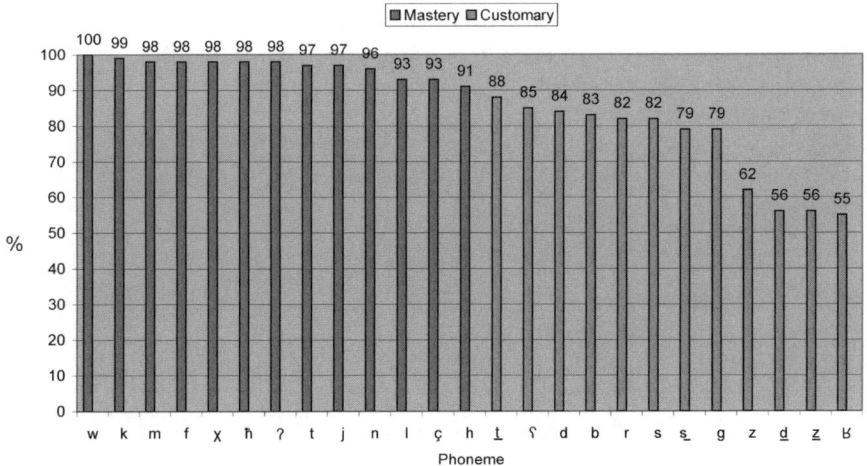

Figure 9.3 Percentage of correct responses of normal children (3–4 years old)

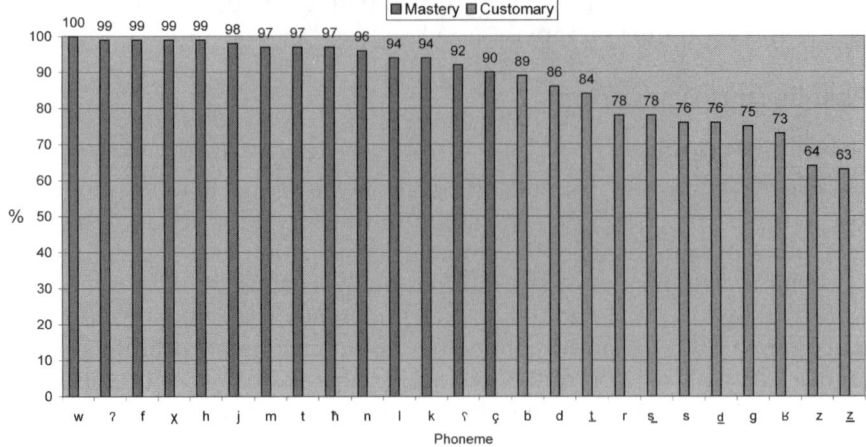

Figure 9.4 Percentage of correct responses of normal children (4–5 years old)

except for devoicing in four subjects, /r/ deviation and sibilant deviation in two subjects, cluster simplification and de-emphasisation in one subject. According to the 25% criterion for process identification, the results show that devoicing is the only significant process. Devoicing is considered one of the common errors among English-speaking children (Olmsted, 1971) and previous results (Ammar, 1992) indicate that it persists in the speech of Egyptian Arabic-speaking children after four years (see Figure 9.5).

Group II: Each child uses between one and eight processes. According to the 25% criterion for process identification, the results indicate that all processes have been suppressed. This also agrees with Morsi's results

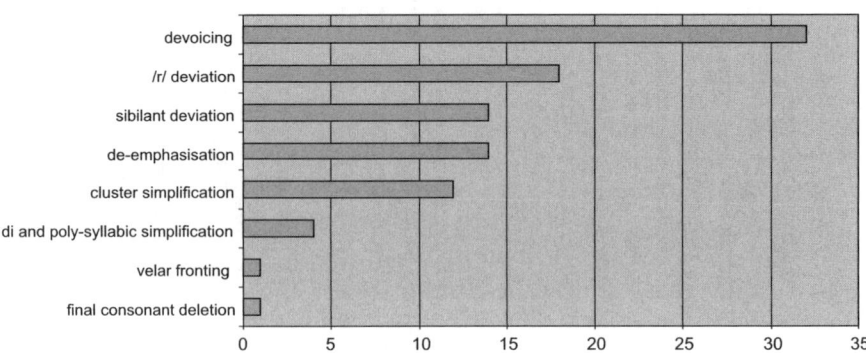

Figure 9.5 Average percentage of occurrence for each phonological process for normal children (3–4 years old)

Phonological Development and Disorders

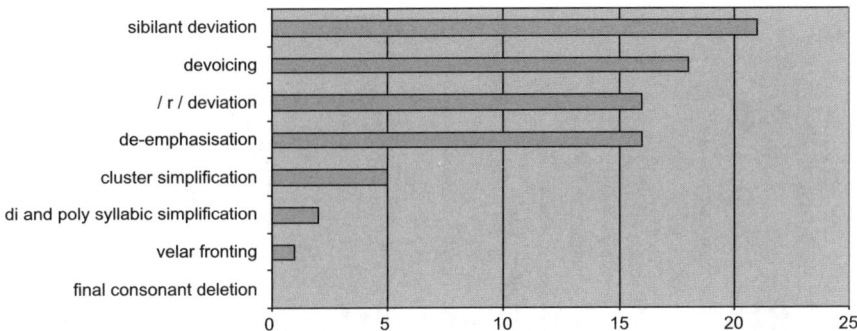

Figure 9.6 Average percentage of occurrence for each phonological process for normal children (4–5 years old)

(2001). Sibilant deviation, devoicing, /r/ deviation and de-emphsisation are the most common processes. Cluster simplification, di- and polysyllabic simplification and velar fronting register 5% or below. Final consonant deletion scores zero (see Figure 9.6).

In both groups, in general, structural processes register lower scores than systemic processes.

Disordered Phonology of Arabic-Speaking Children

Participants

Twenty-two children from different speech therapy clinics in Alexandria participated in the study. Their ages range from 3;10 to 9;2. All children were diagnosed as having delayed speech, mainly in phonology. They have normal intelligence, and no signs of any organic symptoms or adverse medical history. The methodology used for the disordered children is the same as that of the typically developing group. The results are summarised below.

Results and Discussion

Phonemic inventory

The speech of one child is excluded from this analysis as she showed the process of favourite sound, i.e. most consonants are reduced to one. The results are based on data from 21 children. Figure 9.7 shows the percentages of correct responses for the 25 phonemes. The figure indicates that /ʔ/ recorded the highest percentage in its correct occurrence (79%). Eleven phonemes /ʔ, w, ħ, m, h, n, j, t, f, χ, l/ are pronounced correctly on over 50% of responses. Seven phonemes /k, t̪, ʕ, b, s, ç, d/ are pronounced correctly for between 25% and 49% of responses. Seven phonemes /s̪, r, d̪, g, z, ʁ, z̪/ are pronounced correctly in less than 25% of responses.

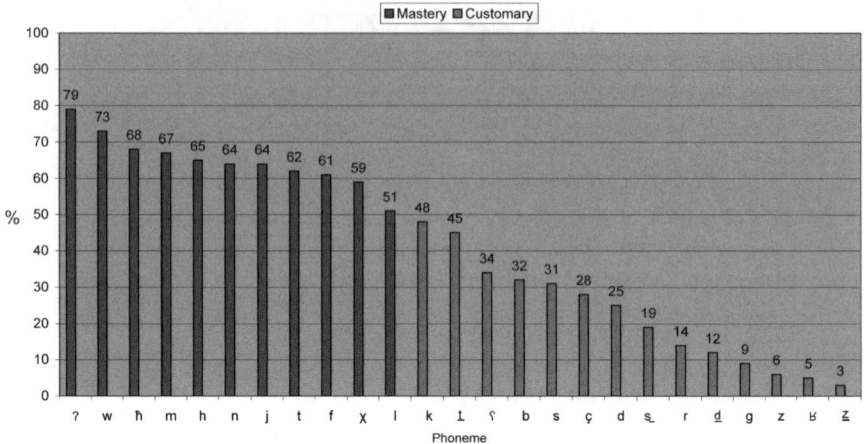

Figure 9.7 Percentage of correct responses of disordered children

The results indicate that children can be categorised as having a moderate to severe or severe phonological impairment according to Shriberg and Kwiatkowski's (1980) scale of severity.

Phonological processes

All 22 children implemented, with different levels of frequency of occurrence, the following processes: di- and polysyllabic word simplification, devoicing, /r/ deviation and de-emphasisation. Sibilant deviation is used by 21 children (95%). Both cluster simplification and velar fronting occur in the speech of 19 children (86%). Final consonant deletion is observed in 15 children (68%) (see Figure 9.8).

Figure 9.9 shows the rank of the average percentage of occurrence for each phonological process. The /r/ deviation process ranks first (85%). This is predictable because /r/ is a phoneme which is not in the range of mastery production. It is followed by devoicing (61%) and then sibilant deviation (52%). Final consonant deletion scores the lowest (11%), i.e. it appears infrequently in the speech of children. For comparison between the disordered group and the typically developing groups in the average percentage of occurrence for each phonological process, see Figure 9.10.

The following paragraphs present some examples and further elaboration on forms of occurrence of the eight processes in the disordered subjects.

Syllable structure processes

Di- and polysyllabic word simplification

This appears in three different forms. The first is the unstressed syllable deletion, where the child omits an unstressed syllable or more,

Phonological Development and Disorders

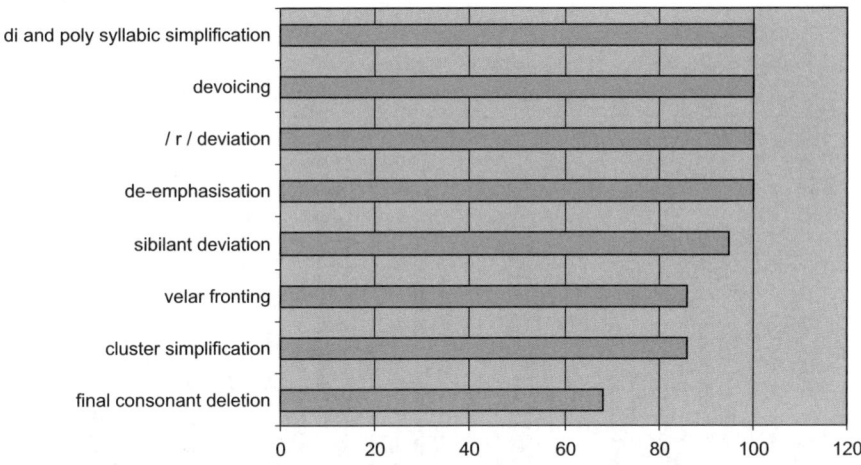

Figure 9.8 Percentage of occurence for each phonological process across disordered children

e.g. [mænæχiːr] 'nose' is pronounced [χiːl] or [mæfætiːħ] 'keys' is pronounced [fætiːħ]. The second is insertion of pause between the syllables, e.g. [ʔʊtʊbiːs] 'bus' is pronounced [ʔʊtʊ—biːθ]. The third is vowel lengthening, e.g. [çæmsɪjjæ] 'umbrella' is pronounced [θæːːbmɪjjæ]. This phenomenon indicates an advanced level in the ability to produce longer words. Most of the children have more difficulty with polysyllabic words but all except one show some reduction in disyllabic words. The

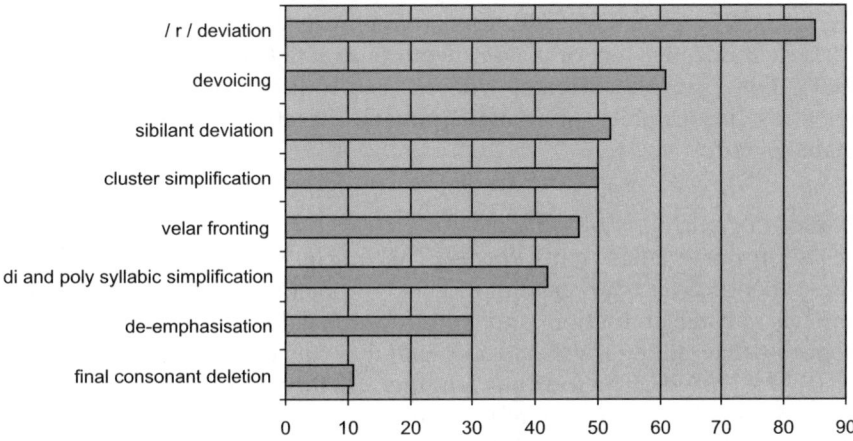

Figure 9.9 Average percentage of occurrence for each phonological process for disordered children

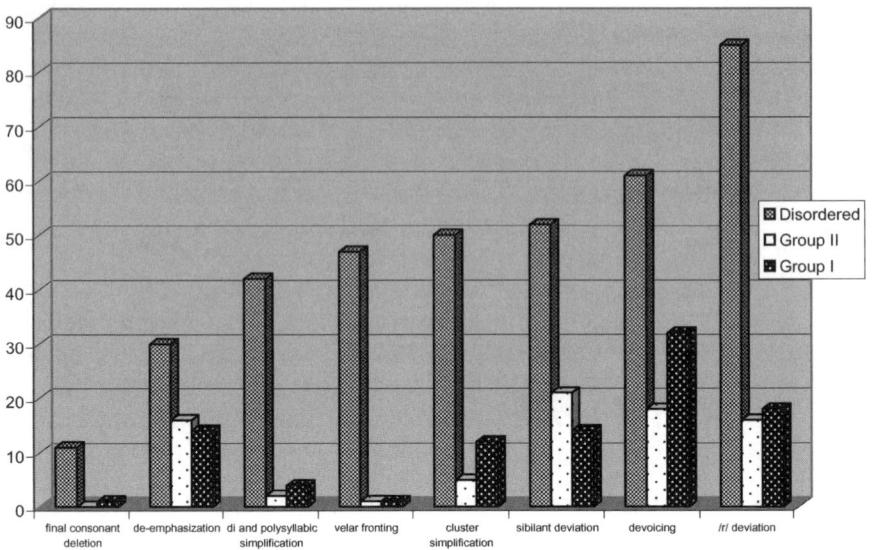

Figure 9.10 Average percentage of occurrence for each phonological process (disordered, group II and group I)

omitted unstressed syllable is usually that which exists in word-initial position. Thus, it might be predicted that disordered children will score lower percentages in initial position than typically developing children, as the process of di- and polysyllabic word simplification is of low frequency of occurrence in the latter group.

Two of the subjects exhibit reduction of disyllabic words such as CV/CV, CV/CVC, CVC/CV, CVC/CVC, which are least liable to deletion in normal children even of a very young age (2;6 to 3;0 years) (Morsi, 2001). For example, [gɪbnæ] 'cheese' is produced as [kɪm], [gæzmæ] 'shoe' as [kæs], [gæs], or [gɪsm], [gaza̱r] 'carrots' as [ka̱s] and [sɪllɪm] 'stair' as [sɪl].

Consonant cluster simplification

This process takes many forms. The first is reduction of the cluster. The second is cluster assimilation, e.g. [mælħ] 'salt' → [mæħħ]. The third is cluster reduction and compensatory lengthening, e.g. [ħæbl] 'rope' → [ħæːp]; lengthening one member of the cluster, e.g. [ʔʊχt] 'sister' → [ʔʊχχt]. The fourth is lengthening the vowel with preservation of the entire cluster, e.g. [çæmʕ] 'candles' → [çæːmʕ]. The fifth form is the insertion of vowel between the two members of the cluster (epenthesis). Cluster assimilation, cluster reduction and cluster reduction with compensatory lengthening are the common forms that occurred frequently in the sample of children. However, the occurrence of different forms for a process in the productions of the same subject may reflect gradual development. In other words, if 'one member deletion' is the only pattern that occurred in the speech of a child, in our opinion, this reflects a degree of severity greater than that of a child who feels that there is a sequence of consonants to be articulated, and when he fails, he tries to compensate by any other technique.

Final consonant deletion
This process does not show any consistency in influencing certain sounds or classes of sounds, e.g. [kıli:m] 'carpet' → [tıli:], [bæsko:t] 'biscuits' → [pæsto:], [mo:z] 'banana' → [mo:], [fi:l] 'elephant' → [fi:], [ħusɑ:n] 'horse' → [sɑ:] and [ʔæsæd] 'lion' → [ʔæsæ].

Concerning syllable and word length, all subjects use open and closed syllables. They all could produce at least two different syllables in sequence. Short syllables are used frequently. Only two subjects have very restricted word shapes. They have never produced more than two syllables, except in few words, for example, [ʁæssæ:læ] 'washing machine' is pronounced [hæθθæjæ]), [ʕægælæ] 'bicycle' is pronounced as [ʕædælæ], [bæʁbæʁæ:n] 'parrot' as [mæmæχæ] and [bɑtɑ:tɪs] 'potatoes' as [bɑttɑ:tɪs]).

Systemic processes

/r/ deviation
This process takes many forms. It may be deleted, assimilated, replaced by/l/and replaced by a vowel or by a glide. A child may show more than one pattern of these forms./l/replacement is the most frequent form that occurred. Examples: [kɑ:sɑ] for [gɑzɑr] 'carrots', [tʊssɪ] for [kʊrsɪ] 'chair', [pɑħl] or [bɑħɑ] for [bɑħr] 'sea' and [ʔæjmæn] for [ʔærnæb] 'rabbit'.

Devoicing
Examples of this process are: [be:dɑ] 'egg' became [pe:tɑ], [sɪggæ:dæ] 'carpet' → [tɪkkæ:tæ], [gæ:mɪʕ] 'mosque' → [kæ:meħ], [bæ:b] 'door' → [pæ:p] and [dɪbbæ] 'bear' → [dɪppæ].

Sibilant deviation
Children use different substitutions for this process. One of the subjects use interdental fricatives to replace sibilants and this form is used more frequent than other forms. For instance, [sɪllɪm] 'stair' → [θɪllɪm], [χɑs] 'lettuce' → [hɑθ], [mo:zæ] 'banana' → [mo:θæ] and [zɑrf] 'envelope' → [θɑlf]. Another subject uses dental stops to replace sibilants. For instance, [sæ:ʕæ] 'watch' → [tæ:ʕæ], [ze:t] 'oil' → [de:t] and [sɑħ] 'correct' → [tɑħ].

Velar fronting

Children substitute dentals for velars. Examples of this process are: [gæzmæ] 'shoe' → [tæzmæ], [mækwæ] 'iron' → [mætwæ] and [gɑzɑr] 'carrot' → [tɑsal].

De-emphasisation

Children replace the emphatic sounds by their non-emphatic counterparts, e.g. [bɑtt] 'ducks' → [pætt], [dɑhr] 'back' → [tæh], [be:dɑ] 'egg' → [pe:tæ] and [sɑħ] 'correct' → [tæħ].

Other processes

There are other processes, apart from the eight examined in this study, which are observed in the speech samples of some children, but as infrequent processes. These are:

- *Metathesis.* It occurred in few words throughout the speech sample, for example, [færχæ] 'hen' was pronounced [χæ:fæ] and [gɑrɑs] 'bell' is pronounced [tɑsal].
- *Backing.* A child used to back the dental fricatives to palatals, for example, [mo:z] 'banana' was pronounced [mo:ç] and [sæ:ʕæ] 'watch' was pronounced [çæ:ʕæ]. Also, he used to back uvular fricatives to pharyngeal or laryngeal fricatives, for example, [χɑru:f] 'sheep' was pronounced [ħɑlu:f] and [færχæ] 'hen' was pronounced [færħæ]. Another child used the same process of backing dental fricatives to palatals but in few examples; producing [sɪtt] 'lady' as [çɪtt] and [sæmækæ] 'fish' as [çæmækæ]. She also used back uvular fricatives for pharyngeal ħ or laryngeal fricatives, but unlike the former case she also used to back pharyngeal fricatives to laryngeal fricative [h]. For example, [ʕe:n] 'eye' → [he:n] and [hʊsɑ:n] 'horse' → [hʊθɑ:n].
- *Stopping.* Few children tended to substitute stops for fricatives, for example, [zærʕ] 'plant' was pronounced [tæħ] and [sæmæk] 'fish' was pronounced [tæmæk]. Sibilant fricatives were the most fricatives that were affected by this process, except one girl who exactly demonstrated in her speech Stoel-Gammon and Dunn's (1985: 43) claim that 'stopping might apply to all target fricatives at first, then only to a subset of fricatives'. This will be discussed in the next section.
- *Glottal replacement.* It occurred in almost all children, but few of them used it frequently.They tended to replace a target phoneme by a glottal stop, for example, [ħæbl] 'rope' was replaced by [ʔætl], [[tɑbɑʔ] 'dish' → [ʔɑbɑʔ]. This process may be misleading in Arabic while testing it, because of the probability of the addition of the definite article [ʔɪl]. So the examiner should be cautious and include verbs and proper nouns in her/his testing word list.

- *Assimilation.* It is very significant process in the speech of children. It exists in all its forms, whether regressive, e.g. [zɪbdæ] 'butter' → [sɪttæ] or progressive as in [mækkæ] instead of [mækwæ] 'iron'. Also, it occurred both contiguous and non-contiguous. There was one subject who assimilated /l/ in the definite article /ʔil/ to the following sound in contexts where assimilation is not allowed in CEA, as /l/ was a problematic sound for him. For example, [ʔɪlfuːl] 'the beans' was produced as [ʔɪffuːʔ] and [ʔɪlmoːzæ] 'the banana' as [ʔɪmmoːsæ].

Interesting cases

While the majority of children who have phonological disorder show a delayed pattern of acquisition, there are two interesting cases that showed deviant development: a case with frequent unusual processes and another one with favourite articulation.

A case with frequent unusual processes

The child had two unusual error patterns. The first was replacing /l/ by [r] which was really deviant and unpredictable error, e.g. [biːr] for [fiːl] 'elephant' and [mærħ] for [mælħ] 'salt', as the /r/ sound is considered a problematic sound to many children and is acquired late compared with the /l/ sound, which is acquired early in Egyptian Arabic (Morsi, 2001). The second unusual pattern was stopping of all fricatives except for the pharyngeals ([ħ,ʕ]) and the laryngeal fricative [h]. The voiced uvular fricative [ʁ] is realized as a stop ([ʔ] or [k]) but realized more as a fricative ([h]). Examples of stopping are: [bænuːt] for [fænuːs] 'lantern', [moːt] for [moːz] 'bananas', [kɑt] for [χɑs] 'lettuce', [rʊt] for [rʊz] 'rice' and [tæːj] for [çæːj] 'tea'. As a result of stopping, seven sounds /f, s, z, s̱, ẕ, ç, χ/ were missing from her inventory and [t] was used most of the time to substitute /s, z, ç/ and [ṯ] to substitute /s̱, ẕ/. The subject also had devoicing which contributed to realising the phoneme /d/ as [t] and the phoneme /ḏ/ as [ṯ], most of the time. As a result, five phonemes /t, d, s, z, ç/ were realised as [t] and four phonemes /ṯ, ḏ, s̱, ẕ/ were realised as [ṯ].

A case with favourite articulation

Ingram (1976) and Weiner (1981) reported the concept of 'favourite articulation' or 'sound preference' as a characteristic of some children with phonological disorders. This kind of children does not follow a particular phonological pattern.

One of the children of this study showed the above phenomenon. This child had a phonetic inventory that contained about 19 sounds, but actually she used /w/ and /j/ in most of her pronunciations, although the /w/ was more dominant in her speech sample. The /w/ was almost always used in the substitutions of consonants in initial position, while the /j/ was used usually in medial position. The phoneme /m/ is a sound that was often preserved even if the structure of the whole word was changed, e.g. [mʊrgeːħæ] 'swing' is pronounced [mæ] and [mʊmsaːr] 'nail' is pronounced [moː]. Also /h/ is observed as a favourite sound but not in the frequency of the /w/ or /j/.

Comparison of Normal and Disordered Children

The 13 speech sounds that are mastered in typically developing children are mostly those that occur in the customary age range for the phonologically disordered children. This shows that the phonological disordered children follow the pattern of normal children but it is delayed, in terms of the acquisition of phonemes (see Figure 9.11).

The most widespread processes, /r/ deviation, sibilant deviation and devoicing, are the same in normal and disordered children. /r/ deviation in normal children does not take as many forms as it does for the disordered participants, but is restricted to /l/ substitution and gliding. Assimilation is significantly realised in the speech of the disordered children, while it is applied to few instances in the speech of the normal children. Cluster simplification, di- and polysyllabic word simplification and velar fronting are insignificant processes in the normal children's speech; they occur in a few instances, but these marginal occurrences support the idea of Ingram (1976) that the phonological processes are common to normal children and persist in disordered children.

Implications for Universality

The results of this study and the previous studies on CEA comply with the implicational universalities of Jakobson (1968). For example:

(1) Children acquire voiceless plosives before their voiced counterparts and use voiceless plosives for both. This is also true for Jordanian Arabic (Amayreh & Dyson, 2000). In CEA, this implication may be extended to cover even fricatives.

(2) In this study, most of the phonemes of CEA that were not mastered yet (90% and above) showed the difficult articulatory features that were described by Olmsted (1971), Bauman-Waengler (1994) and Amayreh and Dyson (2000), for example, voicing, emphasis, sibilance and trilling. This might also show a universal trend.

(3) CEA agrees with Jordanian Arabic (Amayreh & Dyson, 2000) and English (Stoel-Gammon & Dunn, 1985) in the early suppression of the processes of final consonant deletion, di- and polysyllabic simplification and velar fronting.

Phonological Development and Disorders 231

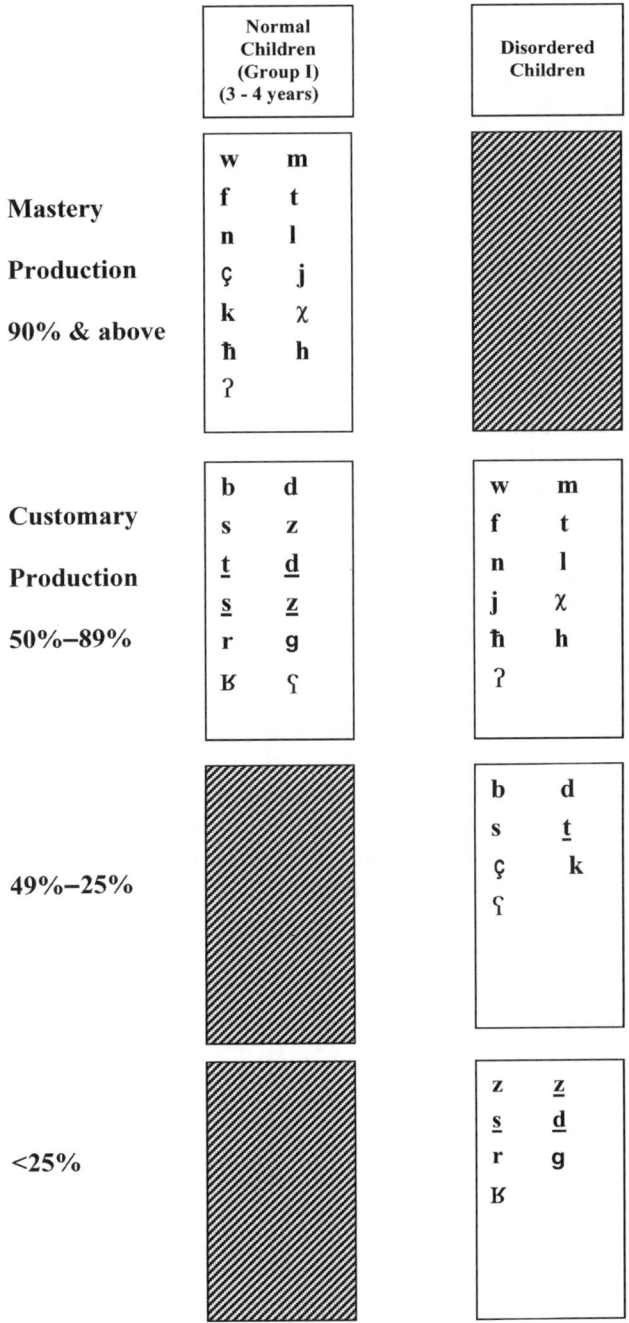

Figure 9.11 Comparison between normal and disordered children in mastery and customary production of phonemes

(4) CEA conforms to the fact that di- and polysyllabic word simplification process is considered a common process across disordered children and that the omitted unstressed syllable occurs word-initially (Weiner, 1979).

As there are universal trends across languages, there are also individual differences between them. For example:

(1) CEA agrees with Jordanian Arabic (Amayreh & Dyson, 2000) in the early mastery of /l/, but it disagrees with English in that /l/ is mastered late (Locke, 1983b).
(2) Back consonants in English are considered among the difficult consonants, but this is not the case in CEA. Voiceless back consonants are among the early mastered phonemes. The early acquisition of back consonants applies not only to CEA but also to Jordanian Arabic (Amayreh & Dyson, 2000).
(3) Cluster simplification process disappears early in CEA compared with final clusters in English.

Conclusion

This chapter constitutes a step for a comprehensive profile of phonological development in Colloquial Egyptian Arabic. It fulfils this aim by two ways. First, it reviews the previous studies on both normal and abnormal phonologies of Egyptian Arabic. Second, it fills the gap in the study of Egyptian Arabic phonological development with an investigation of both normally developing and disordered children of age ranges 3–5 and 3;10–9;2, respectively. Finally, it tries to fit the results of Egyptian Arabic to the universals of phonological development. This study confirms the concept that there are some universal or near-universal patterns of phonological development.

Notes

1. 'Accented' has proven to be different from being stressed. It has been shown that a pitch peak is only associated with stressed syllables and not caused by stressed syllables (Pierrehumbert, 1980). For more details on Egyptian Arabic, see Rifaat (2003).
2. VV as in CVV refers to long vowels, while CC as in CVCC refers to two subsequent consonants in its usual sense.

Chapter 10
Phonological Acquisition and Disorders in Turkish

S. TOPBAŞ and M. YAVAŞ

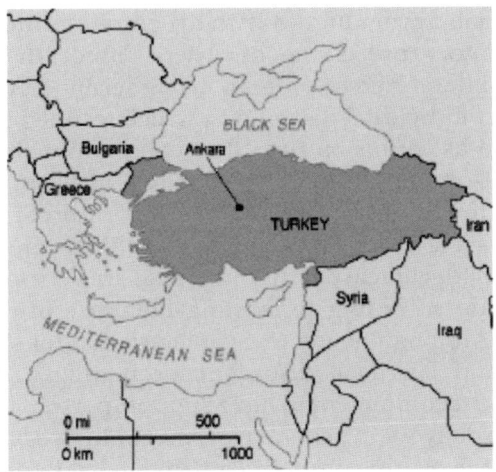

This chapter focuses on the phonological development of Turkish-speaking children. The plan of the chapter is as follows: we will start our exposition with a short history of the field of Speech and Language Therapy in Turkey, which will be followed by a brief sketch of Turkish phonology. We will then present a summary of the previous studies on the acquisition of Turkish phonology by normally developing children and by children with phonological disorders. Next, we will report the findings from the study conducted by the first author in 665 normally developing and 70 phonologically disordered children and discuss the tendencies found in the respective populations.

The Field of Speech and Language Therapy in Turkey

Speech-Language Pathology/Therapy (SLP) is a newly developing profession in Turkey. Currently, in the entire country only seven persons hold advanced (Masters and Doctoral level) degrees in speech-language pathology trained overseas at postgraduate levels mainly in England and the United States. Unlike other countries in Europe or USA, or even in other developing countries, the treating professional for the assessment and treatment services in speech-language pathology is not an SLP. Presently, the vast majority of direct care providers of services are psychologists and special educators who receive three to four weeks of training in communication disorders through the efforts of governmental organisations, mainly the Ministry of Education.

Historically, medical specialists provided most of the rehabilitation services with a special emphasis on diagnosis. Audiologists have been the principal professionals involved in the treatment of individuals with communicative disorders. Speech Language Pathology/Therapy and Audiology were joint programmes with the emphasis more on audiology and related auditory processing disorders. Unfortunately, combining these two related but different professions undermined the development of both as distinct individual disciplines, which resulted in several ethical problems as well as confusion over the scope of practice. Thus, speech and language disorders are rarely recognised in hospitals and usually accepted as occurring secondary to hearing disorders. Standardised, culturally unbiased assessment instruments, which were developed only recently as a basis for clinical decision-making, are very few. Usually comparisons are made according to existing literature in other languages, mainly English. Although newly revised legislation for special education covers speech and language disorders, promoting a 'least restrictive environment' with requirement to have support personnel to provide services, the service delivery in general is restricted to five handicapping categories, which are hearing impairment, mental retardation, autism or pervasive developmental disorders, visual impairment and physical handicap. Consequently, the diagnosis of speech disorders follows a medical classification based on aetiology. Children with speech and language disorders under the age of six years are not differentially diagnosed as having articulation difficulties, phonological delay or phonological disorder. The distinction between phonetic/articulatory and phonological disorders was introduced initially by Konrot (1986) and Topbaş (1994) but it is not recognised by medical professionals or legislation. Rather, the 'wait and see paradigm' still exists. Unless speech and language disorders occur due to a known organic aetiology, they are not recognised as a category of impairment. Nevertheless, public awareness is growing and an increasing number of parents refer their children for assessment and intervention by the few practicing speech-language pathologists.

Due to the scarcity of licensed speech-language pathologists in a country with such a large population, it is unrealistic to expect that qualified speech therapists will be the primary providers of direct services in the near future. But a long-term plan should place a heavy emphasis on training qualified professionals via graduate programmes in SLP. Encouraging signs for such a development are visible. Licensing requirements for the field are beginning to be established and the graduate programme (MSc and PhD) in Speech and Language Pathology at Anadolu University is flourishing. As the profession becomes better established, it will increasingly assume responsibility for the provision of direct care, in-service training of other professionals and research in communication disorders.

A Brief Sketch of Turkish Phonology

Consonants of Turkish (20 in total)

	Bilabial	Labio-dental	Alveolar	Palato-alveolar	Palatal	Velar	Glottal
Stop	p b		t d			k g	
Fricative		f v	s z	ʃ ʒ			h
Affricate				tʃ dʒ			
Nasal	m		n				
Liquid			l, ɾ				
Glide					j		

Obstruents

All obstruents, except /h/, come in voiced and voiceless pairs. With the exception of the voiced non-continuants, /b, d, g, dʒ/, which cannot occur in final position; they can appear in any position in a word. Voiceless non-continuants, /p, t, k, tʃ/ are aspirated in all positions. The velar stops /k, g/ also have palatal counterparts [c] and [ɟ]. In general, palatal [c] and [ɟ] occur in syllables with front vowels /i, e, y, ø/ and the velar [k] and [g] occur in syllables with back vowels /ɨ, a, o, u/. This symmetry is violated in a few words where palatals can co-occur with the low back vowel /a/ (e.g. [caɾir] 'infidel', [ɾyzɟaɾ] 'wind') and can even create some minimal pairs (e.g. [kaɾ] 'snow' – [caɾ] 'profit'). Such examples, not being numerous, have created a dispute over whether these segments should be fully recognized as separate phonemes.

In general, the status of the continuant obstruents (i.e. fricatives) is fairly straightforward; the only exception to this is /v/, which has two allophones: it is a fricative in initial position (e.g. [vahʃi] 'wild'), but in medial or final position it becomes a frictionless continuant, [ʋ], (e.g. [haʋa] 'weather', [haʋlu] 'towel', [aʋ] 'hunt'). Another comment that may be in order here is related to the orthographically preserved (soft-g) old voiced velar fricative, [ɣ], (which survives in some non-standard dialects). In syllable final position, it indicates lengthening of the previous vowel (e.g. tuğla [tuːɫa] 'brick', sağ [saː] 'right'), and is optionally replaced by the palatal glide when occurring after front vowels (e.g. düğme [dy:mɛ]/[dyjmɛ] 'button'). It does not occur at all post-vocalically, in syllable-initial position (e.g. <u>soğan</u> [soan] 'onion', <u>doğu</u> [dou] 'east').

Sonorants

While the nasals and the palatal glide are straightforward, the liquids require some elaboration. The non-lateral alveolar flap /ɾ/ has a voiceless allophone in final position which is produced with friction (e.g. [kaɾ̥]). The alveolar lateral approximant /l/ has two allophones in native words: (a) velarised or 'dark-l', [ɫ], when it occurs with a tautosyllabic back vowel (e.g. [haɫa] 'aunt'), and (b) palatalised or 'clear-l' when it occurs with a tautosyllabic front vowel (e.g. [bilɛ] 'even'). All laterals in word-initial position are borrowings, which are predictably palatalised; laterals are also predictably palatalised when either the immediately preceding or following a front vowel, even if that vowel is not tautosyllabic (e.g. [sɛ.lam] 'greeting'). Furthermore, several laterals in other positions of borrowed words are of the 'clear' or palatalised version regardless of their vocalic environment. This fact creates some (but not many) minimal pairs ([boɫ] 'loose fitting' – [bol] 'punch, cocktail') and opens the discussion as to whether these two laterals should be considered phonemically distinct.

Vowels of Turkish (eight in total)

Although there are phonetically three degrees of height (high, mid, low), phonologically, it is a common practice to analyse Turkish vowels as 'high' (/i, y, ɯ, u/) versus 'non-high' (/ɛ, ø, a, o/).

	Front	*Back*
High	i y	ɯ u
Mid	ɛ ø	o
Low		a

All vowels in Turkish are short. Long vowels occur through the above-mentioned deletion of 'soft-g', or in borrowed vocabulary. All vowels may be followed by /j/ creating diphthong like sounds; /j/ becomes the onset consonant if it is followed by a vowel (e.g. [boja] 'paint').

Finally, vowels in native words are subject to vowel harmony. This can be described as follows: vowels in a word agree in backness (i.e. all 'front' or all 'back'); in addition, high vowels agree in rounding with the preceding vowel, as shown below.

[ɛk.mɛk]	'bread'	vowels: front
[ɛk.mɛk.lɛɾ.dɛn]	'from the breads'	vowels: all front
[ɛk.mɛk.lɛ.ɾin]	'of the breads'	vowels: all front, high V agrees in rounding

[a.ɾa.ba]   'car'   vowels: back
[a.ɾa.ba.ɫaɾ.dan]   'from the cars'   vowels: all back
[a.ɾa.ba.ɫa.rɯn]   'of the cars'   vowels: all back, high V agrees
                                        in rounding

Syllable structure

The syllable structure of Turkish can be described as (C) V (C) (C), in that the vowel nucleus is the only obligatory element. There are no onset clusters; the language does allow certain double codas, which can be described as:

(a) sonorant + obstruent (e.g. [faɾk] 'difference')
(b) fricative + stop (e.g. [tʃift] 'couple')
(c) k + s (e.g. [boks] 'box')

Sequences of two consonants that are not tautosyllabic, which are permissible in Turkish words, have to split up into different syllables following the maximum onset principle (Clements & Keyser 1983), as in [ban.ka] 'bank', [baɫ.kon] 'balcony', and so on. By the same token, an intervocalic consonant is always assigned to the following syllable and there is no question of ambisyllabicity (e.g. [dɛ.miɾ] 'iron', [ka.lɛm] 'pencil').

Stress

Stress, which has the phonetic correlates of loudness and higher pitch in Turkish, in general falls on the last syllable (e.g. [a.ɾa.bá] 'car', [a.ɾa.ba.já] 'to the car', [a.ɾa.ba.mɯ.zá] 'to our car', [a.ɾa.ba.ɫa.rɯ.mɯź] 'our cars', [a.ɾa.ba.ɫa.rɯ.mɯ.zá] 'to our cars').

There are a number of exceptions to the final syllable rule. Among these are:

(a) place names (e.g. [áŋ.ka.ɾa], [sám.sun], [gi.ɾɛ́.sun], [is.tán.bul]. In such words, the addition of affixes does not change the position of the stress (e.g. [án.ka.ɾa.ja] 'to Ankara');
(b) many (but not all) adverbs (e.g. [kɯ́.ʃɯn] 'in winter', [hɛ́.mɛn] 'right now', [ó.ɾa.da] 'there'); and
(c) interjections and vocatives (e.g. [háj.di] 'let's, come on').

Turkish is said to be a syllable-timed language in that all syllables, stressed and unstressed, have more or less equal duration. An example is a seven-syllable word [a.ɾa.ba.la.rɯ.mɯ.zá] 'to our cars'.

Previous Studies on Phonological Development and Disorders in Turkish

In the following, we summarise the studies that have been done on Turkish with normally developing and phonologically disordered children. To combine brevity and clarity, we have chosen a table format for our exposition (Table 10.1). Although there might be some differences

Table 10.1 Review of studies in Turkish phonological acquisition

	Age span	Subject number	Data	Focus	Major findings
Topbaş, 1988	1;0–3;0	20 normal	Cross-sectional	The frequency effect and the acquisition of /k, t, tʃ/ sounds in Turkish. Analysis: PCC, substitution errors	The findings revealed that certain sounds are better at certain ages; /t/, /k/ are acquired early and followed by /tʃ/ at the age of 2;9. The frequency of occurrence of certain sounds was suggested as being one of the significant factors in the acquisition. It is implied that, language-specific factors, such as the syllable structure, the transparency of phonological and morphological system of Turkish might contribute to the early acquisition of phonology.
Topbaş, 1997	1;0–3;0 normal 5;0 PD	22 normal 1 phonologically disordered	Longitudinal and cross-sectional	Phonological acquisition and implications for a disordered system are discussed. Age of phoneme acquisition and phonological process are compared with the PD system of a single child	Phoneme acquisition is very early: speech onset /b, d, k/ and /m/ are acquired before the age of 1;6, followed by n /, /t/ and /j//p/. The fricatives /v, s, ʒ, t/ (in that order) seem to be mastered between ages 2;4–2;8, although some allophonic variation may continue. The flap /ɾ/ is found to be the latest sound to appear. The processes identified include: reduplication, syllable deletion, consonant deletion, assimilation, final cluster reduction, liquid deviation, stopping, fronting, affrication and backing. From a cross-linguistic perspective, the phonological process patterns exhibited coincide broadly with literature, although there were language-specific patterns.

Study	Age	Participants	Design	Aim/Analysis	Findings
Topbaş and Konrot, 1998; Kopkalli-Yavuz and Topbaş, 1998	5;0–8;0	10 phonologically disordered	Cross-sectional	Variability in phonological disorders and the sub-classification of phonological disorders is discussed in comparison to seven languages from the literature. Analysis: Qualitative analysis of phonological7 processes	The processes observed were sub classified as delayed (persisting), unusual-consistent and inconsistent (variable). Delayed processes were typical of normally developing children whereas unusual error patterns such as stopping of liquids were rarely used. Inconsistent patterns were variable and observed as glottal insertion, glottal realisations, 'idiosyncratic velarisation' diosyncratic use of /h/, systematic sound preference. The study presented evidence cross-linguistically for sub-classification of disorders (Dodd, 1993).
Acarlar, 1995	2;0–6;0	20 normal 20 phonologically disordered	Cross-sectional	Comparison of normally developing and disordered children in phonological process usage	Children with phonological disorders used many more process than normally developing children. The most common processes in normally developing children were stopping, fronting, gliding, cluster reduction, assimilation and devoicing. Unusual processes occurring frequently with phonologically disordered children were liquid stopping, glottal replacement, backing and pharyngeal fricatives.
Acarlar and Ege, 1996	2;0–6;0	20 normal	Cross-sectional	Phonological process usage in normal children	Processes usually suppressed by the age of three were final consonant deletion, initial consonant deletion, metathesis and gliding. Syllable deletion, cluster reduction, assimilation, devoicing and stopping persisted after the age of three.

Continued

Table 10.1 *(Continued)*

	Age span	Subject number	Data	Focus	Major findings
Topbaş, 1996	5;0–8;0	10 phonologically disordered	Cross-sectional	Intelligibility of the speech of phonologically disordered children by listener judgments: correlation of average words per utterance, intended words, PCC and suprasegmental aspects as voice (pitch, loudness, quality) and rhythm (phrasing, stress and rate) based on Shriberg and Kwiatkowski, 1982	Some unusual processes observed were initial consonant deletion, metathesis, backing, denasalisation, deaffrication, nasalisation, fricatives substituted for stops and stops substituted for glides. This small group study found significant correlation between suprasegmentals and PCC. It is reported that low performance on PCC may affect child's performance on suprasegmentals. The need for larger studies was suggested.
Topbaş and Kopkallı-Yavuz, 1998	16 months–30 months	30 normal	Longitudinal and cross-sectional	Phonological process of word final devoicing (FD) concerning the /b, d, c, g/ sounds in Turkish	At 16 months children began using inflected forms, which gives evidence for the presence of the FD rule. By 18 months inflected forms become increasingly frequent. Alternations between the voiced and voiceless set of non-continuant obstruents were examined. At 22 months, alternating forms were pretty

					well established although there were a few cases of substitution of non-alternating forms for alternating ones. At 26 months the rule is completely acquired.
Kopkallı-Yavuz and Topbaş, 2000	16 months–30 months 15-50-75 word level	30 normal	Longitudinal & cross-sectional	Children's preferences for syllable/word forms in phonological acquisition	Turkish children attempted disyllabic words more frequently than monosyllabic words. In production, disyllabic words usually were not reduced to monosyllables. As for open/closed syllables, the children did not avoid closed syllables either in monosyllabic or disyllabic words. When closed syllables were reduced to open syllables, the closing consonants were /l/, /r/, /j/.
Topbaş & Dinçer, 2002	4;0–8;0	40 disordered	Cross-sectional	Universal and language specific aspects of variability in phonological disorders: The correct underlying representations (CUR) and the substitution errors to verify incorrect underlying representations (IUR) were analysed according to Dinnsen and Chin (1994), Barlow (1996).	This study adopted the analysis proposed by to Dinnsen and Chin (1994), Barlow (1996). The data showed considerable variation in children's underlying representations. The mean number of substitution errors was 33. And the scores ranged from 6 to 59. As the severity of variability increased, the CUR decreased.

Continued

Table 10.1 (Continued)

	Age span	Subject number	Data	Focus	Major findings
Yavaş and Topbaş, 2004	20–26 months 5;0–7;0 PD	10 normal 10 disordered	Longitudinal and cross-sectional	Liquid acquisition in Turkish: saliency versus frequency	Acquisition of Turkish liquids provided an interesting case to determine which of these two forces, markedness of the environment or frequency of occurrence, is dominant. Results showed that the unmarked word-initial liquids have the highest success rate in acquisition. The study points to the observation that the saliency of the liquids in initial position is the most potent determining factor, and overrides the adverse effect created by the infrequency.

Topbaş & Bleile, 2004	1;3–2;6	30 normal	Longitudinal	Comparison of phoneme emergence in Turkish and English based on Stoel-Gammon (1985)	Almost similar patterns in two languages but more rapid in Turkish:
					 15 Syllable Initial b, d, m, t, j
					          Final p, k, tʃ, t
					 18 Initial k, p, g, tʃ, dʒ, v
					          Final j
					 21 Initial s, ɪ, ʃ, h
					          Final s, ʃ, z
					 24 Initial r, f, z
					          Final r, f

in the terminology used, most of the studies in Table 10.1 followed an approach taken by Ingram (1979), Grunwell (1992), Leonard (1985) was adopted and Dodd's (1993) sub-classification system for speech disorders. Accordingly:

1. *Articulation disorder or phonetic disorder* is an inability to produce or the consistent distortion of a phoneme in isolation or any phonetic context in speech (e.g. lisp) or substitution of another phoneme. Articulation errors could be the result of a peripheral impairment in the planning and execution of gestures of the speech organs (Fey, 1992: 225) or due to organic-structural disorders such as cleft palate.
2. *Phonological disorder*, in contrast, is the inappropriate use of sounds according to the rules of the particular language being acquired. Thus, the error patterns observed reflects an impaired ability to abstract phonological knowledge of the language system. The error pattern are analysed as phonological processes, a well known method of analysing children's phonology according to the target adult language. Phonological disorder is a generic term in which there may be no known aetiology, impoverished language learning environment, general cognitive delay, and slower neurological maturation and can further be sub-grouped (Zhu Hua & Dodd, 2000a; So & Dodd, 1994):
   (a) *Delayed phonological development*: Most phonemes can be correctly realized or imitated in isolation but there are persisting error patterns which are inappropriate for the child's chronological age but appropriate for a younger child,
   (b) *Unusual (disorder) consistent:* The error patterns are either rarely used or atypical of normal phonological development but they are *consistent*. Consistency in these study meant that the error patterns could be explained or interpreted systematically by rules.
   (c) *Inconsistent/variable disorder*: The error patterns are either not used or very atypical of normal phonological development; they are so variable and inconsistent that they can not be described systematically by rules. There may be variable pronunciation of the same phonological features, there are multiple mismatches between the realisation and the target (Grunwell, 1992), and there may be inter-word or intra-word variability (Ingram, 1979). The speech is so unintelligible or idiosyncratic that even the parents cannot detect what the child might say.

To summarise, during the last decade a few researchers have studied different aspects of phonological acquisition and disordered development in Turkish. Most of these studies used small sample data in determining the age of acquisition for each sound and the error patterns analysed both in normal and disordered children were not computed statistically. The longitudinal studies focused only on specific aspects of phonological development. Thus, although previous research made contribution to the field of cross-linguistic acquisition, it failed to provide norms for Turkish children, which are essential to clinical assessment and therapy. In order to provide clinically reliable measures for phonological development, a large-scale study was conducted to develop norms by using both longitudinal and cross-sectional data. It is hoped that large-scale longitudinal data will supplement the information derived from the cross-sectional data such as the order of phoneme acquisition, age of phoneme acquisition and phonological processes used by children.

The Study

Subjects

In this study the speech samples of three groups of children were analysed.

Normally developing children: Longitudinal data

Longitudinal data were obtained from 88 monolingual Turkish-speaking children between 1;3 and 3;0 years of age. Three of these children were observed from birth. The remaining children were divided into three-month cross-sectional age bands from 16 to 36 months of age and were observed longitudinally in their natural home environment at three-week intervals. The children were from middle class families living in Eskişehir, Turkey. Parental reports, verified by family doctors, showed that all children had normal hearing, vision, cognitive function, speech and language, as well as normal oral-motor skills.

Normally developing children: Cross-sectional data

Cross-sectional data were obtained from 577 children aged 3;0 to 8;0 years. The children between 3;0 and 5;0 years old were divided into four age groups in six-month age bands. The rest of the children were divided into four age groups of 12-month intervals. The children in this group came from six metropolitan cities in four geographical areas of Turkey. School files and reports from the class teachers were used to verify that all the children had normal hearing, vision, cognitive function, speech and language, as well as normal oral-motor skills. If the children had any known or diagnosed developmental delay or organic disorder, they were excluded from the normative sample.

The disordered children

Seventy monolingual Turkish-speaking children (38 girls and 32 boys), aged 4;0 to 10;0 years, were the subjects of this group. These children were diagnosed either at university hospitals or other clinics as speech disordered and referred to Anadolu University for detailed assessment. The first author did the phonological assessment. A laryngologist and

Table 10.2 Subject information

Group	Age	n	Girls	Boys	Mean age month	SD	% of total sample
1	1;3–2;0	41	19	22	18	0.27	6.1
2	2;1–3;0	47	22	25	32	0.19	7.0
3	3;1–4;0	41	27	14	38	0.38	6.1
4	4;1–5;0	57	25	32	56	0.27	8.5
5	5;1–6;0	63	33	30	66	0.26	9.4
6	6;1–7;0	159	78	81	78	0.41	23.9
7	7;1–8;0	128	75	53	88	0.44	19.2
8	8;0 > above	129	66	63	97	0.38	19.3
	Total	665	345	320		2.15	100
9	Phonologically disordered	70	38	32	72	1.76	10.0
	Grand total	735	383	352		3.12	

a paediatric neurologist further examined the children and found no audiological or cognitive problems. Thus, all the children included in this study had no organic, sensory disorders or craniofacial anomalies. The Peabody Picture Vocabulary test (Turkish version) was used to measure the children's receptive and expressive language.

Putting all the subjects together, we had a total of 735 children (665 normal, 70 disordered), (383 boys and 352 girls) who participated in this study. Table 10.2 gives the breakdown of the participants. For the purpose of this study, the overall data were combined into yearly age groups, resulting in nine groups, including the phonologically disordered group. The younger group (below 3;0) who were observed longitudinally was further analysed in six-month age bands for descriptive analysis of phoneme emergence.

Data collection procedure

Normally developing children: Longitudinal data

The longitudinal data from the normally developing children were collected in naturalistic home environments. The data were recorded by the first author and a graduate assistant. The mothers or caregivers were always present and were asked to play with their children during the sessions. The mothers were also asked to tape record and keep a diary of the child's speech. They were given a record-keeping file, and were given special instructions for recording the data. These data were used to supplement the formal sample collected by the examiners in order to verify the sequential development of sound/consonant emergence and error patterns. The visits for the data collection lasted an hour: after a brief warm-up period, a 30-minute recording was made during each session. Since the children were young, pictures from the articulation-phonology test and sample toys were utilised to encourage the children to talk. This was done in order both to elicit the target phonemes and to provide consistency between subjects in the study.

Normally developing children: Cross-sectional data

The cross-sectional data from the normally developing children were collected primarily in nurseries and primary schools. Graduate students trained in speech and language pathology made the recordings in a quiet room using Sony MZ-R70 mini-disc digital audio recorders. The children were given SST test (Turkish Articulation and Phonology Test, Topbaş, 2004b/2005 (described below) (based on picture naming and picture description (narration and free conversation). The sessions lasted 45 minutes.

The disordered children

The data from children with phonological disorders were obtained during the assessment phase via SST Test when the children were referred to for diagnosis. All three subtests of SST were given and the assessments lasted about an hour and a half. Graduate assistants in speech and language pathology recorded the data in the phoniatrics speech laboratory with Sony MZ-R70 Mini-disc digital audio recorders. The sessions lasted about one and a half hours.

Materials

Before we discuss the results, some words on the material (SST) used for data collection and analysis are in order. SST is the first detailed standardised (valid and reliable) phonology test for Turkish children. It has three subtests:

Assessment of Articulation (SET) subtest is designed to examine the child's articulatory competence of speech sounds in words and scored as either correct or wrong. It contains 93 pictures based on a picture-naming task. Pictures were mostly nouns and basic colour terms known by young children. The children were asked to say the target words shown in the pictures. If the child failed to produce the target sound in the item or pronounce it wrongly, an imitated response was elicited within three trials. The trials included an isolated form and a form in CV and VC structures of Turkish vowels. If a phone is elicited by imitation, it is included in the consonant inventory and it is noted for stimulability for therapy measures for disordered children. If the sound cannot be produced by either prompts it is not included in the inventory.

Assessment of Auditory Discrimination (IAT) contains 48 pictures, comprised of 24 minimal pairs differing in manner, place or voicing distinction which is designed to assess the perceptibility of the sounds that are in error or not produced. This subtest requires the child to select the picture of the word pronounced by the examiner. The results of this subtest are not included in the current analysis.

Phonological Analysis Subtest (SAT) is based on phonological process analysis. It contains 13 pictures of thematic compositions meant to elicit expressive language samples in continuous speech. The pictures were culturally appropriate for spontaneous data collection based on narration, dialogues and conversation. The children were asked to describe the picture. They were prompted with 'Can you describe what is happening here? What happened? What do you see in this picture?' Additional conversational material was elicited by questions related to the pictures, like, 'When is your birthday? Do you also give parties? Who/what is this? Where does the ambulance go? Have you seen any accidents?' etc. The test includes 18 phonological processes. In the analysis forms of this subtest all the probable target words are listed and the ones which may be subject to a particular process are marked. As an example, there are 71 words which might be subject to a fronting process.

The words in all the SST subtests were chosen to provide a representative sample of Turkish phonology.

Each phoneme occurred in the following positions:

Syllable-initial word-initial (SIWI)	pil	(battery)
Syllable-initial within-word (SIWW) intervocalic	ka-pı	(door)
-C, C-post-consonantal	kar-puz	(watermelon)
Syllable-final within-word (SFWW)		
-C, C-pre-consonantal	şap-ka	(hat)
Syllable-final word-final (SFWF)	top	(ball)
Word-final Clusters	Türk	(Turkish)

Transcription

The transcriptions of the disordered data were first done by graduate (MSc) students in speech-language pathology and then listened and checked independently by four speech-language pathology graduate research assistants who were well trained in phonetic and phonological analysis. The reliability analysis was computed by inter-rater reliability analysis of the first author with the four assistants. This was done on a random sampling of 10 mini-discs. In each disc there were data from four children, so a total speech sample of 40 children was compared for transcription reliability. The inter-transcriber reliability correlation coefficient measure was computed by Cronbach Alpha as alpha = 0.829 (Hotelling's t-squared = 252.21, $F = 124.27\ p < 0.000$).

Data analysis

Measures of the present study

For the present study, the following measures were examined: percentage of consonants correct (PCC) for phoneme emergence, phoneme stabilisation and error patterns as the percentage of phonological processes (PPP).

Phoneme emergence

For the emergence of phonemes, the individual phonetic inventory of each child in the longitudinal data was identified one by one. The term emergence is used as the first appearance of the sound. During this stage, regardless of phonological correctness every phone that occurred twice in a child's repertoire was included in the inventory. A phoneme was considered to be emerging in the overall data, if 90% of the children produced the sound consistently in two words, irrespective of whether the sound was the correct target. When calculating phoneme emergence, the imitated responses were also taken into consideration to determine the child's articulation ability.

Phoneme stabilisation

Each phoneme (except /b, d, dʒ, g/, since they do not occur word-finally) occurred at least four times in the SST articulation sub-test, and several times in the phonology sub-test. The term stabilisation is referred as the consistent use of the target sound. Thus a phoneme was considered stable if it occurred correctly in at least two different syllables positions (SI and SF) of three different words, out of the four possibilities. Thus, a 90% criterion for an age group was used as an overall accuracy rate (when children achieved an accuracy rate of at least 75% (i.e. 3/4) to determine the age of acquisition in each age band In this measure the imitated responses were not taken into analysis. The formula proposed by Shriberg & Kwiatkowski (1982) was used to compute the percentage of consonants correct (PCC): consonants produced correctly divided by the total number of target phoneme × 100).

Percentage of phonological processes

A detailed analysis was performed using the assessment forms of the phonological analysis subtest based on spontaneous language samples. For each child, a process had to be used in at least three different words, and if 10% of the children in an age group used the same error pattern, it was considered as a process. The percentage of occurrence of processes was calculated by the following formula: the number of times a consonant occurs in a process divided by target process × 100. As an example, the number of times /k/ is realised as [t] is divided by the total number of marked words for fronting processes × 100.

Overall data analysis

Besides using descriptive statistics to show general developmental trends, one-way analysis of variance, and regression analysis were used to verify the age and gender effect in comparison with disordered development, the processes.

Results

Acquisition of phonemes

Quantitative analysis of performance in phonemic accuracy by age and gender

Table 10.3 presents the means and standard deviations of the children according to age and gender on percent consonants correct (PCC).

Children aged from 3;1 performed more accurately than the younger children on the PCC. The PCC increased as age increased. However, the performance of the phonologically disordered group was considerably lower on the PCC measure. No significant difference was found between the youngest group (Group 1) and the phonologically disordered group. The result of a one-way ANOVA was computed for the effects of age and gender. There was a significant age effect on PCC scores ($F_{8,726} = 481.865\ p < 0.000$), and post hoc Tukey HSD analysis showed differences between Group 1, 2 and all the other groups. The younger age groups differed significantly from each other but no significant differences were found between Group 3 and Groups 4, 5, 6, 7, 8.

There were no differences for gender among the groups on the PCC, as shown by the ANOVA results ($F_{1,733} = 0.086\ p > 0.770$). The gender effect for phonologically disordered children was analysed separately by t-test for PCC measure but no significant gender difference was found (PCC $t = 1.345\ p > 0.183$).

Qualitative analysis

Emergence of phonemes

The phonetic inventory of each child was determined individually, using the articulation-phonology test. Table 10.4 shows the emergence of phonemes for each age band in the longitudinal data. The consonants that were produced by 90% of the children in each age group were included in the table. By age 3;6 all the sounds seemed to be established in syllable-initial and syllable-final positions. Among the very earliest

Table 10.3 Means and standard deviations by age and gender on PCC in picture-naming task (SET)

	Age																Phonologically disordered (n = 70)		Total (n = 735)	
	1;3–2;0 (n = 41)		2;1–3;0 (n = 47)		3;1–4;0 (n = 41)		4;1–5;0 (n = 57)		5;1–6;0 (n = 63)		6;1–7;0 (n = 159)		7;1–8;0 (n = 128)		> 8 (n = 129)					
	Mean	SD	Mean	SD	Mean	SD	Mean	SD	Mean	SD	Mean	SD	Mean	SD	Mean	SD	Mean	SD	Mean	SD
Boys	41.10	13.21	68.50	12.76	94.88	4.29	98.72	2.26	97.54	3.21	98.52	2.53	99.56	1.31	99.40	1.13	60.02	18.56	90.15	18.69
Girls	44.27	11.80	74.00	8.77	94.78	4.87	97.78	2.53	98.33	2.39	98.80	2.18	99.22	1.76	99.54	1.37	65.96	18.04	90.55	17.52
Total	42.80	12.42	71.42	11.05	94.85	4.44	98.19	2.44	97.92	2.85	98.66	2.35	99.42	1.51	99.47	1.25	62.74	18.43	90.34	18.13

Table 10.4 Emergence of phonemes in 90% of the children in the longitudinal data (n = 121)

Age group		SIWI	SIWW	SFWW	SFWF
1;3–1;6	Stop-plosives Nasals Glide	b, d, m,	b, d, t m, j,	 m, n,	p, t, k, c, m, n,
1;7–2;0	Stop-plosives Nasals Affricates, fricatives Liquids Glide	p, t, g, ɟ, n, ʃ, tʃ, dʒ, j	k, g, n, tʃ, dʒ, ʋ, l, ɫ,	p, k, t, tʃ, l j	tʃ, ʋ, l j
2;1–2;6	Fricatives Liquids Flap	s, f l, ɾ	s, ʃ, ʋ	s, ʃ ɫ	f, s, ʃ, l, ɫ
2;7–3;0	Fricatives Flap	v, z, h,	f, h, z ɾ	f, z	z, h
3;1–3;6	Fricatives Flap			h ɾ	ɾ

sounds produced by 90% of children between the ages 13–15 months were labial, alveolar, and velar stops, nasals and /j/. The voiced labial stop emerged earlier than its voiceless counterpart in word initial position. The voiceless velar stop /k/, and its allophone /c/, first emerged in syllable final word final position, and later in other syllable positions. The voiceless labial stop /p/ first appeared in syllable-final-word-final position as well. The labiodental fricative /v/ (realised as [ʋ] and accepted as an allophone of /v/), appeared in word final and intervocalic positions at early ages. The fricatives emerged at around 2;0 and 2;5. The voiceless alveolar and palato-alveolar fricatives emerged almost simultaneously. The voiced fricative /z/, the glottal fricative /h/ and the flap /ɾ/ and its allophonic variations emerged at around 2;6. Among the clusters, nasal + stop (e.g. /nk/) combinations appeared earlier than flap + stop (e.g. /ɾt, ɾk/) or liquid + stop (e.g. /lp/) combinations. Although the liquids seemed to occur in children's speech much earlier, they were subject to deletion when occurring in clusters.

Stabilisation of SI and SF phonemes

Table 10.5 presents the stabilisation of phonemes for all age groups, drawing from both longitudinal and cross-sectional data. The consonants /b, p, t, d, k, m, n, j/ that appeared early in the children's repertoire were stabilised by the age of 1;11 and used consistently in a lot of different

Table 10.5 Age of stabilisation of phonemes in four word positions for 90% of children ($n = 665$)

Age group	SIWI	SIWW	SFWW	SFWF
1;6–1;11	b, d, k, t, m	b, d, t, m	m, n, j	p, k, t, m, n, j
2;0–2;5	p, g, t, n, ɟ, tʃ, dʒ, j	p, k, g, n, j	p, k, l, j, ʋ	c, n, tʃ, ʋ,
2;6–2;11	s, l, ʃ, f,	s, ʃ, l, ɬ,, tʃ, dʒ,	s, ʃ, tʃ,	s, ʃ, l,
3;0–3;5	v, z, ʒ, h,	f, ʒ, ʋ, z	ɬ, z	f, ʒ
3;6–3;11	ɾ	h, ɾ		z, h
4;0–4;5			h, ɾ	ɾ
4;6–4;11	All	All		Clusters
5;0–5;11	All	All	All	Clusters
6;0–6;11	All	All	All	All
7;0–7;11	All	All	All	All
8;0 > above	All	All	All	All

words with almost no error phonologically. The velar /g, ɟ/, the affricates /tʃ, dʒ/ and the fricative consonants /s, ʒ/ stabilised between the ages of 2;0 and 2;6. The liquid /l/, which emerged earlier, was subject to deletion in within word pre-consonantal positions and thus stabilised around 2;5 years of age. The labiodental fricatives and the voiced fricatives /z/, and /h/ stabilised between 2;8–3;5. The stabilisation of /ɾ/ took a longer period of time although in WI and WF positions it appeared earlier in 50% of children's speech.

Error patterns as phonological processes

Comparison of subtests of the SST showed slight differences in the articulation of sounds in picture-naming tasks and in Spontaneous Speech samples. Although almost all the phonemes were acquired earlier and articulated correctly in the picture-naming task, error patterns were observed in the spontaneous speech of the children. This was obvious in the younger age group. At later ages no significant results were obtained between the two tasks. The error patterns observed are defined by descriptive statistics as structural and systemic phonological processes. Table 10.6 shows the percentage of children from each age group who used these processes in at least four words. The most frequently observed processes were summarised. Most of the processes were suppressed by the age of four. The error patterns were high around two years of age, which might be due to the increase in vocabulary

Phonological Acquisition and Disorders in Turkish

Table 10.6 Percentage of phonological processes by age

Age →	1;6	2;0	2;6	3;0	3;6	4;0	4;6	5;0	5.6	6;0	Most common error types and examples
					Structural simplifications						
Reduplication	41	9	1	–	–	–	–	–	–	–	/doktor/ → [dodo] (doctor)
Syllable deletion	37	30	22	13	2	–	–	–	–	–	/cɛlɛbɛc/ → [cɛbɛc] (butterfly); /portakal/ → [pɔtʌt] (orange); /bisiklet/ → [bitet] or [pɪʃɪc] (bicycle)
Consonant deletion	19	21	11	6	2	–	–	–	–	–	Usually SI and SF /h/ either in WI or WW pre- and postconsonantal positions /horoz/ → [ojoz]; /tʌhtʌ/ → [tʌtʌ] (board) /n/deletion /dondurmʌ/ → [dodumʌ] (icecream)
WF cluster reduction	56	98	71	48	30	4	3	1	1		Liquids in the cluster deleted /rk/ → [k]: /tyrc/ → [tyc] (Turkish) and /or vowel lengthening occurred when the liquid is deleted /rk/ → [:k]: /ʃɔrt/ → [ʃɔːt] Nasals delete: /rɛnc/ → [jɛc]
Assimilation processes	15	22	17	3	1						SI and SF consonants harmonize in place and manner; progressively and regressively. Stop → nasal: /bʌnʌ/ → [manʌ] (to me);

Continued

Table 10.6 (Continued)

Age →	1;6	2;0	2;6	3;0	3;6	4;0	4;6	5;0	5;6	6;0	Most common error types and examples
											fricative → nasal: /mɛjvʌ/ → [mɛjma] (fruit); velar → alveolar: /citʌp/ → [titʌp] (book); alveolar → velar: //kutu/ → [kuku] (box); velar → labial: /kʌpu/ → [pʌpɯ] (door); labial → velar: /pʌrmʌk/ → [kʌːmʌk] (finger); alveolar → labial: /tɔp/ → [pɔp] (ball). An interaction with metathesis was observed with assimilation as well: /citʌp/ → [tipʌt] (book)
Systemic simplifications											
Liquid deviation	76	90	55	42	24	8	3	1	1		SF /l, r/ → either in WF or WW pre- and postconsonantal positions /bir/ → [bi] (one) SI and SF /l, r/ → [jl/ʌrɯ/ → [ʌjɯ] (bee); /ɛrcɛc/ → [ɛjcɛc] (man) SI and SF /r/ → [l] /ʌrʌbʌ/ → [ʌlʌbʌ] (car); /kʌr/ → [kʌl] (snow), SF /l, r/ → deletion by vowel Lengthening /bʌrdʌk/ → [bʌːdʌk] (cup);

Fronting	28	46	10	2		/kɔtuk/ → [kɔtuk] (armchair) Velar fronting: /k/ → [t] /bɛbɛc/ → [bɛbɛt] (doll); Palatal fronting: alveopalatals fronted /ʃ/ → [s] /ʃiʃɛ/ → [sisɛ] (bottle)
Stopping	44	58	36	16	5 1	Stopping of fricatives mostly [s, z, ʃ, ʒ, :/su/ → [du] (water) rarely/f/ → [p]: /fʌrɛ/ → [pʌjɛ] (mouse) Stopping of affricates: /dʒʌm/ → [dʌm] (glass)
Deaffrication	7	13	5	0.5		/tʃitʃɛc/ → [ʃiʃɛc] (flower)
Affrication	8	19	6	1		Rarely observed/kʌʃ/ → [kʌtʃ] (eyebrow)
Voicing (SIWI & SIWW)	38	11	3			/pʌmuk/ → [bʌmut] (cotton); /tɔp/ → [bɔp] (ball)
WF devoicing	21	45	17	1		Usually WF voiced fricatives devoiced/kɯz/ → [kɯs] (girl)
Metathesis	9	11	2			/citʌp/ → [cipʌt] book; /ryjʌ/ → [jyrʌ] (dream),
Backing	3	6	2			Velar backing: /tʃʌtʌt/ → [tʃʌkʌt] (fork) Backing of alveolars palatalization: /kas/ → [kʌʃ] (muscle);/su/ → [ʃu] (water); /sʌtʃ/ → [ʃʌʃ] (hair)

at this age. Children at this age attempted to use larger lexical vocabulary. Due to the agglutinating nature of Turkish they had to use longer strings of utterances in spontaneous speech. It seems that their phonological accuracy is affected by making more error patterns with complex syntactic structures at such an early stage. As can be inferred from the table, the error patterns diminish rapidly after that age. Reduplication, SI voicing, and fronting are among the earliest to be suppressed. Word final devoicing was observed for /z/ only. Assimilatory substitutions, although observed with high frequency, both progressively and regressively disappeared early. The two remaining error patterns observed after age four were liquid deviation and cluster reduction. The deletion of SI and SF consonants /ɾ, l/ which are analysed under liquid deviation were observed mostly in pre-consonantal and post-consonantal within word positions. In pre-consonantal deletions of /ɾ/ usually vowel lengthening was realized. In post-consonantal positions either deleted or /j/ substitution occurred (/bʌjɾʌk/ → [bʌjʌk] 'flag'; /cibɾit/ → [cibit] 'matches'; /jʌpɾʌk/ → [jʌpʌk] or [jʌpjʌk] 'leaf'. The findings of this large data support the findings of Yavaş and Topbaş (2004). The chronology of suppression of processes is given in Figure 10.1.

There were also patterns which are used by less than 10% of children in the sample. These patterns are noted as unusual. Among these were

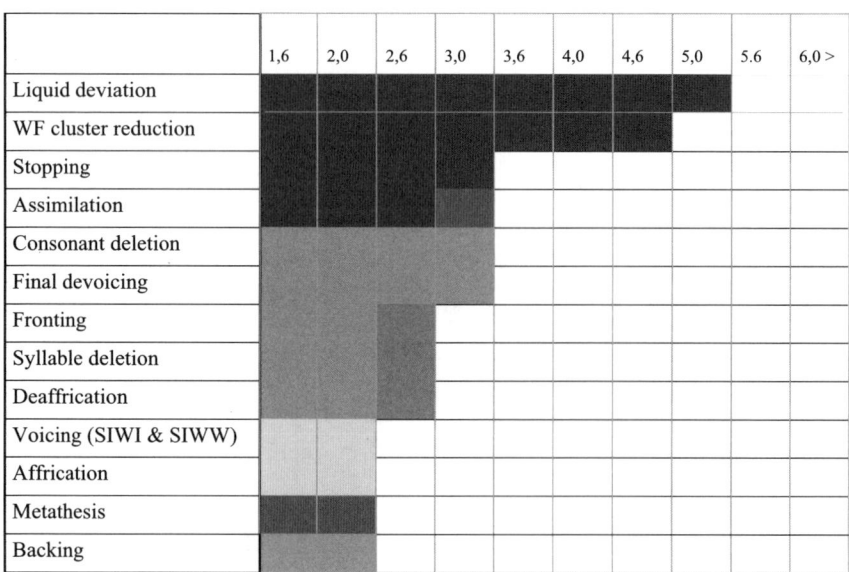

Figure 10.1 Suppression of the most frequent error patterns by age in normally developing children

liquid stopping, gliding of fricatives, nasalisation liquids and fricatives, consonant insertion. Another notable process was frication of liquids (usually SF /ɾ/ → [ʃ] /motoɾ/ → [motoʃ] 'motor'; /kɑɾ/ → [kʌʃ] 'snow') which might be due to the allophonic realisation of the flap in SFWF positions as [ɾ̥] in Turkish. It occurred very rarely and analysed under liquid deviation and not considered as an unusual process. These data needs further research in comparison with disordered data.

Phonologically disordered children

As shown in Table 10.3 above the PCC scores were very low compared to normally developing children. There were more deletions and substitutions in their speech and their phonetic inventories were very restricted (see examples in Appendix 1).

The error patterns used by phonologically disordered children are subdivided into three categories as delayed, unusual inconsistent/variable processes. The processes used by at least 10% of children in the data are presented in Tables 10.7. and 10.8.

The delayed error patterns were typical of developmentally normal children and used by 90% of normally developing children but were used with high frequency and were not suppressed by the expected age. The delayed error patterns were much more predictable when compared with children's error patterns that show unusual and inconsistent patterns. However, the type of sound changes was somewhat different. As an example, an alveolar or labial harmony and a metathesis in the word /citʌp/ → [tipʌt], [cipʌp] (book), was more common in normal children whereas in phonologically disordered children's data a variety of forms was observed as [bipʌp], [pipʌt], [cikʌp], [pipʌp], [titʌt].

The unusual but consistent error patterns observed were stopping of liquids, gliding of fricatives, and nasal stopping. Only the stopping of liquids was observed in a few normally developing children, with very low frequency below the criteria. The inconsistent/variable errors patterns inconsistent velarisation, glottal stop insertion, lateralisation, inconsistent use of /h/ and systematic sound preference. The more severe the children's PCC scores, the more unintelligible they were. A strong negative correlation was found between PCC scores and phonological error patterns ($r^2 = -0.929$ $p < 0.000$, $F_{1,69} = 431.178$ $p < 0.000$).

Conclusion

In this study, we examined the data from 577 normally developing children for normative data. As expected, children's speech became more accurate as they got older. Most consonants were produced correctly around 3;0. The sequence of sound acquisition found in the data was

Table 10.7 Error patterns used by phonologically disordered children

	Mean frequency of errors	Std. Dev.	% number of cases
Delayed processes			
Liquid deviation	16.81	10.08	90
WF cluster reduction	3.65	2.4	71.4
Fronting	8.37	11.90	52.8
Assimilation processes	3.58	4.57	48.5
Consonant deletion (except liquids)	3.18	6.7	41.4
Stopping	4.47	7.91	37.1
Metathesis	1.41	1.39	37.1
Voicing (SIWI & SIWW)	2.47	4.46	34.2
WF devoicing	1.78	2.22	34.2
Deaffrication	1.92	3.77	31.4
Affrication	1.75	4.57	25.7
Backing	1.52	3.90	24.2
Syllable deletion	0.90	1.7	22.8
Unusual consistent processes			
Stopping of /r, l, j/	0.69	0.95	10.9
Nasal stopping (denasalisation)	0.21	0.79	7.1
Nasalisation of fricatives and liquids	0.6	3.87	7.1
Fricative gliding	0.21	0.69	5.7
Unusual metathesis	0.18	0.51	2
Inconsistent processes			
Glottal stop insertion	0.27	1.43	5.7
Idiosyncratic velarisation (k-sation)	0.5	0.65	4.2
Lateralisation	0.45	0.13	3.4
Systematic sound preference	2.14	1.59	3
Idiosyncratic use of /h/	0.31	2.62	1.4
Mean percent phonological process	57.47	31.66	
Mean percent consonants in error in articulation sub-test (SET)	34.95	16.91	
Mean percent consonants in error in spontaneous speech (SAT)	37.30	18.40	

Table 10.8 Error patterns observed in phonologically disordered children ($n = 70$)

Unusual consistent processes		
Stopping of /ɾ, l, j/	/ɾ, l, j/ → [d] realised usually interacting with metathesis and asssimilation	/yilan/ → [dijʌj] (snake) /bʌjɾak/ → [bʌjdʌt] (flag) /jʌpɾʌk/ → [bʌttʌt] (leaf)
Nasal stopping denasalisation)	/m/ → [b, d]	/mɛctʊp// → [bɛtʊt] (letter)
Nasalisation of fricatives and liquids	/l/,/v/ → [n] usually in intervocalic positions but not necessarily	/dɛvɛ/ → [tɛnɛ] (camel) /kʌlɛm/ → [kənɛm] (pencil) /polis/ → [pʰənɪs] (police)
Fricative gliding	Usually SI, SF /v/ → [j]	/ev/ → [ɛj] (house) /tʌʊʊk/ → [tʌjʊk]
Unusual metathesis	Different metathesis forms not seen in normally developing children interacting with other simplification patterns	/ʌɾmʊt/ → [ʌmbʊt] (pear) /tʃɔɾʌp/ → [pojjʌt] (socks) /dɔktoɾ/ → [kotdo] (doctor)
Inconsistent processes		
Idiosyncratic use of /h/	/h/ substituted elsewhere for different consonants	/mʌsʌɫ/ → matah] (tale) /bisiklɛt/ → [həhəhət] (bicycle) /tʃizmɛ/ → [hɛhnɛ] (boots)
Idiosyncratic velarisation (k-sation)	/k/ substituted elsewhere for different consonants	/ʃɛmsijɛ/ → [cɛntɛ] (umbrella) /ʃiʃɛ/ → [cɪcæ] (bottle) /jɛʃil/ → [ɟiɟi] (green)
Glottal stop insertion	[ʔ] inserted or substituted elsewhere for different consonants	/ʌtkɯ/ → [ʌʔtɯ] (scarf) /lʌstic/ → [dʌʔcit] (elastic) /kʌhvɛ/ → [kʌʔvɛ] (coffee) /tɔp/ → [dəʔpʼ] (ball)
Lateralisation	Different lateral realisations of fricatives or liquids	/sɛs/ → [λ ɛ λ] (sound/voice) /lamba/ → [λamma] (lamp) /su/[ɬʉ] (water)
Systematic sound preference	Use of one consonant for different targets	Use of /t, d/ or /p, b/

consistent with previous studies in that stops, nasals and the glide were the earlier ones, which were followed by the affricates, fricatives, the lateral, and the flap, in that order. Liquid deviation and final cluster reduction were found to be the late processes.

We also examined the data from 70 children with phonological disorders. Findings, in general, suggest these children are in many respects similar to younger children; the phonetic inventories are restricted, and the percent correct consonants and the simplification processes used with high frequency. The error patterns of children with disorders were much more variable than those found in normally developing children. In addition to the delayed normal processes they exhibited, children with disorders revealed two other types of errors, which are called 'unusual processes' and 'inconsistent'.

The former are those processes that are infrequently found in normally developing children. In our data 'stopping of liquids' was the most frequent in this group and was followed by 'stopping of nasals', 'gliding of fricatives, and 'nasalisation of fricatives', in that order. Inconsistent errors are those that are not found in normal development and result in high unintelligibility. Inconsistent velarisation (idiosyncratic use of /k/) (errors that cannot be explained or interpreted in any regularity) was the most frequent and was distantly followed in frequency by 'glottalisation', 'lateralisation', and inconsistent use of /h/ (idiosyncratic use of /h/), in that order.

In conclusion, we can say that this study is in agreement with several others showing similar universal and language-specific tendencies and patterns in normally developing children and in children with phonological disorders. Normal development was characterised by the predictable order of acquisition by certain sound classes, and the certain chronology of suppression of the normal simplification error patterns. The speech accuracy increased with the chronological age and gender did not exert an influence on it. Following the trend found in several languages, children with phonological disorders, in addition to the normal simplification processes, revealed some unusual, and some inconsistent, the latter of which was an important source for much unintelligibility.

Acknowledgements

The project was made possible by Anadolu University Research Foundation AUAF003051 and by a Ministry of Education of Turkey grant awarded to the first author.

The first author acknowledges the assistance of Baris Dincer, Bülent Togram and MSc students at DILKOM in data collection, transcription and analysis; as well as to children and parents participating in this study.

Appendix 1: Phonetic Inventories of Phonologically Disordered Subjects S. and F.

Subject S.			Post			
	Bilabial	Labio-dental	Dental Alveolar Alveolar	Palatal	Velar	Glottal
Plosive	p b		t d	c	k g	
Nasal		m	n			
Tap or flap						
Fricative						h
Affricate						
Central approximant		ʋ		j		
Lateral approximant						

Subject F.			Post			
	Bilabial	Labio-dental	Dental Alveolar Alveolar	Palatal	Velar	Glottal
Plosive	p b		t			
Nasal		m				
Tap or flap						
Fricative						
Affricate						
Central approximant		ʋ				
Lateral approximant						

Part 3
Bilingual Context

Chapter 11
Aspects of Bilingual Phonology: The Case of Spanish–English Bilingual Children

M. YAVAŞ and B. GOLDSTEIN

Introduction

Children acquiring one language have to accomplish various tasks. For example, in developing the phonological system, a child has to determine which sounds constitute the phonetic inventory of the language, deduce the set of oppositions, and figure out how sounds can be combined in permissible ways. The task increases considerably in the case of bilingual children, as they have to accomplish the same things in their two languages. Because bilingual children are acquiring two phonological systems, it is likely that patterns of acquisition may be different from monolinguals. Those differences that may be observed may or may not be due to the influence of the dominant language (i.e. interference), because bilingual children, just like their monolingual counterparts, may exhibit speech and/or language disorders. Thus, when a bilingual child reveals developmental patterns that are different from those found in monolinguals, it is crucial to determine whether these nonconforming patterns are due to the influence of the child's other language(s), or if they are indications of a disorder.

The issue of interference is a valid one whether a child becomes bilingual simultaneously (two languages are acquired simultaneously), or successively (one language, generally the home language, is acquired earlier, and the other language is acquired, for example, when the child goes to school). Successive bilingualism is the more commonly observed phenomenon. Although this may suggest that the influence of one language over the other would be more evident, there is hardly any uniformity among bilinguals with respect to the range of interference and thus, patterns may vary from one bilingual to another.

One can easily identify several cases of the influence of the dominant language. For example, if we encounter in the English productions of a five to six-year-old Spanish–English bilingual child forms such as [espik] for speak [spik] etc., whereby the prothetic vowel before the target cluster, we can, with certain confidence, say that this is due to Spanish interference. The reasons for this are as follows. First, the simplification we observe in normal phonological development of monolingual English speaking children is reduction of the cluster to a single consonant (e.g. /spik/ → [pik]). Second, Spanish structure does not allow double onset clusters whereby the first consonant is /s/. When English words with a #sC pattern are borrowed into Spanish, the typical solution is to insert a prothetic /e/ to make it appropriate to the Spanish structure by resyllabifying the word as [es.pik].

There may be, however, some other cases where the dominant native language cannot be held responsible. Such cases come from certain developmental simplification processes that are universally phonetically motivated and shared by many languages. For example, if a Spanish–English bilingual child produces forms such as [bæk] for bag, or [kæp] for cab by devoicing the final stops, these patterns cannot be attributed to Spanish interference, because Spanish does not have any stops, voiced or voiceless, in this position. This devoicing process is universally motivated and thus that pattern is among the commonly occurring developmental processes that occur in the speech of children in many languages, including monolingual English speaking children. It is, however, one of the processes that is 'suppressed' rather early in the development. The reason that this process was not exhibited until this age is due to the fact that it was not demanded by the structure of Spanish (see Yavaş, 1998 for a review of these universal patterns).

Having made the argument that patterns in bilingual development may be different from those of monolinguals, we can now examine some important issues in the phonological development of Spanish–English bilingual children and discuss the points that might be relevant for the practicing therapist to separate children with delay and/or disorder from children with typical development. In doing this, we will first present a general picture of phonological patterns of Spanish in order to note similarities and differences between the source language (Spanish) and the target language (English). After this, we will give a brief summary of the studies on phonological development in monolingual Spanish-speaking children, and then look at the findings of previous studies on phonological development in Spanish–English bilingual children. Then we will report the findings from the specific studies we conducted on the English phonological characteristics of Spanish–English bilingual children. The chapter will conclude with some guidelines for clinicians for the identification of phonological disorders.

Brief Sketch of Spanish Phonology

Consonant and vowel phonemes of Spanish are given in Tables 11.1 and 11.2.

While the status of the vowels is rather consistent across varieties of Spanish, consonants show considerable variation. For example, /θ/, which is not included in Table 11.1, is only used in dialects in Spain. Voiceless velar and glottal fricatives are encircled to indicate that either one or the other, not both, occur in a given variety. Also noteworthy is the fact that the palatal lateral liquid /ʎ/, which is in contrast with the alveolar lateral /l/ in some varieties, is gradually being lost.

Besides the inventories given above, some other features of Spanish phonology are also noteworthy. While all Spanish consonants, are capable of occurring in syllable-initial-within-word (SIWW) position, /ɾ/ and /ɲ/ cannot appear in syllable-initial-word-initial (SIWI) position. As for the occurrences in coda position, there are severe restrictions. While all consonants, except for /x/, /tʃ/, /r/ and /ɲ/, can occur in syllable-final-within word (SFWW) position, only /s, n, ɾ, l/ (and maybe /d/) are allowed in syllable-final-word-final (SFWF) position.

As for the consonant clusters that occur in Spanish, the following restrictions hold. The onset clusters must have a stop or /f/ as their first member, which is followed by a liquid (e.g. <u>frente</u> [fɾente], <u>tren</u> [tɾen], <u>globo</u> [gloβo]). Coda clusters are exclusively within word; they are not allowed word-finally. There are some limited within word codas, which are restricted to combinations that end in /s/ preceded by a stop or a sonorant consonant (e.g. <u>abstracto</u> [abs.tɾak.to], <u>extensor</u> [eks.ten.sor], <u>instintivo</u> [ins.tin.ti.βo], <u>perspicaz</u> [peɾs.pi.kas]).

Differences in the inventory as well as the distribution of sounds between English and Spanish systems create several mismatches, and these may be very important for the SLP/SLT in making the diagnosis of phonological disorder. Although the two languages have the same

Table 11.1 Consonants of Spanish

	Bilabial	*Labio-dental*	*Dental*	*Alveolar*	*Palatal*	*Velar*	*Glottal*
Stops	p b		t d			k g	
Fricatives		f		s		(x)	(h)
Affricates					tʃ		
Nasals	m			n	ɲ		
Liquids				l r ɾ	ʎ		
Glides					j	w	

Table 11.2 Vowels of Spanish

	Front	*Central*	*Back*
High	i		u
Mid	e		o
Low		a	

number of stop phonemes, the following problems are frequently observed. Voiceless stops are always unaspirated in Spanish. Thus, in their production of English, Spanish speakers may show a lack of aspiration in initial position of a stressed syllable, e.g. ton, pay, car. Also, voiced stops /b, d, g/ have fricative allophones [βðɣ] in Spanish. Stop variants occur after pauses, after nasals and /l/; the fricative variants occur in other environments. Thus, in their production of English, Spanish speakers may produce fricatives for voiced stop targets in words such as adore, aboard, ago.

Fricatives are the category that presents the greatest disparity between the two languages. The total lack of interdental and palatal (palato-alveolar) fricatives, and the lack of voiced labio-dentals and alveolar fricatives in Spanish are the causes of several difficulties. The substitutions, to a great extent, are predictable. Interdental targets /θ, ð/ are generally rendered [t,d] initially (thank, those) and [s] finally (both, bathe). While /v/ is rendered as [b], and /z/ is rendered as [s], the common substitute for /ʃ/ is [tʃ]. These differences between the two languages may result in a loss of contrast in word pairs such as vowel–bowel, sip–zip, shop–chop, etc.

As for nasals, only /n/ is allowed in final position in Spanish, and thus is the substitute for any English nasal in this position.

Both languages have the lateral and non-lateral liquids, but the phonetic qualities of them are rather different in the two languages. While the Spanish lateral is always 'clear-l' (i.e. non-velarised), the American-English variant is produced mostly as shades of 'dark-l' (i.e. velarised). The r-sounds of the two languages also exemplify considerable phonetic disparity. The American English r is a retroflex approximant, and the two r-sounds of Spanish are a trill and a flap. These differences are sources of potential difficulties at the phonetic (not phonemic) level.

Regarding the positional freedom of occurrence the following observation needs to be made. While English allows almost all consonants (except for /h/) in final position, because of the restrictions stated above in Spanish (only /s, n, r, l/ (and maybe /d/) can occur in this position), we might encounter several instances of final consonant deletion in the speech of Spanish–English bilinguals.

Finally, consonant clusters are rather different in the two languages. English has all possible double onset clusters of Spanish and many more combinations, and in addition, some triple onsets. A more important difference relates to the coda clusters whereby English, in contrast with the lack of coda clusters in Spanish, presents very rich combinations of double and triple coda clusters. Such mismatches are frequent sources of difficulty, which may result in reductions of clusters or modifications by epenthetic vowels.

Spanish has far fewer vowels (five) than English, and this may prove to be an important source of frequent insufficient separation of English vowels. For example, lack of /i/ versus /ɪ/ contrast may create a confusion between grid and greed, while the lack of /u/ versus /ʊ/ contrast would result in the insufficient separation of fool and full. Similarly, the lack of /ʌ/ versus /a/ contrast would be the source of a neutralisation between buddy and body, and the lack of /ɛ/ versus /æ/ between mess and mass. A comparison of basic phonological features of Spanish and English is given in Table 11.3.

Besides the segmental mismatches noted above, the comparison of the two languages reveal significant differences in the prosodic domain.

Table 11.3 Comparative chart of Spanish and English sound systems

		Spanish	*English*
Consonants			
	SIWI	All except /r, ɲ/	All except /ŋ, ʒ/
	SIWW	All	All except /ŋ/
	SFWW	All except /x, tʃ, ɲ, r/	All except /h/
	SFWF	Only /s, n, l, r/ (maybe /d/)	All except /h/
Clusters			
	Onset	Only: 'stop/f + liquid'	A wide variety of double and triple clusters
	Coda	No, except 'stop/sonorant + /s/' in SFWW	A wide variety of double and triple clusters
	Vowels	i, e, a, o, u	i, ɪ, e, ɛ, æ, ɑ, ɔ, o, ʊ, u, ʌ/ə, ɚ/ɜ·
	Diphthongs	A wide variety including all of those occurring in English	aɪ, aw, ɔɪ
	Syllable struc.	(C)(C) V(C)(C)*	(C)(C)(C) V (C)(C)(C)(C)**

*Possible only in SFWW.
**Possible only if an affix.

Spanish is said to be a syllable-timed language (all syllables, stressed and unstressed, have more or less equal duration) as opposed to English, which is a stressed-timed language, (stressed syllables are longer than unstressed syllables and occur in regular intervals). A cognate word such as probability (Sp. probabilidad) provides a relevant example. This word has five syllables in both languages; it receives the stress on the third (ante-penultimate) syllable in English, and on the last (ultimate) syllable in Spanish. However, the real difference between the two languages lies in what happens to the unstressed syllables. In Spanish, the first four unstressed syllables have almost the equal duration to the last stressed one. In English [pra.bə.bi.lə.ti], on the other hand, the situation is very different. First of all, the second and the fourth syllables are unstressed and have reduced vowels, [ə], which are very short. The first, third and the fifth syllables have full vowels and thus their durations are greater than the second and the fourth syllables. Yet, their durations among themselves are different. The third syllable, which has the primary stress, is the longest; the first syllable, which has the secondary stress, is a little shorter; and the last syllable, which is not stressed but contains a full vowel, has a shorter duration. These differences result in different rhythmic patterns of the languages; it is said that Spanish, because of the equal duration of all syllables, has a 'staccato rhythm' as opposed to the 'galloping rhythm' of English, which is the result of different durations of syllables and vowel reduction processes.

Although the brief account given above is a fair reflection of the general core of formal Spanish spoken within the United States, there are some noteworthy differences that need to be pointed out, as these might be crucial in the therapist's evaluation of children's patterns. It is commonplace to hear the binary split between the 'Conservative dialects' (Guatemala, Costa Rica, Central Mexico, Western Argentina) and 'Radical dialects', which is also known as Caribbean Spanish, (Cuba, Puerto Rico, Dominican Republic, Coastal Venezuela, eastern coast of Mexico) (Guitart, 1978). The majority of the Spanish speakers in the United States are of either Mexican origin (California, Arizona and Texas), or Cuban origin (Florida). The basic difference between the conservative and the radical dialects is that the former generally maintains the syllable final /s/ and /ɾ/ while the latter deletes them. Beyond this, radical dialects reveal some other noteworthy features. Prevocalic word-initial voiced stops may be spirantised (realised as fricatives) in running speech (Hammond, 1976). /d/ is frequently deleted in intervocalic (dedo [deo]) and in word-final position (pared [pare]). In many radical dialects, velar nasal /ŋ/, instead of the alveolar /n/, is the norm in word-final position. There are also some features that are more specific to certain radical dialects. For example, /r/ is often realised as voiced or voiceless velar vibrant in mainly rural Puerto Rican Spanish. In some speakers of Cuban Spanish, liquids (/l,r/) may lose the contrast and both are realised as /h/ in word-final position (Lopez Morales, 1971). It is also possible that the flap totally assimilates to following dentals (verde 'green' [verde] → vedde]), or realised as [l] in word-final position (pintor 'painter' [pintoɾ] → [pintol]).

Phonological Development in Monolingual Spanish-Speaking Children

There are relatively few studies examining phonological development in monolingual Spanish-speaking children. Existing studies have investigated both segmental development and use of phonological patterns. Studies of early phonetic development indicated that typically developing Spanish-speaking children developed most of the phonetic system by two years and six months (e.g. Anderson & Smith, 1987; Gonzalez, 1983; Maez, 1981). In particular, the two-year-old children in those studies exhibited good production of stops, nasals and glides; fair production of voiceless fricatives; and poor production of the affricate, voiced spirants and liquid /l/, flap, and trill. Results of studies examining phonological patterns in two-year-olds demonstrated that cluster reduction and weak syllable deletion occurred greater than 50% of the time; initial, medial and final consonant deletion occurred 25–50% of the time; and velar fronting and assimilation occurred less than 25% of the time (Anderson & Smith, 1987; Mann *et al.*, 1992; Pandolfi & Herrera, 1990; Vivaldi, 1990).

Studies examining phonological development in monolingual Spanish speakers have gathered data mainly from preschool children. Data from segment-based studies have indicated that typically developing Spanish-speaking children mastered all but a few phonemes (/g/, /f/, /s/, /ɲ/, /ɾ/, /r/) by age five (Acevedo, 1993; De la Fuente, 1985; Gonzalez, 1978; Mason *et al.*, 1976). Previous studies examining the frequency-of-occurrence of phonological patterns indicated that Spanish-speaking children suppressed many phonological patterns by age three and a half (e.g. Goldstein & Iglesias, 1996; Gonzalez, 1981; Mann *et al.*, 1992; Stepanof, 1990). Specifically, postvocalic singleton omission, stridency deletion, tap/trill /r/, consonant sequence reduction and final consonant deletion were commonly exhibited, and fronting (both velar and palatal), prevocalic singleton omission, assimilation, and stopping were less commonly exhibited (e.g. Goldstein, 1996; Gonzalez, 1981).

It is important to add that the particular dialect background seems to influence the substitutions. For example, while Mexican background children in Jimenez (1987) used [ɾ], [d] or [l] for /r/, the Puerto Rican children in Anderson and Smith (1987) showed [l] or [h] for the same target. The two populations also differed for /s/ targets; Mexican children's substitutions varied among [t], [θ], [tʃ] (or deletion), whereas Puerto Rican children used [ʃ] or [h] for this target.

Phonological Development in Spanish–English Bilingual Children

The number of studies examining phonological development in monolingual Spanish speakers is relatively extensive compared to the few studies that have examined the phonological skills of bilingual children. Gildersleeve *et al.* (1996) examined the English phonological skills of typically developing, bilingual (English–Spanish) three-year-olds. The results indicated that the bilingual children showed an overall lower intelligibility rating, made more consonant and vowel errors overall, distorted more sounds, and produced more uncommon error patterns than either the monolingual English or monolingual Spanish speakers in the study. The bilingual children also exhibited error patterns found in both languages (cluster reduction, stopping and gliding) and evidenced phonological patterns that were not exhibited by either monolingual Spanish speakers (e.g. final consonant devoicing) or monolingual English speakers (e.g. initial consonant deletion). Gildersleeve *et al.* (1996) and Gildersleeve-Neumann and Davis (1998) also found higher percentages-of-occurrence for typically developing, bilingual children (in comparison to their monolingual peers) on a number of phonological processes including cluster reduction, final consonant deletion, and initial voicing. As for the influence of one language over the other, limited data do not allow us to make conclusive statements. While it is expected that the dominant (first) language would influence the weaker (later) language, there are conflicting cases. Yavaş (2002), examining the acquisition of voiceless stops in 10 Spanish–English bilingual children, found that although two subjects realised English /p, t, k/ as unaspirated (Spanish L1 influence), two others, unexpectedly, did the reverse by realising Spanish voiceless stops with aspiration.

Goldstein and Washington (2001) examined the English and Spanish phonological skills of typically developing, four-year-old simultaneous bilingual (Spanish–English) children and found that there were no significant differences between the two languages on percent consonants correct; percent consonants correct for voicing, place of articulation, manner of articulation; or percentage-of-occurrence for phonological processes. With the exception of interdental sounds in English, all other places of articulation either exceeded or approached mastery (greater than or equal to 90% correct) (Smit *et al.*, 1990). The results indicated that the phonological skills of these bilingual four-year-olds were similar overall to monolingual children. The bilingual children, however, were much less accurate than monolingual speakers on a few sounds classes.

Previous studies examining the phonological skills of bilingual children indicate that bilingual phonological development is somewhat different from monolingual phonological development. In the following sections, we will report data on some specific studies we conducted on some English phonological skills of Spanish–English bilingual children. We will then compare the results obtained with monolingual populations for the same targets.

Study I

The first study reported here, conducted by the second author, had the objective of examining the development of liquids and double onsets in the English productions of Spanish–English bilingual children.

Method

Participants were 15 typically developing bilingual (Spanish–English) children ranging in age from 4;1–6;2. To examine developmental trends, participants included five four-year-olds (mean age = 4;3), five five-year-olds (mean age = (5;1), and five six-year-olds (mean age = 6;1). All children were speakers of Carribean Spanish (either Puerto Rican or Dominican Spanish) or Mexican Spanish.

All bilingual children in the study received input in and used both languages at home and in school. According to parent report, output in each language was at least 25% of the time for each child at home and in school. Average output in English was 65.5% for four-year-olds, 41.2% for five-year-olds and 57.3% for six-year-olds. Finally, in terms of age of acquisition of both languages, all the bilingual children were considered sequential bilinguals (i.e. acquiring the second language (L2) after the first language), and in terms of functional ability, the children would be described as incipient bilinguals (i.e. 'beginning to acquire L2') (Valdés & Figueroa, 1994: 11).

For all 15 children, there was no parental or teacher concerns about phonological, language, or cognitive development. None of the children in the study had been diagnosed with a communication disorder, and thus none had received previous intervention for a communication disorder. Moreover, according to teacher report, each child exhibited normal functioning in the classroom (e.g. able to follow classroom routines and directions). Finally, each child passed a hearing screening at the child's school and passed an oral-peripheral mechanism screening (St. Louis & Ruscello, 1981).

Procedures and analyses

The Phonological Assessment of Latino Children (Goldstein, 1999), a single-word phonological assessment, was used to gauge children's speech sound productions. The assessment contains 26 separate target items for English and 29 separate target items for Spanish. The assessment was designed to assess the Spanish and English phonological skills in bilingual (Spanish–English) Latino children. For the current study, only the data from the English items are reported. This assessment tool has been used previously to assess the phonological skills of bilingual children (e.g. Goldstein & Washington, 2001).

Phonological data from the samples were transcribed and analysed with the computerised Logical International Phonetics Program (Oller & Delgado, 2000). The samples were analysed for (1) percent correct segments, consonants and vowels, (2) percent correct by manner class, (3) percent correct for /ɹ/ and /l/, and (4) percent correct for initial and final clusters. Inter-judge and intra-judge reliability for transcription were completed on the sample. Both inter-judge and intra-judge reliability were greater than 90%.

Results

The first analysis considered the children's overall segmental (consonants + vowels), consonant, and vowel accuracy, as shown in Table 11.4.

The results indicated a developmental trend in the children's accuracy on segments, consonants and vowels. Percent correct segments increased from 89% in four-year-olds to 94% in five-year-olds to 95% in six-year-olds. Percent correct consonants rose from 86.3% in four-year-olds to 91.9% in five-year-olds to 95.1% in six-year-olds. Percent correct vowels increased from 94.2% in four-year-olds to 98.1% in five-year-olds but dropped slightly to 95.3% in six-year-olds.

The data also indicated that the youngest children (four-year-olds) evidenced more variability than the older children (five- and six-year-olds) on segmental, consonant and vowel accuracy. The range of scores was larger for the four-year-olds than for either five- or six-year-olds. For example, percent correct consonants ranged from 72.9% to 98.9% for the younger group, from 88.5% to 94.5% for five-year-olds, and from 90.1% to 97.3% for six-year-olds. Thus, the standard deviations were much larger for the younger children than they were for the older children across all three measures. For example, the standard deviation on percent correct consonants for four-year-olds was 11.39 but decreased dramatically to 3.55 and 2.88 for five- and six-year-olds, respectively.

Table 11.4 Percent correct segments, consonants, vowels

	C1	C2	C3	C4	C5	Mean (SD)
			Four-year-olds			
Percent correct segments	92.59	80.56	76.51	99.33	95.07	89.04 (9.79)
Percent correct consonants	89.04	75.34	72.92	98.97	93.55	86.34 (11.39)
Percent correct vowels	100	91.43	83.02	100	97.96	94.22 (7.31)
			Five-year-olds			
Percent correct segments	96.3	93.52	98.15	92.57	91.28	94.04 (2.81)
Percent correct consonants	94.52	90.41	97.26	90.53	88.54	91.95 (3.55)
Percent correct vowels	100	100	100	96.23	96.23	98.1 (2.07)
			Six-year-olds			
Percent correct segments	96.3	96.3	88.68	96.0	97.33	95.18 (3.53)
Percent correct consonants	95.89	97.26	90.14	94.85	96.91	95.13 (2.88)
Percent correct vowels	97.14	94.29	85.71	98.11	98.11	95.26 (5.25)

In order to judge the children's phonological skills in more detail, percent correct by manner class was measured. The results are given in Table 11.5.

The findings indicated a development trend across the three age groups for each manner class. There was one exception to this trend, however. Affricates showed a developmental trend for four-year-olds (percent correct = 73.3%) and five-year-olds (percent correct = 86.7%) but dropped somewhat for six-year-olds (percent correct = 80%).

As noted above, one of the objectives of this study was to determine how bilingual children produced liquids, a later-developing sound class. The children in this study showed a developmental trend in their production of liquids. Percent correct for liquids was 73.3% for four-year-olds, 88% for five-year-olds and 93.2% for six-year-olds. The individual variation in the production of liquids, particularly for four- and five-year-olds should be noted, however. Percent correct for liquids ranged from 33.3% to 100% in the four-year-old group and from 69.2%

Table 11.5 Percent correct by manner class

	C1	C2	C3	C4	C5	Mean
Four-year-olds						
Stops	93.3	96.67	83.78	100	100	94.8
Nasals	100	90.91	93.33	100	92.31	95.38
Fricatives	92.86	50	72.22	94.44	94.12	81.48
Affricates	66.67	66.67	33.33	100	100	73.33
Liquids	69.23	38.46	50	100	77.78	68.75
–/ɹ/	100	0	0	100	66.67	53.85
–/l/	42.86	71.43	100	100	88.89	82.93
Glides	100	100	66.67	100	100	92.31
Five-year-olds						
Stops	90	96.67	96.67	91.67	97.3	94.48
Nasals	100	100	100	100	80	95.24
Fricatives	100	85.71	92.86	83.33	83.33	88.46
Affricates	66.67	100	100	66.67	100	86.67
Liquids	100	69.23	100	94.44	77.78	88.0
–/ɹ/	100	100	100	88.89	55.56	86.11
–/l/	100	42.86	100	100	100	89.74
Glides	100	100	100	100	100	100
Six-year-olds						
Stops	100	100	96.43	100	100	99.39
Nasals	90.91	100	100	100	100	98.41
Fricatives	92.86	100	78.57	77.78	88.89	87.18
Affricates	66.67	66.67	66.67	100	100	80
Liquids	100	92.31	84.62	94.12	94.44	93.24
–/ɹ/	100	100	100	87.5	88.89	94.29
–/l/	100	85.71	71.43	100	100	92.31
Glides	100	100	100	100	100	100

to 100% for five-year-olds. The range was slightly smaller for six-year-olds, from 84.6% to 100%. The children also showed variation in the production of the two members of the liquid class. Five- and six-year-old children showed much greater accuracy on both /ɹ/ and /l/ than did four-year-olds. Accuracy on /ɹ/ was only 53.9% for four-year-olds

Table 11.6 Onset cluster accuracy

	C1	C2	C3	C4	C5	Mean
Four-year-olds	84.62	46.15	23.08	100	84.62	69.23
Five-year-olds	92.31	69.23	100	76.92	92.31	86.15
Six-year-olds	100	100	100	92.31	92.31	96.9

but increased dramatically to 86.1% for five-year-olds and to 94.3% for six-year-olds. It should be noted, however, that two of the four-year-olds produced /ɹ/ with 100% accuracy. Accuracy on /l/ was also lower for four-year-olds (mean = 82.9%) than for either five-year-olds (mean = 89.7%) or six-year-olds (92.3%). The range of scores for both sounds was large, especially for four- and five-year-olds. Accuracy for /ɹ/ ranged from 0% to 100% for four-year-olds and from 55.6% to 100% for five-year-olds. Accuracy for /l/ ranged from 42.9% to 100% for four-year-olds and from 42.9% to 100% for five-year-olds.

The children's accuracy in producing word initial clusters was also measured, and the results are given in Table 11.6.

Overall, the children again showed a developmental trend. As would be expected, four-year-olds exhibited less accuracy (mean = 69.2%) than did five-year-olds (mean = 86.2%). Mean accuracy for six-year-olds was almost 97%. As was found for the analyses presented previously, there was variation within age groups (not unexpected given the limited number of children in the study), particularly for four- and five-year-olds. Accuracy for word initial clusters ranged from 23.1–100% in four-year-olds and from 69.2–92.3% in five-year-olds. Not surprisingly, accuracy for clusters showed a more narrow range for six-year-olds, 92.3–100%.

Study II

The second study, conducted by the first author, examined the development of two-member final consonant cluster targets in light of sonority sequencing principle (SSP hereafter). In this study, the objective was to see if the paths of development, rather than the age norms, were different from monolingual children. Stated simply, SSP requires the segments preceding and/or following the nucleus of the syllable to be progressively decreasing in sonority values. For example, in print [prɪnt] we have the nucleus /ɪ/ preceded by /pr/ and followed by /nt/, and in these sequences, segments closer to the nucleus, i.e. /r/ and /n/ are higher in sonority than the segments that are at the outer ends of these sequences (i.e. /p/ and /t/). Two factors seem directly related to the sonority index of a sound. These are (a) the degree of opening of the oral cavity in producing the sound and (b) the sound's propensity for voicing. The more open articulation a sound has, the greater its sonority level should be. Also, if two sounds have the same degree of opening, the voiced one will have greater sonority than its voiceless counterpart. The following scale is adopted from Hogg and McCully (1987).

Sounds	SI (sonority index)
Low vowels	10
Mid vowels	9
High vowels	8
Flaps	7
Laterals	6
Nasals	5
Vd. fricatives	4
Vs. fricatives	3
Vd. stops	2
Vs. stops	1

Sonority sequencing principle has been shown to be influential in several aspects of developmental patterns in first and second language phonologies including onset and coda acquisitions (Yavaş, 2003). The appeal to sonority is not only to separate what is natural (expected) from unnatural (unexpected), but also to distinguish the relative degree of naturalness. The greater the sonority distance is between the members of a cluster, the more natural the sequence is. With respect to two-member codas, a sequence such as –rk# (e.g. park), which has a sonority distance $7 - 1 = 6$, is more natural than –nd# (e.g. sand), which has a sonority distance of $5 - 2 = 3$. The generalisations stated above must be interpreted within the context of optimal syllable shape, CV, cross-linguistically. Thus, syllables can be characterised by a maximal rise in sonority at the beginning and minimal or no descend in sonority at the end. Thus, no coda is the maximal, single coda is the next best (in the order of glide, liquid, nasal, obstruent), then the double-coda, etc.

The study reported here focuses on the development of two-member English coda clusters in Spanish–English bilingual children. It was hypothesised that if the child produced the target unsuccessfully and reduced it to a single coda (e.g. CVCC → CVC) s/he will follow the

SSP and delete the segment with the lower sonority index so that the one retained will provide the minimum descent in sonority from the nucleus to the coda. Evidence for this tendency, in monolingual acquisition, is given by (Ohala, 1999). It was also hypothesised that the greater the sonority distance is between the first and the second member in the coda cluster, the more natural (i.e. easier to acquire) it would be. Thus, the ultimate goal was to determine if bilingual children follow the same path of universal dictum of sonority sequencing as their monolingual counterparts in developing the two member coda clusters of English.

Subjects

Sixty-two bilingual children (ages: 4;0–5;10) participated in the study. The population, although not identical to that of the first study, was very similar in many respects. All children were speakers of Caribbean Spanish (Cuban). They all used both languages at home and in school, and all were at the beginning stages of sequential bilingualism. There was no reported abnormalities regarding their language or cognitive development by their teachers or parents, nor was there any concern about their hearing.

Method and analysis

The following 12 target words with different coda cluster combinations were elicited via picture descriptions.

Target words	Sonority distance between the members of the coda
[fɪst] [dɛsk] [lɛft]	2
[sænd] [hænd]	3
[læmp] [tɛnt] [hɔrs]	4
[bɛ·d][2] [sɔlt] [mɪlk]	5
[park]	6

Thirty-four subjects were excluded from the analyses; 30 were faultless, and four could not complete the task. The data from the remaining 28 subjects showing differential productions were analysed with respect to sonority effects.

Results

Results, in general, confirmed the hypotheses, as subjects had much more difficulty (i.e. incorrect productions) with the target codas when the sonority distance between C1 and C2 was smaller. They had greater success with the coda clusters with greater sonority distance.

Number of children who had difficulty with different targets					
Sonority distance in the cluster	2	3	4	5	6
Number of children	23	17	5	2	0

It is also worth noting that an implicational relationship regarding the in/correct renditions was found. When a subject had difficulty with a coda cluster of X (where X = sonority distance between C1 and C2), s/he had difficulty with a cluster of the type X-1. That is, when a subject had difficulty with a coda cluster with the sonority distance from C1 to C2 is '4', s/he had difficulty with the clusters with the sonority distance of '3' and '2', but not vice versa. This implicational relationship was valid for 20 out of 28 subjects.

Erroneous coda productions as a function of the sonority distance of the targets	
	Number of subjects
4 > 3 > 2	4
3 > 2	7
2	9

The eight subjects who did not follow this implicational line showed deviations of a minimal nature.

Simplification patterns in target cluster reductions were also in conformity with the universal tendency of minimal descent in sonority from the nucleus to the coda. The tendency of deleting the lower sonority consonant in the cluster provides the minimal descent in sonority from the nucleus to the single coda. The explanation of modifications could not have come from first language influence, as we have productions (e.g. [lɛft] → [lɛf]) that are not possible in Spanish. Thus, we can conclude that the results obtained from this limited study support the view that bilingual phonology, like monolingual phonologies, incorporates the universal patterns.

Discussion

The purpose of these studies was to begin to determine how phonological development in bilingual children compares to phonological development in monolingual speakers. Currently, placing the phonological skills of bilingual children into a developmental context is difficult because there are relatively few studies of bilingual phonological development. Moreover, comparing the phonological skills of bilingual children with monolingual children is difficult because of the inherent methodological differences between studies. There are some existing comparison data, however, for both percent accuracy for sound classes and phonological patterns.

Overall, the English phonological skills, as measured by accuracy on sound classes, of the bilingual children in the first study appear to be commensurate with those of monolingual children (Templin, 1957). In comparing Templin's data from same-aged children of lower socioeconomic backgrounds (to match the demographic characteristics of the children in the current investigation), the bilingual children's accuracy for sound classes was similar to or even exceeded that of monolingual children. Templin reported comparable data on percent accuracy for stops, nasals, fricatives, /ɹ/ and /l/. With few exceptions, the bilingual children exhibited higher accuracy on those elements than did the monolingual children. The exceptions to that overall trend related to the liquids /ɹ/ and /l/ in four- and six-year-olds. Accuracy in the four-year-old bilingual group for /ɹ/ (mean = 54%) and /l/ (mean = 83%) was lower than in Templin's four-year-old monolingual group (mean = 78% for /ɹ/ and 86% for /l/). Accuracy for /l/ in the six-year-old bilingual group (mean = 92%) was slightly lower than in the six-year-old monolingual group (mean = 95%).

Accuracy for /ɹ/ and /l/ may have been lower generally for the bilingual children because of their task of acquiring two phonological systems. In their attempt to master sounds in two languages, the bilingual children may be focusing, unconsciously of course, on earlier developing sound classes in both languages while not concentrating as much on later developing sound classes. Goldstein and Washington (2001) found such a trend for the Spanish phonological skills of four-year-old Spanish–English bilingual children. In their study, accuracy on earlier developing sound classes (e.g. stops, nasals, glides) was similar for both bilingual and monolingual children. Accuracy on later developing sound classes (flap and trill), however, was significantly lower for bilingual children than for monolingual children. These data indicate that bilingual children may not exhibit an 'across-the-board' delay in phonological acquisition, but the data show that any 'difficulty' they are having in acquiring two phonological systems is concentrated in later developing sound classes.

Accuracy on word initial two-member, consonant clusters for the bilingual children in the current study also was commensurate with and sometimes greater than that of monolingual English-speaking children (Templin, 1957). Mean accuracy for the four-year-old bilingual children was identical to that of the four-year-olds in Templin's study (mean = 69%). Accuracy on word initial clusters for five- and six-year-old bilingual children was higher (86% and 97%, respectively) than that of monolingual children (77% and 87%, respectively). Discrepancies between the studies may be the result of two primary characteristics of the methodology of the two investigations. The number of participants was disparate in the studies; Templin included 60 children in each age group as opposed to only five in each age group in the current study. Also, three times as many cluster types were elicited in Templin's study as in the current one. Templin measured the accuracy of 41 different word initial cluster compared with only 13 in the present investigation (albeit the most commonly occurring ones in the language). Despite the methodological differences, it appears that accuracy on word initial consonant clusters are similar for both monolingual and bilingual children.

As for the second study, the patterns bilingual children showed for the target double codas were very much in line with those that are found in the monolingual data. The sonority driven simplifications of the targets are further proof that bilingual acquisition, like its monolingual counterpart, integrates the universal constraints, as well as other factors.

Although these studies begin to shed light on the phonological skills of bilingual children, there are a number of limitations that should be rectified in future studies. Future research will need to focus on both the English and Spanish phonological skills of bilingual children and include a larger number of children. In addition, comparisons of phonological development in bilingual children to that of monolingual children will need to be made with children from same community using the same methodology.

Bilingual Children with (Suspected) Disorders

Due to very small number of studies on bilingual children with disorders we are not in a position to make any conclusive statements regarding the phonological characteristics of these children. This difficulty is exacerbated by the lack of bilingual acquisition norms. Before we can suggest any guidelines with certainty, we would need developmental norms and assessment procedures unique to these individuals. Language skills in bilinguals have almost always been appraised in terms of monolingual standards. As Grosjean (1992) states, this assumes that a bilingual is two monolinguals in one person. However, due to the constant interaction of the two languages, each phonological system of a bilingual child may, and in most cases, will not be necessarily acquired identically to a monolingual child (Watson, 1991).

Despite these immense difficulties, we can offer the following observations. The available data suggest that many of the differences revealed between typically developing monolingual and bilingual children are also seen in children with phonological disorders. Compared to their monolingual peers, bilingual children with phonological disorders show that they have overall lower intelligibility rating, make more errors overall, distort more sounds, exhibit error patterns found in both languages (e.g. 'cluster reduction' in both Spanish and English), as well as those (e.g. 'liquid gliding') that are typical in one language (English), but atypical in the other (Spanish) (Dodd et al., 1997). More significantly, they are likely to produce more uncommon error patterns, and are likely to suppress the substitution patterns more slowly than typically developing children.

Earlier we noted that the 'delay' seen in normally developing bilingual children in comparison to their monolingual counterparts was exhibited more significantly in later developing sounds (e.g. fricatives, liquids). Limited data we have from pilot studies point in the same direction with respect to the difference between typically developing and phonologically disordered Spanish–English bilingual children. Although there is an overall delay in all sound classes in the latter group, the delay is significantly greater with respect to later developing sounds such as fricatives and liquids.

Phonological Assessment Tools for Children who Speak Spanish

Finally, we would like to offer some information on the assessment of Spanish phonological skills. Although there is a general lack of bilingual norms and assessment tools, these are the tools that SLPs/SLTs often use for Spanish–English bilingual children. In assessing the phonological skills of children who speak Spanish, SLPs/SLTs typically use both formal (i.e. published tests) and informal measures (i.e. connected speech samples). It is quite likely, however, that the published test will neither be standardised nor include normative data (Goldstein, 2001; Yavas & Goldstein, 1998).

There are five commonly used published assessments for Spanish-speaking children used by SLPs in the United States: Austin Spanish Articulation Test (Carrow, 1974); Assessment of Phonological Processes-Spanish (Hodson, 1986); Medida Española de Articulación [Measurement of Spanish Articulation] (Mason *et al.*, 1976); Spanish Articulation Measures (Mattes, 1995); Southwest Spanish Articulation Test (Toronto, 1977). Although some of these tests have associated normative data, SLPs must be cautious in applying them to bilingual children. Normative data obtained from monolingual speakers (of either Spanish or English) cannot be applied to bilingual speakers, because, as reviewed above, bilingual phonological development is different from monolingual phonological development in either language. To our knowledge, there are no published assessment tools designed specifically for Spanish–English bilingual children.

In attempting to assess the phonological skills of children who speak Spanish (be they monolingual or bilingual), SLPs/SLTs should make an effort to assess in both languages, regardless of the child's purported proficiency. If the SLP/SLT does not speak the language of the child, support personnel should be utilised. For a detailed discussion of using support personnel, including interpreters and translators, see Roseberry-McKibbin (1994) and Langdon and Cheng (2002). In order to appropriately assess children who speak Spanish, SLPs/SLTs might use the services of bilingual diagnosticians, interpreters, translators or assistants. For example, bilingual SLPs/SLTs might be hired as consultants or diagnosticians, an itinerant bilingual SLP/SLT might be hired by a group of school districts or programmes, or University and work settings might cooperate to help recruit bilingual speakers into the workforce (ASHA, 1985). Regardless of the person who is performing the assessment, that individual should be prepared to ask a number of questions regarding the child's phonological skills.

> First, does the child sound like other children of the same age? Second, what consonants does the child produce (front vs. back, syllable-initial vs. syllable-final)? Third, what vowels are produced (all, some, none)? Fourth, how intelligible is the child? Finally, do the child's parents, family members, teachers, and friends understand the child all, some, or none of the time? In addition, information from support personnel might be supplemented with client observations with siblings, peers, and/or parent(s). (Yavas & Goldstein, 1998: 51)

Completing these modifications of the typical assessment procedure will help to ensure a least-biased assessment. In addition, as more research delineates phonological acquisition and development in bilingual children, more specific recommendations can be made concerning its assessment.

Notes

1. The second author gratefully acknowledges the assistance of Leah Fabiano in data collection and analysis.

2. The appropriateness of the item bird may be questioned on the grounds that it has an r-coloured vowel rather than a coda cluster. The simplification patterns observed with this target word was the deletion of the final /d/, which was not in any way different than the other items with sonority distance 5 (i.e. salt, milk). Thus, the inclusion or exclusion of this item does not alter the results.

Chapter 12
Phonological Development and Disorder of Bilingual Children Acquiring Cantonese and English

A. HOLM and B. DODD

Introduction

The monolingual phonological development of both Cantonese and English has been well documented. Contrasts between monolingual and bilingual development for each language are therefore possible. Table 12.1 outlines the differences in the phonological systems of Cantonese and English. Despite the very different phonological structures in the two languages, monolingual developmental error patterns are very similar. Where phonemes occur in both languages, the sequence of Cantonese phoneme acquisition is similar to that of English, although the rate of acquisition is more rapid. While syllable-final consonants are rarely in error in Cantonese, both English- and Cantonese-speaking children's errors are characterised by assimilation, cluster reduction and simplification of the system of phoneme contrasts (e.g. fronting and stopping). Phonologically disordered monolingual children's error patterns are also similar, irrespective of language (So & Dodd, 1994).

The primary objective of the current study was to describe the successive phonological development of Cantonese–English bilingual children. A previous group study of Cantonese–English bilingual children has shown that error processes atypical for monolingual children in either language may be more prevalent in the speech of bilingual children (Dodd et al., 1996). The current study investigates these differences in more detail with larger speech samples and with a larger group of children. A longitudinal case study will also be presented. Factors that might have affected the children's phonological acquisition are investigated. Finally, a treatment case study of a child with articulatory and phonological errors will be presented that examines the effect of disorder and treatment across languages.

Table 12.1 Comparison of the phonological structure of English and Cantonese

	English	*Cantonese*
Vowels and diphthongs	21 + 5 trithongs	8
Consonants	24 + 49 clusters	17 + 2 clusters
Syllable/word structure	$[C_{0-3}]$-V-$[C_{0-4}]$ Polysyllabic	[C]-[G]-V-[C/G] Mostly monosyllabic
Tones	None	6 + 3 allotones
Stress	Complex	Simple

Study 1: Cross-Sectional Group Study

Method

Subjects

The phonological development of 40 children acquiring Cantonese and then English will be presented. The children were recruited from childcare centres located in areas of Brisbane, Australia, with strong Chinese immigrant communities.

A questionnaire was completed by 36 of the children's parents. The questionnaire provided information about each child's general developmental and medical history. Specific information regarding type and amount of exposure to and use of each language was also collected. The questionnaire was provided in both Chinese and English. All of the children were acquiring Cantonese at home and were attending child care centres where English was the only language spoken. All of the children had started to speak Cantonese prior to exposure to English. The children included in the study had not had significant exposure to any other languages. Children with intellectual or hearing impairment or a history of speech or language disorder were not included in the study. Equal numbers of boys and girls were included. Table 12.2 provides group subject information.

Procedure

Data collection

Each assessment session lasted for approximately two hours. All of the assessments involved an adult interacting with the child. The assessment sessions involved two speech pathologists experienced in eliciting speech samples: one was a native Cantonese-speaker, the other a native English-speaker. The data included spontaneous speech samples collected while playing with toys and looking at picture books. Single word naming was also elicited using standardised speech assessments. The Cantonese Segmental Phonology Test (So, 1992) was used to elicit all the phonemes

Table 12.2 Subject information in age bands

	26–39 months	40–54 months	55–67 months	Whole group
Number of children	13	15	12	40
Gender				
Female	7	6	7	20
Male	6	9	5	20
Exposure to English				
Mean (months)	10.23	19.75	25.7	18.14
SD	3.8	9.3	10.5	10.3
TACL difference*				
Mean (months)	0.8	−7.1	−8.7	−5.5
SD	2.2	5.8	7.3	6.8

*TACL difference = TACL age equivalent score − child's chronological age.

of Cantonese, and the Goldman Fristoe Test of Articulation (Goldman & Fristoe, 1987) was used to assess the English phonemes. Three additional words were consistently elicited in English: *quack, queen* and *quiet*. These words were included because /kw/ is the only legal cluster in Cantonese. Because of some of the children's shyness when speaking English and their limited vocabularies, some of the words on the Goldman–Fristoe were only elicited in imitation.

The assessment sessions were split into two distinct sections with a break in the middle: this was done to create two separate language environments. Often the English and Cantonese data was collected on different days because of fatigue, time restrictions or unco-operativeness. The data collections were always within three days of each other in these instances.

The transcription used for the analysis was based on the audio-recording taken during each session. The recorder used was a Marantz CP130 recorder and Sony lapel microphone. Transcription of the data was conducted as soon as possible to ensure accuracy. The samples were transcribed by experienced speech language pathologists who were native speakers of the language. The reliability of the transcribers was examined. Two independent judges, both native speakers of the language, were asked to transcribe the standardised tests. Ten English samples were transcribed with 89% agreement. Five Cantonese samples were transcribed with 92% agreement. The most consistent disagreement between the two transcribers of each language were of vowel productions and voicing/aspiration contrasts. The English transcribers also occasionally disagreed about syllable-final consonant deletion versus unreleased final consonants. For this reason aspiration/voicing, and final consonant deletion/unreleased final consonant were combined for phonological analysis.

The Test of Auditory Comprehension of Language – Revised (TACL-R) (Carrow-Woolfolk, 1985) was administered to each child to monitor comprehension development in English. A TACL Difference Score was calculated (TACL age equivalent score – child's chronological age) to provide a gross measure of English language competence. For example, a child aged 39 months with a TACL age equivalent of 32 months would have a TACL Difference Score of −7 indicating slightly delayed language competence in comparison to normal monolingual English acquisition. This measure was used instead of using the standard scores within the assessment due to the non-standardised nature of the children's language exposure. However, a rough estimate of the child's language comprehension was required.

Data analysis

The Cantonese and English data were analysed separately and then compared. The speech samples were analysed to provide data on the children's phonetic inventories and phonological processes for each language. A phone was considered to be part of the phonetic inventory if (a) there were two productions of the sound in non-imitated speech; and (b) at least one production of the phone correctly (even if it occurred in imitation). Due to the large number of phonological processes evident in some of the children's spontaneous speech the phone was not required to be consistently used *correctly* to be included as part of their *phonetic* inventory. However, to allow comparison to published normative data, correct production in at least imitated speech was also required.

Phonological processes were classified, according to monolingual normative developmental data reported by Grunwell (1982) – English; and So and Dodd (1995) – Cantonese, as either:

- appropriate – occurring in the speech of normally developing monolingual children of the same age;
- delayed – occurring in the speech of normally developing monolingual children of a younger age; or
- atypical – used by less than 10% of the normally developing monolingual population.

Phonological processes were identified if there were at least five examples of the process in spontaneous speech. Counter examples of processes were also noted (e.g. when a child inconsistently applied a phonological process and therefore also used phonemes correctly at times), however, the process was still considered to be part of the child's system if there were examples of the process on five different lexical items. Phonetic transcriptions of the raw data from a study reported by Dodd *et al.* (1996) (16 Cantonese–English successive bilingual pre-school children with comparable linguistic backgrounds to the children in the current study) were reanalysed and included with the data from the 40 children in the current study for the detection of phonological process use. Therefore, the phonological processes reported are from a sample of 56 children. Appendix A includes examples of all of the phonological processes identified in the study.

The percent phonemes correct (PPC: number of correct phonemes ÷ total number of phonemes in sample) was calculated. The PPC samples were the responses to the standardised assessments, and provided quantitative information about the children's accuracy on a controlled word list. PPC data was further analysed into percent consonants correct (PCC).

The bilingual children were compared to individually matched (by age and sex) groups of monolingual children. The bilingual children's accuracy (PPC and PCC) was compared to data from children assessed by So and Dodd (1995) in their description of monolingual Cantonese phonological acquisition. The bilingual children were also individually matched to data (PPC and PCC) for monolingual English speaking children in the development of the DEAP (Dodd *et al.*, 2002).

Results

Phonetic acquisition

The phonetic repertoires of only 33 of the 40 bilingual children were age-appropriate compared to monolingual norms (cf. English: Prather *et al.*, 1975; Cantonese: So & Dodd, 1995). However, a single pattern of English plosive acquisition accounts for four of the group not meeting English monolingual norms. Four of the five children under 2;6 years were using the voiced but not the unvoiced plosive of plosive pairs (i.e. /b/ but not /p^h/).

Monolingual English speaking children acquire /p^h/ by 2;6 years. Three other children were missing one or two of the later developing English phonemes (e.g. /ʧ, r, ʃ, θ, ð/). The phonetic repertoires of three representative children are outlined in Appendix B. Thirty-one of the children made vowel errors and five children made tone errors. However, all of the children were using the complete range of Cantonese and English vowels and Cantonese tones contrastively.

The phonemes shared by the two languages were generally evident in both languages simultaneously. Cantonese and English share 12 phonemes. Only four of the 40 children were using a shared phoneme (expected to be present for their age in one of the languages) in only one language. All of the other children were using all of the shared phonemes that they had acquired in both languages.

Speech accuracy

Whole group

The speech accuracy (percent phonemes correct: PPC) of the bilingual children was compared to the data available for matched monolingual children. Figure 12.1 shows the differences between the monolingual and bilingual children over the entire group. Independent samples t-tests with Bonferroni corrections indicated that:

- There was no difference in the Cantonese accuracy between the monolingual and bilingual speakers ($t = -1.67$, $df = 78$, $p > 0.05$);
- The bilingual children's English accuracy was significantly lower than the monolingual children's ($t = -5.03$, $df = 78$, $p < 0.001$).

Comparison of the bilingual children's Cantonese and English speech accuracy using a t-test for paired samples indicated that the children's Cantonese accuracy was significantly better than their English accuracy ($t = 8.55$, $df = 38$, $p > 0.001$).

Accuracy development over the age groups

An analysis of variance (group: bilingual versus monolingual children × condition: three age bands) of the children's Cantonese speech accuracy (PPC) revealed a significant group effect ($F_{1,73} = 5.36$, $p < 0.05$). There was also a significant effect of age ($F_{2,73} = 28.96$, $p < 0.001$). However, the interaction term (group × condition) was not significant. Post hoc analysis using independent t-tests with Bonferoni corrections showed that although there was an overall group effect there was no significant difference between the bilingual and monolingual children's Cantonese speech accuracy at any specific age band (see Figure 12.2).

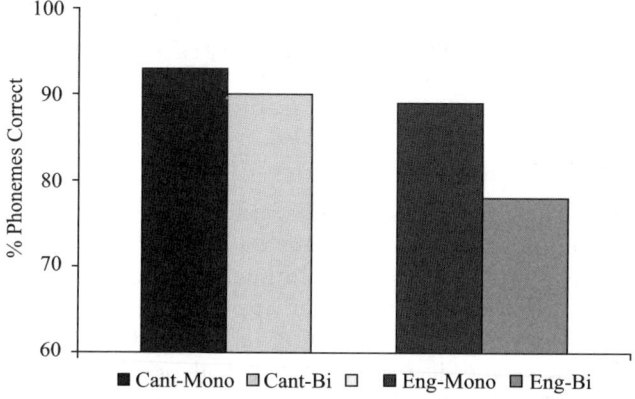

Figure 12.1 Speech accuracy – whole group

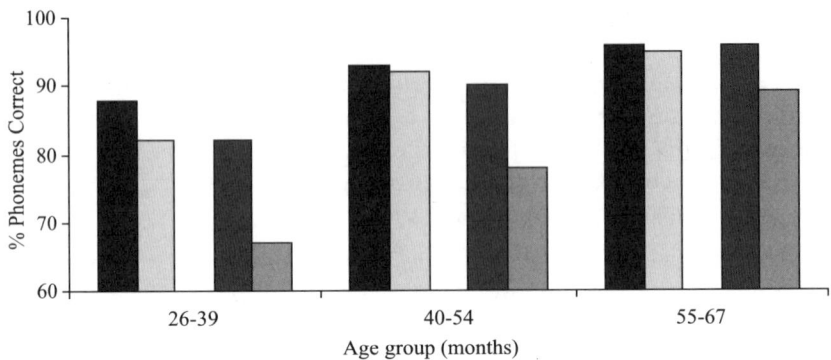

Figure 12.2 Cantonese and English speech accuracy – by age group

In contrast, at each age level there was a significant difference between the monolingual and bilingual children's English PPC scores ($p < 0.001$). The analysis of variance revealed a significant effect of group ($F_{1,73} = 55.62$, $p < 0.001$) and condition ($F_{2,73} = 51.32$, $p < 0.001$). However, the interaction effect was not significant (see Figure 12.2).

Step-wise multiple regression revealed that age was the only significant factor to affect English speech accuracy ($r^2 = 0.73$; Adjusted $r^2 = 0.68$; $F_{5,27} = 14.36$; $p < 0.0001$; Age variable $t = 3.16$; $p < 0.01$) and Cantonese speech accuracy ($r^2 = 0.42$; Adjusted $r^2 = 0.31$; $F_{5,26} = 3.74$; $p < 0.01$; Age variable $t = 2.92$; $p < 0.01$). The effect of the other factors entered in the regression will be discussed later.

Partial correlations controlling for age indicated there was no relationship between the overall speech accuracy scores in each language ($r = 0.27$, $p > 0.05$). However, when restricted to consonants correct scores there was a rather weak relationship between the PCC scores in each language ($r = 0.32$, $p < 0.05$). There was no significant relationship between vowel accuracy across languages. However, there was a relationship between the accuracy of vowel and consonant accuracy within language: English ($r = 0.34$, $p < 0.05$); Cantonese ($r = 0.59$, $p < 0.001$).

Phonological processes

Phonological process analysis of the Cantonese–English bilingual children's spontaneous speech was conducted. The phonological processes identified were compared to monolingual developmental norms for each language and classified as either appropriate/delayed or atypical (used by less than 10% of the monolingual population). Table 12.3 provides a summary of the atypical phonological processes evident in the speech samples of both languages. Table 12.4 summarises the appropriate and delayed (for monolingual speakers) phonological processes used by

Table 12.3 Number of children using each atypical error pattern ($n = 56$)

Cantonese		English	
Backing	27*	Backing	19*
Voicing	15*	Voicing	12*
Initial consonant deletion	12*	Initial consonant deletion	14*
Addition	4	Addition	12*
Aspiration	10*	Affrication	10*
Gliding	7*	Frication	6*
Tone errors	5	Nasalisation	7*
		Transposition	4

*More than 10% of bilingual population (i.e. six or more children).

the bilingual children. Appendix A provides examples of the Cantonese and English phonological processes referred to in this chapter.

The children's use of atypical phonological processes was rarely consistent: only a few children applied an atypical process in most of the phonetic contexts in which it could be evident. However, words that were elicited more than once were usually produced in the same way each time.

The use of normal and delayed phonological processes was more routinely applied. For example, a child who was fronting sounds was more likely to front a range of back sounds in a variety of words and phonetic

Table 12.4 Number of children using appropriate (A) and delayed (D) error patterns ($n = 56$)

Cantonese	A	D	English	A	D
Cluster reduction	21	5	Cluster reduction	14	24
Final consonant deletion	5	7	Final consonant deletion	4	16
Stopping	8	3	Stopping	21	19
Fronting	9	5	Fronting	6	17
Deaffrication	6	14	Deaffrication	6	0
Affrication	9	10	Gliding	30	0
Deaspiration	10	9	Weak syllable deletion	6	5
Consonant harmony	0	6	Consonant harmony	4	8
Continuant variation	0	9	Voicing	9	22
Reduplication	0	10			

contexts. However, a child who was affricating was less likely to be affricating a whole class of sounds, but would occasionally affricate a few fricatives. The process was required to be identified in at least five lexical items to be considered evident in the child's phonological system.

There was evidence that the bilingual children were not using a single phonological system to process both languages. The bilingual children were not using identical processes in each language (i.e. if they were stopping in English they were not necessarily stopping in Cantonese). Over the whole group of children the mean number of shared processes (processes evident in both languages) was 2.1 (SD = 1.2). The mean number of processes evident in the bilingual children's speech was 3.9 (SD = 1.7) in Cantonese and 4.4 (SD = 2.4) in English. Contradictory processes were also common (e.g. fronting /k/ ⇨ /t/ in English but backing /t/ ⇨ /k/ in Cantonese).

Partial correlation coefficients, controlling for age (which multiple regression showed to have an independent effect on speech accuracy), were calculated to determine whether there was a relationship between the use of different process types and speech accuracy. There was a correlation between Cantonese speech accuracy and the number of atypical processes ($r = -0.65$, $p < 0.001$) and appropriate processes ($r = -0.49$, $p < 0.01$). There was also a correlation between English speech accuracy and the number of atypical processes ($r = -0.48$, $p < 0.01$) and appropriate processes ($r = -0.36$, $p < 0.05$). There was not a significant correlation between the number of delayed processes and speech accuracy in either language.

Influential factors

Partial correlation coefficients (controlling for age) were calculated to investigate the influence of the variables targeted in the parental questionnaire on the bilingual children's speech development. The multiple regression results, described earlier, showed that the only overall significant factor to affect speech development was the children's age. Controlling for age, therefore, allowed the effects of the other variables to be determined.

The effect of six other variables was investigated:

(1) Age first exposed to English – there was no significant correlation between the age of first exposure to English and the children's English accuracy (PPC) ($r = 0.27$, $p > 0.05$), Cantonese accuracy ($r = 0.05$, $p > 0.05$), or language development (TACL differences scores) ($r = -0.35$, $p > 0.05$).

(2) Time in childcare – an estimate of the total number of hours the child had spent in childcare was determined from the parent

questionnaires. There was no significant correlation between the time spent in childcare and the children's English accuracy ($r = 0.13$, $p > 0.05$), or Cantonese accuracy ($r = -0.18$, $p > 0.05$). However, there was a correlation to the children's language comprehension development ($r = 0.36$, $p < 0.05$).

(3) Gender – there was no significant correlation between gender and the children's English accuracy ($r = -0.26$, $p > 0.05$), Cantonese accuracy ($r = -0.06$, $p > 0.05$), or language comprehension development ($r = -0.24$, $p > 0.05$).

(4) Siblings – there was no significant correlation between number of older siblings and the children's English accuracy ($r = -0.08$, $p > 0.05$), Cantonese accuracy ($r = -0.12$, $p > 0.05$), or language comprehension development ($r = 0.19$, $p > 0.05$).

(5) Comprehension – the children's English comprehension scores were correlated to their English speech accuracy ($r = 0.37$, $p < 0.05$), but not to their Cantonese accuracy ($r = 0.17$, $p > 0.05$).

(6) Television exposure – the children's daily exposure to English language television was not correlated to the children's English accuracy ($r = 0.10$, $p > 0.05$), or language comprehension development ($r = -0.11$, $p > 0.05$). However, there was a correlation to the children's Cantonese accuracy ($r = -0.45$, $p < 0.05$). Although there was no overall correlation to the children's English accuracy, the children who watched more television used fewer atypical phonological processes in their English speech ($r = -0.48$, $p < 0.01$).

Study 2: Longitudinal Study

The primary objective of the second study was to describe the successive phonological development of a Cantonese–English bilingual child during her first year of exposure to English. The group study of Cantonese–English bilingual children showed that error processes atypical for monolingual children in either language were more prevalent in the speech of bilingual children. Therefore, a longitudinal study was undertaken to establish when and how these atypical error patterns were used, and to monitor changes in the phonological systems. Monolingual developmental data allowed comparison of each language to monolinguals, as well as comparisons across each child's two languages.

Method

Subject

Catherine was aged 2;3 years when she was first assessed. She lives in Australia and is the daughter of immigrants from Hong Kong who moved to Australia when Catherine was six months old. Catherine's parents are both native speakers of Cantonese and are fluent speakers of English as a second language. Her father is a university lecturer and her mother is a housewife. Catherine has two older brothers, aged 16 and eight years. Both of her brothers are fluent, proficient bilingual Cantonese–English speakers. Catherine had been raised in an almost exclusively Cantonese-speaking environment until she was two years old. Although the primary language spoken outside the home is English, her parents decided to establish Cantonese as her first language.

At two years of age Catherine started to attend a childcare centre for approximately 18 hours per week. The language spoken in the childcare centre was exclusively English. Prior to attending the childcare centre Catherine's exposure to English had been minimal and she was not using any English words apart from her name and residential address. Her parents considered her Cantonese development up until this age to be normal. When Catherine started attending childcare the family began to include some English in their home language environment. In particular Catherine's brothers began to use some English with her. Her parents claimed that the language mostly spoken at home remained Cantonese. Catherine watched approximately two hours of English language television and videos (e.g. Play School, Lion King) each day.

Catherine's birth and medical history were without incident. Her hearing had been assessed and was within normal limits. Her developmental milestones were appropriate.

Procedure

Data collection

Catherine was assessed at approximately one-month intervals, although there was one month when no data were collected. She was assessed on 10 occasions over an 11 month period between the age of 2;3 years and 3;1 years. She was not assessed in the month that she was 2;7 years. Data collection began when Catherine had been attending the childcare centre where she was first exposed to English for three months.

The same assessment procedure as outlined in Study 1 was used to collect the longitudinal data. The first two assessment sessions involved two speech pathologists experienced in eliciting speech samples: one was a native Cantonese-speaker, the other a native English-speaker. The child's parents were also present at the assessment sessions. The Cantonese speech pathologist demonstrated the assessment procedures to the parents. For the remaining assessment sessions throughout the longitudinal study the parents elicited the Cantonese speech samples.

Data analysis

The Cantonese and English data were analysed separately and then compared. The speech samples were analysed to provide data on the children's phonetic inventories and phonological processes using the same criteria as in Study 1.

The Peabody Picture Vocabulary Test – Revised (PPVT) and the Reynell Developmental Language Scales – Revised (RDLS) were also administered on two occasions to each child to monitor vocabulary and comprehension development in English.

Results

Catherine's language use and the error data suggest that there were three stages within the period her speech was monitored.

Stage I: 2;3–2;6 years

Catherine's initial response to her new language environment in the childcare centre was silence. For the first eight months she did not talk to anybody in the centre. She was cooperative and participated in activities willingly, she appeared to understand instructions, and took turns in games, however, she did not speak to either children or teachers. She did however, begin to respond to the limited amount of English stimulation she was receiving at home, and began trying out English words. During the assessment sessions Catherine willingly participated in the Cantonese sections but required more persuasion to attempt speaking in English. The majority of the words elicited in the English assessment were imitations of the examiner.

Stage II: 2;8–2;11 years

When she was 2;8 years she first produced some spontaneous English within the childcare environment. In a game of 'Who stole the cookie from the cookie jar?' she responded 'Who me? Couldn't be!' appropriately and clearly when she was accused of the wicked deed. From that point on Catherine slowly became more willing to use English with the other children and adults at the centre. A large proportion of the English speech data remained limited to imitated words, although Catherine's spontaneous utterances increased at each assessment session.

Catherine's previous unwillingness to offer any spontaneous speech made the teachers and her parents concerned about her language development. The language assessments were first administered at age 2;8 years when she had been attending the centre for eight months. Her age equivalent on the RDLS was 2;5 years and standard score on the PPVT was 91. These assessments indicated that Catherine's receptive vocabulary and comprehension were developing well. The language assessment were readministered when Catherine was 2;11 years. Her RDLS age equivalent had improved to 2;10 years and her PPVT standard score was 98. Her performance on these assessments indicated that her English language skills were age appropriate.

Stage III: 3-3;1 years

The final two assessment sessions saw an increased willingness to interact in English, with occasional English words being offered within the Cantonese assessment session. The majority of the English speech data was spontaneous. Catherine's Cantonese errors were minimal during this stage.

Comparison of Cantonese and English Speech Accuracy

Figure 12.3 shows the changes in Catherine's Cantonese and English speech accuracy, as measured by percent consonants correct, over the period of the study. As Catherine acquired more phonemes and suppressed the use of phonological processes, her speech accuracy improved. Catherine's Cantonese was more accurate than her English. Although there was a slight decline in the rate of speech accuracy improvement, concurrent with the use of atypical processes in Catherine's Cantonese, the changes were minimal. Possibly the quantitative PCC scores were not sensitive to qualitative differences in Catherine's speech. The sample used to calculate PCC consists entirely of single named or imitated words. The evidence for phonological process use and phoneme acquisition was based on the entire sample of speech collected at each assessment session. This sample included single words and connected speech.

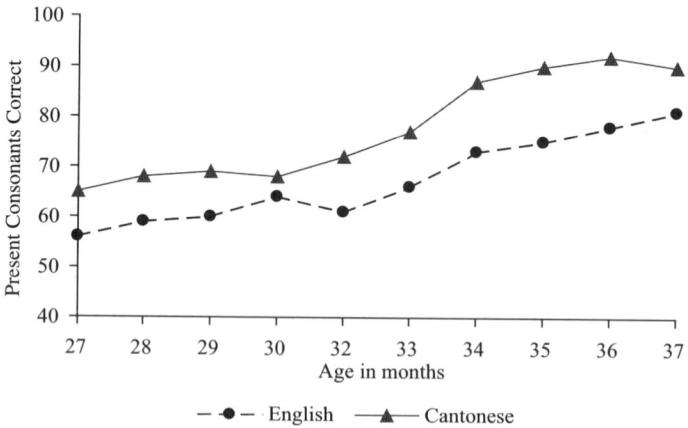

Figure 12.3 Percent consonants correct – Catherine aged 27 to 37 months

Phonetic inventory

Cantonese

Catherine had already acquired nine of 17 Cantonese consonants at 27 months. She was also able to produce five other consonants in imitated speech. She was not able to produce /kʰ, s, l/ at her first assessment. By 30 months Catherine had acquired five more consonants and was able to use another two in imitated speech. She remained unable to produce /s/. Catherine consistently substituted a lateral alveolar fricative for /s/. Table 12.5 outlines the order of Catherine's Cantonese consonant acquisition. All consonants were evident in spontaneous speech at age 37 months. Catherine acquired the unaspirated stops before the aspirated stops.

Table 12.5 Phonetic acquisition of Cantonese: Catherine aged 27–37 months

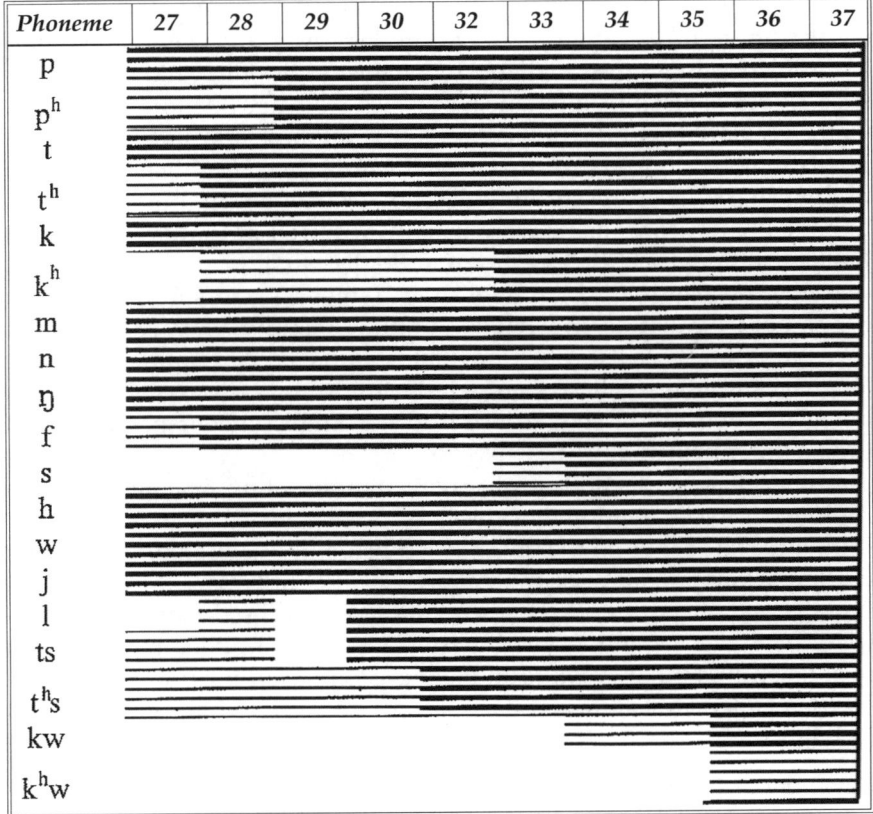

Notes:
(1) Dark shaded areas indicate phone evident in spontaneous speech sample.
(2) Light shaded areas indicate phone evident only in imitated speech sample.
(3) No measures were taken in the month Catherine was 31 months of age.

English

The speech data collected in the first three assessment sessions was mainly imitated speech. It is difficult to identify which speech sounds Catherine could have been using in spontaneous speech. In imitated speech, Catherine was using nine consonants at age 27 months. The assessment session at age 30 months resulted in more spontaneous speech, although the majority of the sample collected remained imitated. However, in the spontaneous speech produced Catherine used nine consonants. A further seven consonants were also evident in her imitated speech. Table 12.6 outlines the order of Catherine's English consonant acquisition. At age 37 months, Catherine was using 20 consonants in spontaneous speech. She did not use /θ, ð, ʒ, r/ in any context over the period of the study.

Comparison of Cantonese and English phonetic acquisition

Cantonese and English share 12 consonants (plosives: /p^h, t^h, k^h/; nasals: /m, n, ŋ/; fricatives: /f, s, h/; glides: /w, j, l/). Due to the differences in speech samples available for analysis, it is only valid to compare speech sounds used in spontaneous speech from age 30 months onward. Of the 12 shared sounds, 10 were used in Cantonese and six were used in English. Four consonants had been acquired in Cantonese but not in English, one was absent in both, one was evident in imitated speech in both. Shared consonants were usually acquired in Cantonese prior to English, although /k^h/ was evident in English first.

Catherine acquired /ʃ/ in English at 30 months and substituted it for /s/ in both Cantonese and English until 34 months when she acquired /s/. Stops and nasals were the first sounds to be acquired in both languages. Catherine had acquired /f/ in Cantonese at age 28 months, however, she did not start to use it in her English spontaneous speech until 33 months.

Catherine's acquisition of plosives was interesting. She acquired the aspirated, voiced before the voiceless of plosive pairs in English. In Cantonese she acquired the unaspirated before the aspirated. Catherine's cluster development was systematic: /k^hw/ ⇨ [p]; /kw/ ⇨ [p] until 32 months and then /kw/ ⇨ [f]. Catherine never realised singleton /k/ to [p] or [f], it was usually fronted to [t]. Catherine simplified most clusters in English in similar ways to monolingual children including the /kw/ words elicited in each session. Catherine reduced /k^hw/ and /k/ ⇨ [t] in English.

Summary of Catherine's phonetic development

Catherine phonetic development was similar to monolingual children of each language. Phonetic acquisition data for monolingual children of each language (Cantonese: So & Dodd, 1995; English: Prather *et al.*, 1975) indicates that the order of acquisition for each

Table 12.6 Phonetic acquisition of English: Catherine aged 27–37 months

Phoneme	27	28	29	30	32	33	34	35	36	37
p										
b										
t										
d										
k										
g										
m										
n										
ŋ										
θ										
ð										
f										
v										
s										
z										
ʃ										
ʒ										
h										
w										
j										
l										
r										
tʃ										
dʒ										

Notes:
(1) Dark shaded areas indicate phone evident in spontaneous speech sample.
(2) Light shaded areas indicate phone evident only in imitated speech sample – most speech data collected from age 27–29 was imitated speech.
(3) No measures were taken in the month Catherine was 31 months of age.

language was generally the same for the bilingual children. Shared phonemes were usually acquired in Cantonese first, but could usually be elicited in imitated speech in both languages at the same time.

Catherine's phonetic development data is not clear because of her reluctance to offer any spontaneous English speech for the first few months of the study. It is also difficult to ascertain when sounds have been acquired when consistent phonological processes are in use. For example, it is interesting that Catherine was using /f/ in imitated Cantonese two months before she used it in imitated English. However, Catherine was stopping most fricatives in English. Catherine's articulatory distortion of /s/ was identical in both languages. The phoneme was acquired simultaneously in each language, and the distortion was the same in each language. When Catherine's production became more accurate at 33 months, the change was evident in both languages.

Catherine acquired English plosives in a different pattern to monolingual English-speaking children. She acquired aspirated, voiced plosives before their voiceless counterparts. This pattern was consistent across all plosives. Monolingual English-speaking children usually acquire voiceless plosives prior to voiced (Prather *et al.*, 1975). In Cantonese she acquired the unaspirated plosives before aspirated in the same way as monolingual children (So & Dodd, 1995). The only shared phoneme that Catherine acquired in English before Cantonese was /k^h/. She acquired all of the other shared aspirated plosives in Cantonese prior to English.

Catherine's phonetic development suggests that because the acquisition of phonemes is due to articulatory maturation, the emergence of the sounds is approximately simultaneous in both languages. The articulatory development and the suppression of phonological processes can be seen in her speech accuracy data of both languages. The quantitative data does not give a very good indication of the qualitative changes that were evident in the phonological processes and atypical errors evident in each language.

Phonological processes

Cantonese

The phonological processes Catherine used between ages 27 and 37 months are outlined in Table 12.7. Although Catherine was often using a number of processes simultaneously, cluster reduction, stopping and fronting were the most frequent and consistently used processes. None of the atypical processes were frequent or consistent, however, there was evidence of their use.

The use of atypical processes in Catherine's Cantonese coincides with her use of spontaneous English speech. Catherine only started having difficulty with aspiration/deaspiration/voicing contrasts when she started using spontaneous English at 32 months. The process of addition was mainly restricted to final consonants, although there were also examples of initial consonant addition. When a consonant was added, it was always phonotactically acceptable (e.g. /tsi/ to [tsip] not [tsif] because /p/ is a

Table 12.7 Cantonese Phonological Processes: Catherine aged 27–37 months

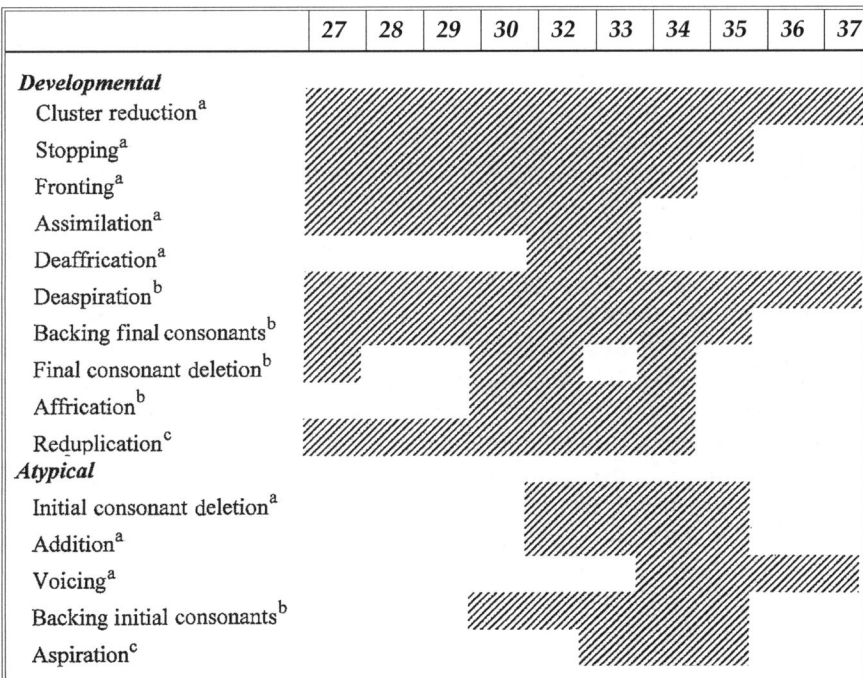

Notes:
(1) Shaded areas indicate process evident in speech sample.
(2) No measures were taken in the month Catherine was 31 months of age.
(3) Catherine first started spontaneously speaking English at age 32 months.
(4) Affrication/deaffrication only evident after suppression of stopping.
(5) [a]Process used in both languages and normal or atypical in both.
(6) [b]Process used in both languages but atypical for one language.
(7) [c]Process only used in one language.

legal final consonant but /f/ is not). Initial consonant deletion was evident over four months from 32 to 35 months. In Cantonese it is sometimes acceptable to omit initial /ŋ/ and initial /h/ deletion is a normal developmental process. Catherine, however, was deleting a range of initial consonants. The presence of atypical processes was transient: only errors involving voicing were still evident at age 37 months.

Catherine used a number of phonological processes common to monolingual Cantonese-speaking children. Many of these processes were suppressed over the period of the study. Affrication and deaffrication processes only became evident following the gradual suppression of stopping. The process of gliding covered all examples of variation involving /j, w, l, n/. Cantonese variation between /l/ and /n/ is sometimes appropriate. However, Catherine had extended the variation to these other sounds (e.g. /j/ to [n], or /w/ to [l]). The majority of errors for these phonemes however, involved variation between /j/–/w/ and /l/–/n/. Catherine's use of final consonant deletion was inconsistent. In the first assessment she occasionally omitted final sounds. She did not show any evidence of this process again until she was 30 months, and then only for a few months before the process was again suppressed.

English

The phonological processes Catherine used in English between ages 27 and 37 months are outlined in Table 12.8. Catherine used a number of processes simultaneously. However, similarly to her Cantonese, cluster reduction, stopping, fronting and gliding were the most frequent and consistently used processes. Again, none of the atypical processes were frequent or consistent, however, there was evidence of their use.

The two atypical processes in Catherine's English that were the most obvious were backing and initial consonant deletion. Although Catherine had acquired the appropriate front phones she commonly substituted a back phone. Initial consonant deletion was evident even though the initial phone was often within Catherine's repertoire. Voicing errors were also evident in unusual contexts. Final consonant devoicing, and intervocalic voicing are normal processes used by monolingual children. However, in addition to these, Catherine sometimes voiced final consonants and devoiced prevocalic sounds. Affrication errors only became evident after Catherine had acquired the affricate phones. Addition of sounds was also evident in Catherine's English. Often Catherine added a sound to make an initial cluster instead of an initial single phoneme. She also sometimes added initial and final sounds, however the sounds were always phonotactically appropriate. At 37 months the only atypical processes evident were backing and voicing.

Catherine used a number of phonological processes common to monolingual English-speaking children. Most of these processes were still evident at the end of the period of the study. Affrication and deaffrication processes only became evident following the gradual suppression of stopping.

Comparison of Cantonese and English phonological processes

Catherine had 13 processes that were evident in both her languages. However, not all of these shared processes were evident in both languages simultaneously. Five developmental processes were shared across both languages. Three atypical processes were evident in both languages. In addition, five other process were used in both languages but were considered atypical for one of the languages. Three processes were only evident in one language. The developmental processes used in Cantonese

Table 12.8 English phonological processes: Catherine aged 27–37 months

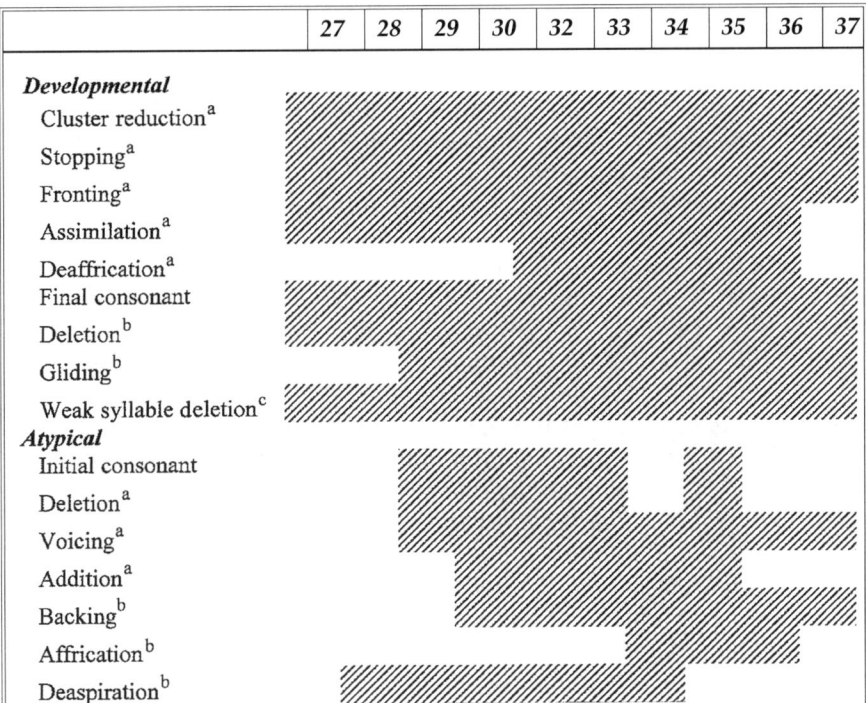

Notes:
(1) Shaded areas indicate process evident in speech sample.
(2) No measures were taken in the month Catherine was 31 months of age.
(3) Voicing errors included normal processes evident in monolingual children and also unusual errors.
(4) De-/affrication errors only became evident following production of fricatives and affricates.
(5) [a]Process used in both languages and normal or atypical in both.
(6) [b]Process used in both languages but atypical for one language.
(7) [c]Pprocess only used in one language.

decreased over the period of the study as Catherine's speech became more accurate. However, the majority of the developmental processes evident in English were still in use at 37 months.

The presence of atypical processes was evident in Catherine's Cantonese only following the increase in spontaneous use of English at 32 months. Atypical processes in Catherine's English were evident as soon as she started using non-imitated speech. The presence of atypical processes in Catherine's English also persisted longer than in her Cantonese (e.g. backing initial consonants suppressed at 35 months in Cantonese but still evident at 37 months in English).

Summary of Catherine's phonological process use

Most of Catherine's processes were shared by both languages. Her speech included the use of atypical phonological processes for monolingual speakers of each language. However, all of the atypical processes were also evident in the speech of a group of bilingual Cantonese–English speaking children, indicating that for this group the use of these error patterns is normal.

Catherine's phonological process use followed a clear pattern. When she first started using English spontaneously, atypical processes became evident in her Cantonese. However, the atypical processes were inconsistent, had only a small impact on overall intelligibility, and were transient. Unlike the results of the group cross-sectional study of Cantonese–English bilingual children, Catherine's atypical processes were nearly all evident in both her languages. Atypical aspiration and gliding were evident in her Cantonese but not in her English. The majority of the bilingual children in the group study shared some atypical processes, but usually the processes were language-specific. Catherine's speech was simplified by a wide range of processes evident simultaneously but not consistently.

Although Catherine often used the same processes in both languages there was also clear evidence that she had discrete phonological systems. She did not necessarily simplify shared phonemes in identical ways. For example, cluster reduction (evident in both languages throughout the study): Cantonese: /k^{h}w/ ⇨ [p^h]; English: /k^{h}w/ ⇨ [t^h]. When Catherine added a phoneme it was always phonotactically appropriate (e.g. English: /blu/ ⇨ [bluf]; Cantonese: /ji/ ⇨ [jik]).

Discussion of Studies 1 and 2

In Study 1 the speech development of 40 Cantonese–English bilingual children was described and compared to monolingual development in each language. The results indicated that there were quantitative and qualitative differences between monolingual and bilingual development in both languages.

The differences resulted from the use of a larger number of delayed and atypical phonological processes when compared to monolingual normative data. In general, the phonetic (articulatory) development of the bilingual children did not differ from monolingual children. The acquisition of speech sounds appeared to be independent of phonological development:

- phonemes were acquired in similar sequences and at similar times in both languages
- shared phonemes were stimulable in both languages.

Although the bilingual children appeared to use a single articulatory system in both languages, there was clear evidence that the bilingual children used separate phonological systems. This evidence included both error types and phoneme use:

- phonemes acquired in one language but not used in the other language (although they were stimulable in imitation);
- language-specific phonemes not used in the 'wrong' language;
- the same phoneme simplified differently in each language (e.g. stopping /s/ ⇨ /d/ in English but affricating /s/ ⇨ /ts/ in Cantonese);
- addition only of legal sounds (e.g. /tsi/ ⇨ [tsip] not [tsif;] because final /f/ is illegal in Cantonese);
- use of contradictory processes (e.g. backing in one language and fronting in the other);
- use of processes specific to only one language (e.g. stopping fricatives in one language but not in the other).

The bilingual children's speech accuracy was better in Cantonese than English. The bilingual children's Cantonese speech accuracy was not different to the monolingual children's at any of the age bands. All the bilingual children in the study were monolingual Cantonese speakers for at least their first year and often until they were three years of age. Therefore, it is not surprising that the children's Cantonese speech development was more advanced than their English.

The differences between the monolingual and bilingual speech accuracy development decreased with age. This pattern showed that the bilingual children were 'catching up' to the accuracy levels of their matched monolingual peers. Therefore, it appears that within a couple of years of exposure to their second language the bilingual children's speech accuracy is comparable to monolingual development in each language.

In addition to the quantitative differences in the children's speech accuracy, there were also differences in the error patterns used by the bilingual children in comparison to normal monolingual development. Table 12.3 shows that there were seven processes evident in English, and five processes evident in Cantonese, that were used by more than 10% of the bilingual group. These processes were all considered to be atypical for monolingual children of each language (i.e. used by less than 10% of the monolingual population). The fact that many bilingual children used these processes indicates that they are 'normal bilingual' processes. However, there were also many age-appropriate and delayed phonological processes in use.

Bilingual children's use of phonological patterns considered to be atypical for monolingual speakers has been previously reported by

Gildersleeve *et al.* (Spanish–English: 1996; cited by Yavas & Goldstein, 1998: 53). This study concluded that 'compared with their monolingual peers, normally developing bilingual children showed an overall lower intelligibility rating, made more errors overall (on both consonants and vowels), distorted more sounds, and *produced more uncommon errors patterns*' (italics added for emphasis). The quantitative and qualitative data reported in this chapter supports most of these findings. However, the Cantonese–English bilingual children did not distort more sounds (presumably the authors mean articulatory distortion) in their speech in either language.

One of the confusing factors in the bilingual children's data was the great variation in the children's ages and their language backgrounds. For example, the children varied greatly in age, the amount of time they spent in childcare, the age they were first exposed to English, and their English comprehension development. Investigation into the relationships between these variables showed that age was the most significant factor in determining speech accuracy. Even when age was controlled for the other factors did not appear to play important roles in the children's development. When controlling for the effect of age the only significant relationships between variables were:

- the more time spent in childcare, the better the child's development of English comprehension;
- the better the child's English comprehension skills, the higher their English speech accuracy scores;
- the better the child's Cantonese speech accuracy, the better their English speech accuracy;
- within each language, fewer consonant errors are related to fewer vowel errors;
- both Cantonese and English speech accuracy were higher when there were fewer atypical and normal processes used;
- there were fewer atypical processes evident in the speech of the children who watched more English language television;
- the age at which the child was first exposed to English, gender, the amount of time spent in childcare, the amount of time spent watching television, and the number of older siblings were relatively unimportant factors in speech accuracy development.

The normative Cantonese–English bilingual group data show that there are clear differences between the acquisition of phonology in bilingual and monolingual children. However, the large number of variables within the data made it difficult to determine clear patterns that may indicate what the individual pattern of development of the phonological systems may be. For example, it is not clear from the group data whether the use of atypical processes is transient or persistent. It is also impossible to determine at what point atypical processes are first evident. The longitudinal study presented in Study 2 monitored the development of the two phonological systems in the first year of exposure to the second language to clarify these issues (see Holm & Dodd, 1999a for a more detailed discussion of the data and an additional case study).

The developmental data raises a primary question: Why do successive bilingual children acquire the phonology of each of their languages in ways that are different to monolingual children who acquire their language in isolation? The types of speech errors and pattern of use (i.e. atypical errors evident in Cantonese only following acquisition of English) suggest that the phonological systems of the two languages were interacting. The successive bilingual children's acquisition of the phonology of each language was slightly qualitatively different to the phonological acquisition for monolingual children of either language. The longitudinal case study indicated that as the child was exposed to a second phonological system there was an effect on their first phonological system. The lack of atypical errors in the child's initial assessment of her Cantonese showed that she was developing normal phonological skills for a monolingual child. However, atypical errors (in addition to the normal developmental process) became evident following exposure to the second language (Holm & Dodd, 1999a).

Most of the atypical errors can be plausibly explained as overgeneralisations of language-specific rules (e.g. Cantonese: initial consonant deletion acceptable for /ŋ/; /l/ and /n/ act as allophones; English: aspiration not contrastive). It is possible that the emergence of atypical errors (although they are only atypical for monolingual children, the data presented in this chapter indicates that these errors are normal for successive bilingual Cantonese–English children) results from underspecified phonological rules.

Vasanta and Dodd (1991) proposed a model of the speech processing chain. Realisation rules are key components of this model. When children generate speech, they select a word that expresses their ideas from their lexicon, and then the lexical phonological specification is fed through the existing set of realisation rules that forms a phonological plan for production (Dodd, 1995). Realisation rules are derived from information in the lexicon, reflecting children's implicit understanding of the nature of the phonological structure of the ambient language (Dodd *et al.*, 1989; Leonard, 1985; Macken & Ferguson, 1983).

Leonard (1985) suggested that children with phonological disorder might have an impaired ability to abstract knowledge about the nature of the phonological system to be acquired. Unusual errors occur when children select the wrong parameters of the perceived speech signal as salient to their native phonology (Grundy, 1989). The successive bilingual children in the current study were not phonologically disordered, yet they made errors that are considered atypical for monolingual children.

Possibly, the cause of the atypical errors may be an inability to adequately process both phonological systems in enough detail to derive all the appropriate language-specific realisation rules. The longitudinal case study data indicated that the atypical errors were generally transient and inconsistent in nature. This suggests that as each child was exposed to more English they were able to differentiate more clearly the realisation rules for each phonological system. For example, a child may hypothesise that final consonants are unreleased because that is the case in Cantonese. Limited exposure to English may not have allowed the child to identify that a salient characteristic of the phonology is that final consonants are usually released, so the child simply used the realisation rules governing the release of final consonants extracted from exposure to Cantonese phonology.

The children's use of atypical processes in Cantonese is particularly interesting considering the successive acquisition of English on top of an already (at least partially) established Cantonese phonology. The overgeneralisation of phonological rules appears to have been both across languages and within each language. Perhaps the burden of differentiating each system, and abstracting two sets of explicit rules, means that for a short period the established rules of the first phonological system are temporarily confused. The children were marking differences between the systems. However, occasionally the precise, specific detail of the realisation rules was inaccurate or absent, resulting in unusual speech errors.

Watson (1991) suggests that the process of successive bilingual phonological acquisition involves superimposing one system on the other or mixing the two phonological systems together (averaging). The data presented in this chapter suggest that neither process is totally accurate. The bilingual children did not simply use their Cantonese phonological system when they spoke English (superimposing) nor did they start mixing the two phonological systems together (averaging).

Cross-linguistic comparisons

The phonological development of children bilingual in Mirpuri/Punjabi/Urdu and English has been reported by Holm *et al.* (1999) and also by Stow and Pert (this volume: Chap. 13). The normally developing successive bilingual children investigated all showed evidence of differences in their acquisition patterns when compared to monolingual children. This pattern is consistent with the Cantonese–English children described in this paper. The differences appeared to be related to the ambient phonology of the two languages for both language-combination groups.

These results suggest that the bilingual children's use of atypical error patterns (different to monolingual children's) is an intralingual effect (a more general process of bilingual language development) rather than an interference effect (specific to the two languages involved). However, the specific error patterns themselves (e.g. initial consonant deletion in Cantonese) is an interference effect. In other words, although bilingual children appear to use unusual error patterns (intralingual effect) the types of errors are determined by the nature of the two phonological systems interacting (interference effect).

Ellis (1994) suggested that intralingual effects might be due to rule learning and applications: faulty generalisation, incomplete application of rules, and underspecified rules. We have argued that the Cantonese–English children's error patterns could be due to the bilingual children's use of underspecified rules. It was suggested that the underspecification might be due to the burden of differentiating and processing two separate phonological systems. The Punjabi–English data appear to support this hypothesis. The nature of the specific rules can be determined by analysing specific aspects of the two target phonological systems. However, the specific difference between bilingual children and monolingual children is the inability to abstract the specific details about the rules that govern the target phonological system. The patterns of over-generalisation and under-specification stem from the development of two phonological systems.

Further cross-linguistic research into successive bilingual children acquiring different language combinations is required to examine this hypothesis further. It is possible that the patterns described are unique to the two language-combination groups investigated. The phonological systems of Punjabi and Cantonese are dramatically different from each other and they are different to English. It may be that languages that have very similar phonological systems (e.g. Dutch and German) will not have any intralingual effects but will still have some interference effects.

Yavaş (1998) suggested that we go beyond examining the similarities and differences between the two phonological systems. He noted the importance of considering universal markedness constraints when accounting for the speech patterns of bilinguals. The error patterns observed in the bilingual children were also affected by universal markedness constraints. These patterns were generally evident in the normal developmental error patterns used by all the children (e.g. cluster reduction, more difficulty with liquid realisation and predominant final devoicing patterns). However, the use of atypical error patterns could not be explained in terms of universal constraints. They are accounted for more plausibly by interaction effects between the two languages.

Failure to identify the normal patterns specific to a certain bilingual group may lead to inaccurate identification of disorder. Therefore, assessment of children with disorder requires: (a) investigation of whether the bilingual child *has* differentiated his/her phonological systems; and if so (b) identification of the phonological error patterns for each language; and then (c) comparison of these patterns with normal *bilingual* developmental data for the child's specific language group.

Study 3: Intervention for a Bilingual Cantonese-English Child

Background information: Case J.L.

J.L. was initially assessed when he was 5;2 years. J.L. was born at full term after a normal pregnancy. He has had no serious illnesses or accidents, and no serious ear infections or hearing problems. He has occasional asthma attacks. His parents reported that his developmental milestones were normal. J.L.'s parents are fluent speakers of Cantonese and English. Cantonese is the only language spoken at home. J.L. acquired English through 10 hours a week attendance, from age 3;3 years, at a child care centre where English is the only language spoken. When he turned four, J.L. began attending the centre for 25 hours per week. J.L.'s only other exposure to English has been through television. His parents reported no concerns about his development of speech or language in either Cantonese or English.

Pre-intervention Assessment

A detailed description of J.L.'s articulation errors and pattern of phonological processes was reported by Dodd *et al.* (1996). His language comprehension and oro-motor skills were considered to be developing appropriately. His speech was assessed by native-speaking Speech Pathologists using the Cantonese Segmental Phonology Test and the Goldman–Fristoe Test of Articulation. Picture books and toys were used to elicit 30 minute spontaneous language samples in both languages. Table 12.9 summarises J.L.'s articulation and phonological errors in Cantonese and in English.

Dodd *et al.* (1996) discuss J.L.'s assessment results in comparison to other normally developing monolingual children as well as normally developing bilingual (Cantonese/English) children. Their conclusions are listed below.

- Comparison of J.L.'s performance with norms for monolingual Cantonese-speaking children of the same age showed that he made many more errors. J.L.'s phoneme repertoire lacked one phoneme, /l/, usually acquired by four years by monolingual children. His articulation of the phonemes /s, ts, ts^h/ was distorted. In contrast, monolingual Cantonese-speaking children have

Table 12.9 Summary of error data

	Cantonese	*English*
Words in error (%)	29	70
Consonants in error (%)	14	42
Phones missing	/l/	/θ, ð, r/
Phone distortion	/s, ts, tʰs/	/s, z, ʃ/
Phonological processes	Cluster reduction*	Cluster reduction*
	Consonant harmony*	Gliding
	Affrication*	Stopping of affricates
	Nasalisation^	Final consonant deletion*
	Backing^	Voicing*
	Blending of two words^	Fronting*
		Deaffrication^

Notes:
(1) Quantitative data is based on the 31 words from the Cantonese Segmental Phonology Test and 43 words from the Goldman–Fristoe Test of Articulation.
(2) Five of the items from the Goldman–Fristoe were imitated.
(3) Qualitative data is based on the spontaneous samples as well as the articulation test responses.
(4) Expected and delayed* processes were determined to be present if there were at least five examples of the process on different lexical items. Atypical^ processes were noted if there were at least three examples of the process.

acquired adequate articulation of all phones by five years. J.L. used three atypical error patterns in Cantonese – patterns either *not* occurring, or evident for less than 10% of the large monolingual sample (So & Dodd, 1995). J.L. also used three developmental error patterns that were inappropriate for his chronological age.
- Comparison of J.L.'s performance with norms for monolingual English-speaking children indicated that his speech was poor. He was producing 70% of words in error at an age when most monolingual English children produce intelligible speech and have acquired a complete phone repertoire, with errors confined to stopping of /θ ð/ and gliding of /r/. Vowels are rarely in error. While J.L.'s English phone repertoire was missing only /r, θ, ð/, he misarticulated /s/ and /ʃ/. J.L.'s English included one atypical error pattern (Dodd & Iacono, 1989) and four developmental error patterns that were inappropriate for his chronological age. Two error patterns were appropriate for J.L.'s chronological age (Grunwell, 1981b).

- Comparison with children from the same linguistic background indicated that he produced slightly more words in error (29%) compared to the group mean for a normative bilingual group (24%) (Dodd et al., 1996). However, J.L.'s score was high, particularly when compared to the older children in the group. J.L.'s percentage of Cantonese phonemes in error was comparable to the group mean. J.L.'s Cantonese phoneme repertoire was not limited compared to other children from the same linguistic background, although unlike any children in that group, his articulation of /s/ was distorted.
- The percentage of English words J.L. produced in error was high compared to the group mean for the normative bilingual group (13%) as was his percentage of English phonemes in error compared to the group mean (5%). Although J.L.'s English phoneme repertoire was almost complete, unlike any children in the normative sample, his articulation was characterised by distortion of two phonemes. All but two of J.L.'s phonological error patterns that were atypical of monolingual Cantonese-speaking and English-speaking children's phonological development, were evident in the speech of the normative bilingual sample. The exceptions were J.L.'s nasalisation of the phoneme /l/ and his blending of two distinct words into one.
- J.L.'s phonological patterns were quite distinct in each language. Only one developmental pattern (cluster reduction) was evident in both Cantonese and English. Seven of the younger children in the normal bilingual sample had one or two shared developmental error patterns. No atypical pattern was evident in both languages. Although J.L. consistently substituted /n/ for /l/ in Cantonese, when he was speaking English, initial /l/ was correct while he substituted /w/ for /l/ in other word positions. Another example of the distinction of J.L.'s phonological systems is that he used the atypical process of consistently backing /t/ to [k] word finally in Cantonese but not in English. The only phoneme distorted in both languages was /s/ with J.L.'s distortion of this phoneme perceptually the same.
- J.L. made articulation errors in Cantonese and English: such errors are atypical of both monolingual and normal bilingual development.
- J.L. made some phonological errors in Cantonese and English that were different to normally developing bilingual Cantonese/English speaking children. That is, his errors cannot simply be attributed to interference between the two developing phonological systems.

Baseline data

To establish the stability of J.L.'s phonological system, baseline data over the month prior to intervention were collected. J.L.'s speech sound systems were relatively stable prior to intervention, with no notable differences between the error profiles (PCC English: 58%, 63%, 61% – two-weekly intervals; PCC Cantonese: 86%, 88% – month interval).

Phase I: Articulation therapy

An articulation programme was used to elicit correct /s/ production. Individual 20-minute therapy sessions were given twice a week in English and homework was done each day. The articulation programme involved progressive stages: production of /s/ in isolation; in syllables; in words; in phrases and sentences; and in conversation. A criterion of 90% accuracy was reached before progression to the next stage. Initial position /s/ words were targeted first, then word-final /s/ words, then words with intervocalic /s/. A different set of 10 words were targeted in each session. The sessions usually involved five minutes revising the previous session, five minutes targeting the new words, and then the rest of the session was used to do an activity or game involving the new words.

A set of 20 words not targeted in therapy were elicited at the end of every second session in order to monitor generalisation of /s/ production to untreated words; generalisation to /ʃ/; and the stability of the phonological processes of gliding and cluster reduction.

Progress during articulation therapy

J.L. required two sessions of practice and feedback before he was able to produce /s/ accurately and consistently in isolation. The next two sessions of therapy targeted initial /s/ in nonsense syllables. Sessions 5–8 focused on initial /s/ single syllable words and introduced final /s/ nonsense syllables. Session 9 involved using the core words in carrier phrases. J.L. then missed two weeks due to asthma. Sessions 10–11 continued to use carrier phrases and introduced final /s/ words. Sessions 12–14 involved longer sentences with initial /s/ words, final /s/ words in short phrases and the introduction of medial /s/ words. Session 15 was a reassessment of J.L.'s speech in both Cantonese and English. Following a four-week break from therapy, J.L. was reassessed to monitor the stability of his productions.

Figure 12.4 shows J.L.'s accuracy on the 10 /s/ targets within the 20 words elicited to measure generalisation. Over the 14 sessions of articulation therapy J.L.'s ability to produce an acceptable version of the /s/ phoneme in various positions in single words improved. His production accuracy of /ʃ/ also improved even though it was not targeted directly in therapy. The lack of change in the pattern of phonological processes that

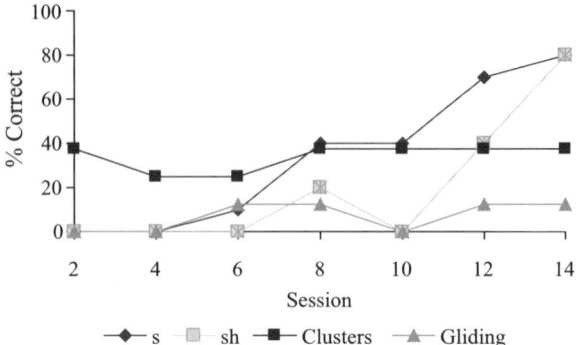

Figure 12.4 Generalisation during articulation therapy. *Notes*: (1) Quantitative data collected from 20 untreated words elicited at every second therapy session. (2) Clusters were counted as correct if both elements of the cluster were marked. (3) There was a two week interval between Sessions 9 and 10

were monitored indicated that J.L.'s phonology was not developing spontaneously.

Changes in consonant accuracy following articulation therapy and after a break from therapy

Pre-treatment and post-treatment accuracy of consonants in Cantonese and English elicited by the standardised speech assessments were compared to consonant accuracy following a four-week withdrawal from therapy (see Figure 12.5).

An improvement in accuracy of consonants in the standardised assessments was observed during the therapy period. This improvement was maintained over the four-week break from intervention. This improvement was evident in both J.L.'s languages, even though the therapy was only given for English words. In the assessment session immediately following articulation therapy J.L. produced /s/, /z/, and /ʃ/ with 90% accuracy in the Goldman–Fristoe Test of Articulation and /s/, /ts/ and /tsʰ/ with 87.5% accuracy in the Cantonese Segmental Phonology Assessment.

A spontaneous sample was not elicited during the assessment immediately following therapy. However, in the assessment following the break from therapy an English sample was elicited while looking at books at the beginning of the session. J.L. did not consistently produce /s/ correctly in spontaneous speech. From an 80 utterance sample, J.L. correctly articulated /s/ with 72% accuracy.

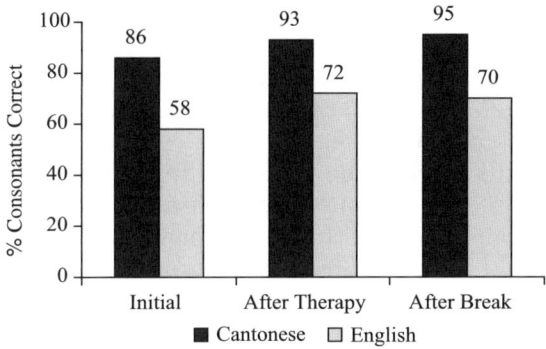

Figure 12.5 Consonant accuracy before and after articulation therapy. *Notes*: (1) Quantitative data collected from the Goldman–Fristoe Test of Articulation and the Cantonese Segmental Phonology Test. (2) The only changes in qualitative error patterns were correct articulation of the phonemes targeted in therapy. Other errors patterns were still evident

Phase II: Phonological therapy

Cluster reduction was the only process that J.L. was using in both Cantonese and English. For this reason it was chosen as one of the targets for phonological therapy. The other process targeted was gliding of /r/ and /l/ to [w]. This process was chosen because baseline data had been kept on the stability of this process during the articulation therapy. Both cluster reduction and gliding were consistent and stable processes in J.L.'s speech.

Data from the assessment following the break from articulation therapy showed that J.L. was reducing 62% of all clusters in English to one element. The main exceptions were clusters with the structure /plosive/ +1 (e.g. plane, blue) which he simplified to [plosive + w] and /kw/ clusters (e.g. queen) which he would occasionally produce correctly although they were rarely elicited. In Cantonese J.L. less consistently reduced clusters to one element. The only legal cluster structures in Cantonese are /kw/ and /k^{h}w/. J.L. reduced these clusters to one element on 36% of opportunities.

The phonological therapy involved weekly 45-minute sessions. Phonological contrast therapy, based on the concept of making the child aware that speech sounds convey meaning, was used to target J.L.'s phonological processes. Minimal pairs and triplets were used as stimuli. The first stage of therapy involved highlighting the differences between the words, ensuring that J.L. could discriminate both the sounds and the meaning between them (e.g. lip versus whip or ski versus sea versus key). Each target process used 10 sets of words. The next stage involved the production of the target words in order to signal appropriate meanings. Words in phrases were then targeted. A 90% criterion was reached before progression to the next stage. Both cluster reduction and gliding were targeted in each session. Activities were provided for J.L.'s mother to do with him at home.

The same words used as the generalisation probe in the articulation therapy were used to monitor generalisation of the phonological therapy to untreated words. This also meant that J.L.'s production of /s/ and /ʃ/ could be monitored. These words were elicited at every second therapy session.

Progress during phonological therapy

J.L. required only one session of discrimination training. Sessions 2–4 concentrated on single word production discrimination between the words. Sessions 5–8 consolidated accurate single word production and the production of the target words in carrier phrases and sentence construction activities. This therapy approach was successful in targeting cluster development and accurate production of /r/ and /l/. Generalisation to untreated words and clusters occurred (see Figure 12.6). The production of /s/ and /ʃ/ also remained stable reflecting the specificity of the intervention method. A spontaneous speech sample was collected at the end of the eighth session. J.L. was assessed on the standardised tests following a three-week break from the phonological therapy. Spontaneous speech samples were also collected at this session.

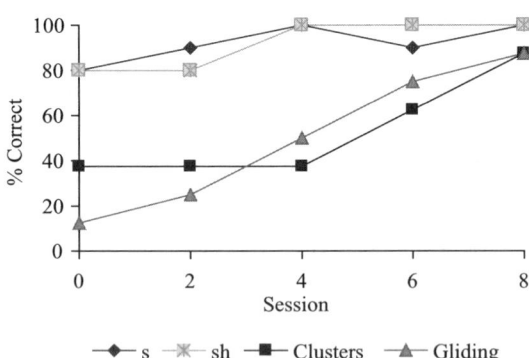

Figure 12.6 Generalisation in English during phonological therapy. *Notes*: (1) Quantitative data collected from 20 untreated words collected at every second therapy session. (2) Clusters were counted as correct if both elements of the cluster were present. (3) The words in the generalisation probe only contained one /s/ cluster. (4) Six of the eight /r/ and /l/ sounds probed for evidence of gliding were also in clusters

Changes in consonant accuracy following phonology therapy

Specific consonant accuracy scores can be compared between spontaneous speech samples collected following the break from articulation therapy and immediately following the phonological therapy (see Figure 12.7). Overall consonant accuracy scores can also be compared between J.L.'s productions on the standardised assessments and in spontaneous speech in both languages following the break from articulation therapy and following the break from phonological therapy (see Figure 12.8).

The data shows that J.L.'s English consonant accuracy improved following the phonological therapy. However, unlike the generalisation to Cantonese observed from the articulation therapy, there was no notable change in J.L.'s Cantonese consonant accuracy following phonological therapy. J.L.'s only shared phonological process, cluster reduction, was suppressed significantly in English, but he showed no notable change in the accuracy of his clusters in Cantonese (see Figure 12.7).

Figure 12.7 also shows the clear distinction between J.L.'s phonological systems in regard to the phoneme /l/. In Cantonese J.L. continued to substitute [n] for /l/ consistently, even though after therapy he achieved correct /l/ production in English. The other processes evident in J.L.'s initial assessments in Cantonese and English were still present following phonological therapy.

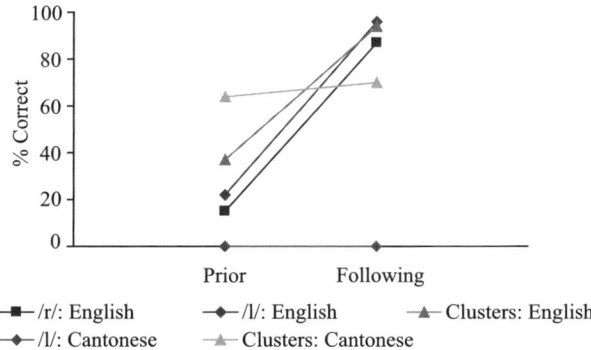

Figure 12.7 Accuracy in spontaneous English before and after phonological therapy. *Notes*: (1) Quantitative data collected from an 80 utterance spontaneous speech collected following the four week break from articulation therapy and a 50 utterance sample collected at the end of Session 8 of phonological therapy. (2) Clusters were counted as correct if both elements of the cluster were marked even if one of the elements was simplified

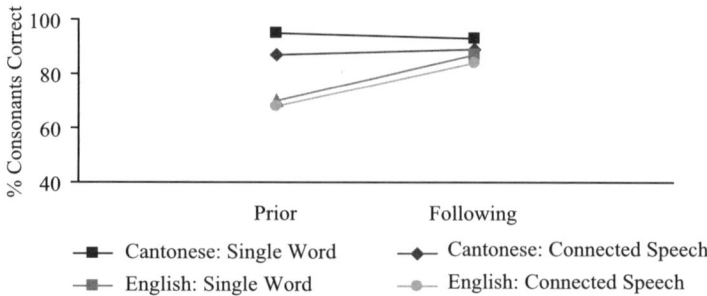

Figure 12.8 Consonant accuracy before and after phonological therapy. *Notes*: (1) Quantitative single word data collected from the Goldman–Fristoe Test of Articulation and the Cantonese Segmental Phonology Test. (2) Quantitative spontaneous connected English speech data collected from an 80 utterance sample collected following the four-week break from articulation therapy and a 50 utterance sample collected following the three week break from phonological therapy. (3) Quantitative spontaneous connected Cantonese speech data from the 20 utterance sample following the four-week break from articulation therapy and following the three week break from phonological therapy

Discussion of Intervention Case Study

The treatment case study presented shows clear evidence concerning two important issues: the difference between articulation and phonological disorders; and the existence of two separate phonological systems in bilingual children. Articulation therapy, targeting /s/, conducted in English and only with English target words, generalised into the correct production of /s/ in Cantonese. Phonological therapy, targeting a shared phonological process across Cantonese and English, cluster reduction, did not generalise from English to Cantonese. Phonological therapy in English did not have any effect on consonant accuracy in Cantonese.

Over the last 15 years the distinction between phonology and articulation and the relationship between them has been discussed widely. Dodd (1995) clearly differentiates between articulation and phonological disorders. Phonology is the cognitive, rule-based system that organises sounds within language, while articulation is the motor skill required to produce the sounds.

Dodd (1995) defined articulation disorders as an inability to produce a perceptually acceptable version of particular phones, either in isolation or in any phonetic context. J.L. was unable to produce an accurate /s/ in either Cantonese or English. His distortion of the sound was the same in both languages. He appeared to have learned the wrong motor programme, in that he used a labiodental lip position with palatalisation of the tongue for both /s/, /z/ and /ʃ/. Articulation disorders in bilingual children are easily identifiable for phonemes shared by the two languages – by definition the child must produce the same phoneme in the same way in both languages or it is not simply a motoric error but governed by phonological constraints.

Therapy that corrected J.L.'s motor programme, through feedback about tongue and lip position, resulted in a generalised remediation in both his languages. There has been very little research into the effects of intervention across languages in bilingual children. A similar pattern to J.L.'s, of generalisation across bilingual children's languages, has been previously reported. McNutt (1994) reported evidence from seven bilingual French/English speaking children. A motor based articulation therapy programme provided in English, generalised into French for all of the children. The children in the study had phonetic errors that were identical across their languages. Intervention successfully resolved the motoric errors – indicating that the errors were peripheral and not embedded in language-bound constraints.

Phonological disorders, however, are not the result of motor program errors. Consistent non-developmental errors might be due to an impaired ability to abstract knowledge about the nature of the phonological system to be acquired (Dodd, 1995). J.L.'s phonological systems were not identical, and the processes he was using in each language were different, which shows that he was having trouble abstracting knowledge about both of the systems. The errors he was making were not normal for bilingual Cantonese/English speaking children either, so it cannot be suggested that his errors were due to normal interference between the languages.

It would be expected that a bilingual child would have disordered phonology in both languages because the underlying process of developing a phonologically appropriate system requires the ability to abstract the relevant information about that system from the input they receive. It follows therefore that the phonological errors need not necessarily be the same if the child is developing and storing two separate sets of phonological parameters from the two different input sources. If a bilingual child only had disordered phonology in one language there would have to be careful consideration of the theories behind the causes of disordered phonology. The data clearly shows that J.L. had a combination of articulation and phonological errors, and that these errors had different underlying causes.

The other theoretical issue that this case study involves is the issue of the separateness of bilingual children's phonological systems. There are two pieces of evidence that suggest that J.L. had two separate phonological systems. The first is that the phonological error patterns were different in each language. The example, previously cited, of J.L.'s backing /t/ to

[k] in Cantonese but not in English is a clear illustration of a phoneme that had been acquired and was used appropriately in one language and yet in the other language an incorrect process was evident. The second piece of evidence is the lack of generalisation across languages following phonological therapy.

The basic goal of phonological therapy is to 'facilitate cognitive reorganisation of the child's phonological system and his phonologically-oriented processing strategies' (Grunwell, 1985: 99). The phonological therapy given was successful in re-organising J.L.'s system, but only in one of his languages. Phonological therapy did not generalise from English to Cantonese. In fact, phonological therapy had no effect on J.L.'s Cantonese. J.L. must have had separate phonological systems otherwise you would expect the error patterns to be identical in each language and you would expect that intervention would resolve errors in both languages not just one.

Clinical Implications

Any conclusions drawn from limited case data must be extremely tentative. However, the treatment case study presented suggests important clinical implications for speech language pathologists:

- Bilingual children's speech needs to be assessed in both of their languages for a clear profile of the nature of their errors.
- Articulation errors, common to both languages due to incorrect motor planning, might be remediated in both languages by providing therapy in only one language.
- Bilingual children appear to have two separate phonological systems for their two languages. This is not to suggest that the two languages are *completely* independent and do not interact or influence each other in any way. The results of Studies 1 and 2 clearly show that the process of acquiring two phonological systems bilingually is different to the process of acquiring each system as a monolingual.
- The deficits underlying phonological disorder are not language specific; they are the product of a general inability to abstract the phonological rules specific to that language accurately. This inability results in different error pattern profiles across the two languages. Phonological assessment in only one language is not sufficient.
- In contrast to articulation therapy, although phonological errors can be remediated in the language that therapy is provided in, this therapy probably will not affect the child's other phonological system. Phonological therapy does not generalise across languages indicating that therapy will need to be carried out in each language separately.

The nature of phonological development and disorder of bilingual children requires far more research. Important theoretical and clinical issues can be explored by studying this linguistically significant group. Bilingual acquisition can show us the potential parameters for language learning, as well as identify the boundaries for intervention.

Appendix A: Examples of Cantonese and English Normal Monolingual Developmental and Non-developmental Processes (cf: Grunwell, 1982; So & Dodd, 1995)

Process	Cantonese		English	
	Example	Status	Example	Status
Cluster reduction	/kwa/ [ka]	Dev	/stɛp/ [tɛp]	Dev
Final consonant deletion*	/suk/ [tsu]	Atyp	/kʌp/ [kʌ]	Dev
Stopping	/si/ [ti]	Dev	/ʃu/ [du]	Dev
Fronting	/kam/ [tam]	Dev	/kʌp/ [tʌp]	Dev
Gliding/ continuant variation*	/lɛj/ [wɛj]	Atyp	/rɪŋ/ [wɪŋ]	Dev
Deaffrication	/tsi/ [si]	Dev	/tʃɪp/ [ʃɪp]	Dev
Affrication*	/sy/ [tsy]	Dev	/ʃak/ [tʃak]	Atyp
Deaspiration*	/pʰiŋ/ [piŋ]	Dev	/pʜɪn/ [pɪn]	Atyp
Aspiration*	/tɐŋ/ [tʰɐŋ]	Atyp		
Voicing*	/pɛŋ/ [bɛŋ]	Atyp	/tɪp/ [dɪp]	Dev
Weak syllable deletion*			/bənana/ [nana]	Dev
Assimilation	/ŋan/ [ŋaŋ]	Dev	/bɛd/ [bɛb]	Dev
Reduplication	/ji/ [jiji]	Dev	/bʌtʌ/ [bʌbʌ]	Dev
Backing	/tin/ [kin]	Atyp	/fʊt/ [kʊt]	Atyp
Initial consonant deletion	/mat/ [at]	Atyp	/tɔi/ [ɔi]	Atyp
Tone errors*	/fa₁/ [fa₄]	Atyp		
Addition	/ap/ [tap]	Atyp	/bæk/ [bæŋk]	Atyp
Nasalisation	/lɛj/ [nɛj]	Atyp	/tɪp/ [mɪp]	Atyp
Transposition	/pa si/ [sa pi]	Atyp	bʌtən/ [tʌbən]	Atyp

*Indicates different status across the two languages: atypical (Atyp) or not possible in one and developmental (Dev) in the other.

Appendix B: The Phonological Profiles of Three Typical Children

	Subject 1: 2;6 years		Subject 2: 3;8 years		Subject 3: 4;10 years	
	English	Cantonese	English	Cantonese	English	Cantonese
Consonants						
Present	b, m, n, ŋ, h, j, l, w, f unaspirated t, k	p, t, k, m, n, ŋ, h, j, l, w, f	pʰ, b, tʰ, d, kʰ, g, m, n, ŋ, h, j, l, r, w, f, s, ʃ, tʃ, dʒ, θ	All	All	All
Absent	pʰ, tʰ, d, kʰ, g, s, r, ʃ, tʃ, dʒ, ʒ, θ, ð, v, z	pʰ, tʰ, kʰ, s, ts, tsʰ	ʒ, ð, v, z			
Vowels	All	All	All	All	All	All
Tones		All		All		All
PPC	61	74	71	93	91	95
PCC	45	54	64	86	88	90
Processes						
Expected	Weak syllable deletion Final cons deletion Stopping Fronting Gliding Cluster reduction					

	Deaspiration Fronting Cluster reduction	Cluster reduction Stopping Gliding	Stopping	Stopping Gliding	None
Delayed	None	Initial /h/ deletion	Fronting Final cons deletion	Deaspiration	Cluster reduction	Deaffrication Stopping
Atypical	Backing Voicing/ aspiration Initial consonant deletion Frication Nasalisation	Backing Gliding Tone errors	Backing Addition Affrication	Voicing/ aspiration Initial consonant deletion	Backing Deaspiration	Addition Voicing/ aspiration

Subject Information:
Subject 1: aged 2;06 years. First exposed to English at age 1;07 years. TACL Age Equivalent Score 2;08 years.
Subject 2: aged 3;08 years. First exposed to English at age 3;00 years. TACL Age Equivalent Score 2;10 years.
Subject 3: aged 4;10 years. First exposed to English at age 2;09 years. TACL Age Equivalent Score 4;06 years.

Chapter 13
Phonological Acquisition in Bilingual Pakistani Heritage Children in England

C. STOW and S. PERT

Introduction

Pakistan is a country of approximately 148 million people (Pakistan Government, 2003) which was created out of the partition of the South Asian sub-continent in 1947. There are 69 languages listed as being spoken in the country (Ethnologue, 2003) with Urdu as the official national language. Pakistan has a long history of migration both internally and externally (Saifullah Khan, 1979) and the 2001 Census (National Statistics Online, 2003a) reveals that there are approximately 747,000 Pakistani heritage people in the United Kingdom making up the second largest minority ethnic group in the country. This population is particularly clustered around the old manufacturing centres in the north of England, for example, around Bradford and Greater Manchester. There is also a sizeable community in Scotland around Glasgow.

The Population Being Studied

The data reported here were collected from a population of Pakistani heritage children living in Rochdale, UK. Rochdale is an old textile manufacturing town in the north of England with a total population of approximately 205,000 (Rochdale, 2003). Of this total, approximately 16,000 (i.e. 7.7%) describe themselves as of a Pakistani heritage and originate from the Mirpur District of Azad Kashmir and the west Punjab. This region is predominantly one of poor farming areas with some larger towns and small cities. There has been a long history, over several centuries, of both internal and external migration driven by economic, political and social factors (Saifullah Khan, 1977). During the 1950s and 1960s the textile towns of Lancashire and Yorkshire sent recruitment officers to the area in response to labour shortages in the United Kingdom (Khan, 1991) and this was the original source of the population being reported. Today the population contains both third generation children, born to parents who were themselves born and raised in England and also many members who are recently arrived from Pakistan, often arriving as marriage partners.

It is acknowledged that minority ethnic families in the United Kingdom suffer disproportionately high rates of poverty (Department for Education and Employment, 1999) and it should be noted that the children whose data are reported here live in electoral wards rated on the Index of Multiple Deprivation as being in the 10% most deprived wards in England (Rochdale, 2003): this index combines information about income, employment, health, education and housing. The link between socio-economic deprivation and delayed language skills is well established (Whitehurst, 1997; Locke et al., 2002) and needs to be borne in mind when considering the data presented below.

The population tends to cluster together within discrete geographic areas which also contain shops and supermarkets run by members of the community. Satellite television allows access to Pakistani television programmes and there are local radio stations broadcasting in mother tongue. In addition BBC radio broadcasts separate programmes in all the three languages under discussion here. The community retains strong links with their families and villages in Pakistan and extended visits to Pakistan are routine.

Acquisition of English

The pattern of language use within families varies considerably. Some children live in extended families with grandparents who have few or no English speaking skills. The majority of family units have one parent with no or very limited skills in English. As they progress through school and acquire English skills children often choose to use English with their peers, and indeed may reply in English to a parent, even when that parent has spoken to them in mother tongue and has little ability in English. The factors outlined above ensure that the majority of children from this community currently enter nursery provision at the age of three with little or no knowledge of English. Nursery places, consisting of half day placements, are offered to all children for one school year. There are very few qualified teaching staff from this community employed in Rochdale schools but support staff who speak Pakistani heritage languages are employed within classrooms both during the nursery year and the following Reception class year (the first year of full time education). As the majority of the community live within a relatively small, well defined, geographic area the majority of children attend schools with a very high proportion of minority ethnic pupils. Lessons and instructions are delivered in English and children are expected to acquire English rapidly: there is little mother tongue support available within the classroom beyond the age of five.

Pakistani Heritage Languages

General background

Three main languages are spoken within the community under discussion here: Mirpuri, Punjabi and Urdu. Previous literature published regarding languages spoken by people from a Pakistani heritage background has often used confusing, conflicting or poorly defined terminology. Indeed there has been some difference about how to spell the language name Punjabi, some authors (usually describing Indian Sikh communities) preferring to use Panjabi. It would seem that this confusion has arisen from varying pronunciations of the word and the fact that there is no standardised written form. There have been conflicting reports of whether Mirpuri is a language in its own right or is a dialect of Punjabi. The difference between language and dialect is the subject of much discussion amongst linguists and useful overviews have been published by Crystal (1997) and Baker and Prys Jones (1998). The three languages under discussion here all come from the same Indo-European origin, have a basic Subject + Object + Verb sentence structure and share many lexical items. The current authors recognise that grammatical variations mean that Mirpuri and Punjabi speakers are not necessarily mutually intelligible. Furthermore whilst Punjabi speakers might refer (in a pejorative manner) to Mirpuri as a dialect of Punjabi, Mirpuri speakers have a clear sense of their language as different. Taking all these factors into account the current authors will refer to Mirpuri, Punjabi and Urdu as separate languages. In an effort to clarify the language community described here each language under consideration in this chapter is outlined below in some detail.

Mirpuri

Mirpuri is spoken in the rural areas of Azad Kashmir, in particular around the city of Mirpur. The region is regarded as economically poor in comparison to many areas of Pakistan (Saifullah Khan, 1977).The language is also sometimes referred to as Potohari and Pahari. There is no written form, although some activists are currently attempting to create an Arabic-based phonetic script (Rahman, 1998). As there is no tradition of literacy, books (other than the Qur'an) are not usually found in Mirpuri speaking homes. Some commentators have incorrectly described such families as 'illiterate': as literacy is not an option it would be more appropriate to use the term 'pre-literate'. It is estimated that there are at least 500,000 speakers of Mirpuri in the United Kingdom (Rahman, 1998).

Punjabi

This language is spoken in the prosperous Punjab province in the north of Pakistan. It is related to the Punjabi spoken in India but unlike that language it is rarely written. Mother tongue Punjabi speakers dominate the government of Pakistan (Rahman, 1998) and so the language is viewed as of a higher status than Mirpuri. Many mother tongue Punjabi speakers (in both Pakistan and the United Kingdom) would encourage their children to use either Urdu or English.

Urdu

Urdu is the official national language of Pakistan and as such is viewed as a high status language. It has a written form and a strong literary tradition to reinforce its high status. In fact in Pakistan less than 8% of the population speak it as their mother tongue, the majority acquiring it as an additional language (Rahman, 1998). Due to the high status of Urdu, some Pakistani heritage parents in the United Kingdom for whom Mirpuri or Punjabi is their mother tongue, but who have some knowledge of Urdu, are bringing their children up to speak Urdu. There are thus some households where the parents are speaking Mirpuri or Punjabi to each other but Urdu to their children.

Religion and Language

The three languages Mirpuri, Punjabi and Urdu are the three mother tongue languages spoken by the community reported here but it is important to recognise that in addition to these languages (and English) children in this community are also exposed to a further language; Arabic. The community is predominantly (but not exclusively) Muslim. From the age of seven (and increasingly from the age of five) Muslim children in Rochdale attend their local mosque for approximately two hours a day to receive religious instruction and learn the Qur'an. This is learnt, by rote, in Arabic, with children often unaware of the meanings of individual words and indeed not necessarily perceiving word boundaries.

Phonemic Inventory

No previously published data could be traced regarding the phonemic inventory of Mirpuri and the current authors postulate that Mirpuri shares the same inventory as Punjabi. Information has been collated from Bhatia (1993), Bhardwaj (1995), Campbell (1995), Matthews and Dalvi (1999) and Bhatia and Koul (2000) regarding the phonemic inventories of Punjabi and Urdu and is set out below. The use of three tones in Punjabi is reported by some authors (Bhatia, 1993; Bhardwaj, 1995; Campbell, 1995). This appears to be related to written script and has not been recorded in the population reported here. When the present authors asked adult members of the population to recognise examples of tone variants quoted in the literature, they all reported that they were relying on the semantic context to establish meaning rather than recognising the presence of a tone variant.

Punjabi consonants

Nasals	m n ṇ ɲ ŋ
Plosives	p pʰ b t̪ t̪ʰ d̪ t tʰ ḍ k kʰ g q
Fricatives	f v s z ʃ x h
Affricates	tʃ tʃʰ dʒ
Flaps	ɾ r ɽ
Laterals	l ɭ
Semi-vowels	j w

The phonemic inventory for Urdu is essentially the same as for Mirpuri and Punjabi with the addition of a uvular fricative.

Urdu consonants

Nasals	m n ṇ ɲ ŋ
Plosives	p pʰ b t̪ t̪ʰ d̪ t tʰ ḍ k kʰ g q+bʰ d̪ʰ ḍʰ gʰ
Fricatives	f v s z ʃ x h ɣ
Affricates	tʃ tʃʰ dʒ dʒʰ
Flaps	ɾ r ɽ ɽʰ
Laterals	l ɭ
Semi-vowels	j w

Vowels

Front				Central	Back	
Close (tense)	i				u	
Close (lax)	ɪ				ʊ	
Half-close	e				o	
Half-open			ɛ æ		ə	ʌ
Open				a		ɑ
All vowels may be produced with nasalisation						

Previous Studies

There has been little previous research published on the phonological acquisition of these languages. Literature searches identified two previous publications reporting data apparently relating to the languages under discussion.

Khan (1984) reported on the phonological development of ten Urdu speaking children aged between 20 and 30 months over a six-month period. Her key findings included:

- The first initial consonants are labial then dental plosives. Velar plosives did not appear before 28 months.
- Aspirated forms appear in initial position at 28–30 months.
- Fricatives appeared after 28 months and are commonly substituted by stops.
- /r/ was acquired very late, generally after 28 or 29 months and was either deleted or replaced by /l/.

Although the data reported are detailed, certain important factors are not reported: no information is given concerning which country the children were in, their socio-economic background, nor the country of origin of their parents. Caution therefore needs to be exercised in concluding that the children are from a homogeneous background to that of the children reported here.

Holm *et al.* (1999) reported on 35 children aged 4;8–7;5 who spoke Mirpuri, Punjabi and Urdu. These children spoke the same languages and came from the same background as the children reported in the data below: they can be viewed as forming a homogeneous group. Key findings reported included:

- When assessed in mother tongue the most frequent (occurring in a minimum of 25% of the sample) processes found were: voicing, stopping, backing, cluster reduction, weak syllable and initial consonant deletion. Gliding of /ɾ/ to /l/ was also noted.
- When assessed in English the most frequent (occurring in a minimum of 37% of the sample) processes found were: cluster reduction, stopping, final consonant deletion glottalisation or non-release, voicing and aspiration and gliding.

Two processes were reported as occurring in the English sample which would be viewed as unusual in monolingual English speakers:

- the reduction of consonant clusters by the insertion of a schwa (/ə/) was observed in 100% of the sample;
- the stopping of syllable final nasals was observed in 51% of the sample.

Normal Phonological Acquisition

Rationale for amalgamation of data

Whilst speakers of each language can be clearly identified within the community, acknowledgement must be made that many speakers will mix Mirpuri and Punjabi together, largely depending on their exact geographic origins in Pakistan, where speakers of the two languages come into close contact. Furthermore the Urdu speaking children in this sample all came from homes where their parents' mother tongue was either Mirpuri or Punjabi. Codeswitching between Mirpuri, Punjabi, Urdu and English was widely observed, occurring in language samples elicited from a sub-group of the children (see Pert & Letts, 2003). In the light of these factors, the data collected were amalgamated and refer to the language development of children of Pakistani heritage.

Subjects

A total of 246 children aged between 1;4 and 7;11 were assessed: 122 females and 124 males. For data handling purposes the children were grouped in to age bands at six-month intervals (Table 13.1). Relatively larger numbers of children aged 3;0 to 4;5 were seen as these are the ages represented in nurseries: the time when most of the children are

Table 13.1 Subject information

Age	Age band	Frequency	Female	Male
0–2;5	0	13	7	6
2;6–2;11	1	11	6	5
3;0–3;5	2	21	10	11
3;6–3;11	3	58	27	31
4;0–4;5	4	41	23	18
4;6–4;11	5	17	9	8
5;0–5;5	6	15	6	9
5;6–5;11	7	21	10	11
6;0–6;5	8	12	5	7
6;6–6;11	9	12	5	7
7;0–7;5	10	17	10	7
7;6–7;11	11	8	4	4
	Totals	246	122	124

first exposed to, and expected to use, English. These ages are also those at which children are first likely to come into contact with the education and health officials who would be expected to identify any speech sound difficulties.

Parents gave informed consent for their children to be included in the data collection. This consent was gained with the help of bilingual speech and language therapy assistants who explained the process to parents. As adults within the community do not always accurately report the language they speak (many speakers will report their mother tongue as Urdu, the highest status language) this opportunity was used to note what language the parent used. Parents were also asked to report what language they viewed as their child's mother tongue. In some cases where mother tongue was stated as Urdu by their parents children were noted to use Mirpuri during assessment: they were then moved to this category for data analysis. Of the 246 children a total of 129 (52%) spoke Mirpuri, 63 (26%) spoke Punjabi and 54 (22%) spoke Urdu.

Methodology of data collection

A screening tool was developed which consisted of 21 words. These words assess a wide variety of phonemes from all the main classes i.e. plosives, fricatives, nasals and affricates. Aspirated and retroflex variants were included. Some phonemes were assessed more than once and in more than one word position. The words were all easy to depict in pictorial form and were words considered to appear early in a child's lexicon. Consideration was also given to using words which had no or only minimal variation in realisation across the three languages.

Children were presented with a series of partially coloured, ethnically appropriate, line drawings and asked to name the picture. Where no response was elicited children were encouraged to respond with a phonemic cue. Where necessary this was followed by a forced alternative choice, before children were (if necessary) encouraged to repeat the target after the tester. Responses were transcribed contemporaneously by one of the authors. A sample of 10% of recordings was then re-transcribed by the other author to measure reliability of transcription. As many of the younger children came from families where they were unlikely to have previous experience of books, real objects were used with all children under the age of three and with those older children who were felt to be responding poorly to the picture material. A bilingual speech and language therapy assistant from the Pakistani heritage community was present during the majority (69%) of assessments. One or both of the two authors was present during the majority (74%) of assessments; both have enough expertise in Mirpuri, Punjabi and Urdu to elicit the target responses. Two student speech and language therapists who had been trained to administer the test collected data from 63 children: these transcriptions were also checked to ensure accuracy.

Assessments were carried out in six schools, a playgroup in a community centre, children's own homes and at two community health clinics. The child's mother was present during all assessments in the youngest age band.

Results

The data collected were analysed under three main headings:

- The number of items completed and the number of consonants correct (see Table 13.2).
- The age by which consonants were acquired (see Table 13.3). The criterion used to categorise a phoneme as acquired was one realisation on target. This is a lower threshold than might normally be applied. Higher thresholds were inappropriate given the nature of the data collection tool which did not elicit all target sounds on more than one occasion.
- The presence of phonological processes (see Tables 13.4–13.6).

Discussion

Number of items completed

Only in age band six (i.e. age 5;0–5;5) did all the children name every item. Whilst it could be predicted that the younger children might not name all the items it was surprising in the older children. The background of deprivation, with its associated language delay, and culturally determined child rearing patterns may well have influenced the number of items that the younger children attempted. Children from this community are expected to show respect for adults, this being demonstrated by silence in their presence. The assessment environment, where unfamiliar adults were attempting to elicit speech from the child, was therefore an unusual experience for that child. This may have been compounded for the very young children by the unusual presence of a white adult; one, furthermore, who was using their mother tongue. This finding, that young children are reluctant even to name simple objects, has important implications for the clinician attempting to elicit speech samples for diagnostic purposes. It is interesting that age bands six and seven (i.e. ages 5;0–5;11) had the smallest range of items completed but that the range again expanded thereafter. It may be that the older children, with extended exposure to English, were becoming less confident in their

Table 13.2 Items completed and consonants correct by age band

Age band	Completed items: Mean	Completed items: Range	Percentage spontaneous attempts: Mean	Percentage spontaneous attempts: Range	Consonants attempted: Mean	Consonants attempted: Range	Consonants correct: Mean	Consonants correct: Range	Percentage consonants correct of attempted: Mean	Percentage consonants correct of attempted: Range
0	4.0	0–18	70%	0–100%	10.5	0–38	6.9	0–32	73%	38–100%
1	14.7	0–21	71%	33–100%	38.9	13–45	27.1	0–40	79%	64–89%
2	15.8	0–21	63%	6–100%	40.9	27–46	32.8	21–41	80%	56–91%
3	18.5	0–21	61%	0–100%	39.5	2–47	33.8	2–44	88%	58–100%
4	17.0	0–21	65%	0–100%	40.0	9–46	36.7	9–45	92%	77–100%
5	18.5	0–21	63%	0–100%	44.7	38–48	42.2	34–48	94%	76–100%
6	21.0	21–21	54%	0–100%	44.3	42–47	41.9	37–45	95%	87–100%
7	21.0	20–21	59%	19–100%	44.5	41–48	43.2	40–47	97%	89–100%
8	20.2	16–21	53%	10–100%	42.4	33–46	41.5	31–46	98%	93–100%
9	20.7	19–21	71%	0–100%	43.1	39–48	42.3	39–47	98%	93–100%
10	20.4	18–21	79%	38–100%	42.7	37–47	42.2	36–45	99%	91–100%
11	20.4	19–21	87%	71–100%	42.9	39–45	41.8	39–45	97%	93–100%

Table 13.3 Development of consonant inventory

	0	1	2	3	4	5	6	7	8	9	10	11
/f/	<50%	50%	50%	50%	70%	70%	90%	90%	90%	90%	90%	90%
/s/	<50%	<50%	<50%	50%	50%	70%	70%	90%	70%	70%	90%	70%
/ʃ/	<50%	<50%	<50%	50%	50%	70%	90%	90%	90%	90%	90%	90%
/h/	<50%	50%	50%	50%	<50%	70%	70%	90%	70%	70%	90%	90%
/dʒ/	<50%	<50%	<50%	<50%	50%	70%	70%	90%	90%	90%	90%	90%
/ɾ/	<50%	<50%	50%	50%	50%	70%	90%	90%	90%	90%	90%	90%
/t/	<50%	50%	50%	50%	70%	70%	90%	90%	90%	90%	90%	90%
/l/	<50%	50%	70%	70%	70%	70%	90%	90%	90%	90%	90%	90%
Age band	n = 13	n = 11	n = 21	n = 58	n = 41	n = 17	n = 15	n = 21	n = 12	n = 12	n = 17	n = 8
Age	0–2;5	2;6–2;11	3;0–3;5	3;6–3;11	4;0–4;5	4;6–4;11	5;0–5;5	5;6–5;11	6;0–6;5	6;6–6;11	7;00–7;5	7;6–7;11

KEY: <50% | 50% | 70% | 90%

Table 13.4 Process present in more than 10% of age band

	0	1	2	3	4	5	6	7	8	9	10	11
Gliding		27%	38%	19%	29%		27%		17%			
Front		27%	14%	29%	29%	23%						25%
WSD	15%	27%	14%	12%			13%					
Stop	46%	18%		33%	17%	23%	13%					
CD: I		18%		15%			13%					
CD: M				12%	15%							
CD: F	15%	18%		15%								
Back							13%					
Voicing		27%	14%	29%	12%	12%		19%				37%
Reduplication	30%	45%				23%						
Assimilation	15%	45%	14%									
Intrusive C				26%	12%		27%			17%		
De-nasalisation	15%											
De-retroflex		18%	33%	19%	12%		13%					
De-dentalisation			19%	26%	17%	18%	13%				12%	
Other	15%	45%	52%	50%	24%	23%	27%	33%				
Age band	0 n=13	1 n=11	2 n=21	3 n=58	4 n=41	5 n=17	6 n=15	7 n=21	8 n=12	9 n=12	10 n=17	11 n=8
Age	0–2;5	2;6–2;11	3;0–3;5	3;6–3;11	4;0–4;5	4;6–4;11	5;0–5;5	5;6–5;11	6;0–6;5	6;6–6;11	7;0–7;5	7;6–7;11

Table 13.5 Examples of processes

Process	Examples		
Gliding	ʈona → lona	mʊɾa → mʊla	ʃeːɾ → ʃel
Deaffrication	dʒabi → ʃabi	dʒabi → zabi	
Fronting	fʌɾɪʃ → fʌɾis	ẽnək → ẽnet	kʊkəɾi → tʊtəli
Weak syllable deletion	kʊkəɾi → ɾi		
Stopping	saːf → taː	dʒabi → dabi	ʃer → del	hʌɳɖi → kændi
Consonant deletion: Initial	saːf → aː	ʈona → ona	dʒabi → abi
Consonant deletion: Medial	mʌʈa → mʊa		
Consonant deletion: Final	ɖʊɖ̥ → dʊ		
Backing	pʰul → gʰul	atʰi̥ → aki	pʰʊl → pʊ
Voicing	kela → gela	kæn → gæn	ʌɳɖi → ʌŋgi
Reduplication	ɖʊɖ̥ → ɖʊɖʊ		murgi → mʊrki
Assimilation	dʒabi → babi ʈopi̥ → popi	ẽnək → nẽə nk saːf → faːf	ak → kak	ʈona → nona
Intrusive consonant	ʃer → ʃert	kæn → kænd	saːf → saːft	saːf → staːf

Table 13.6 Examples of less common errors present in less than 10% of age band

Age	Error	Example
0–2;5	Error on aspirated consonant	pʰʊl → pfʊl
	Retroflex → dental	aṭa → ata̪
2;6–2;11	dʒ → j	dʒabi → jabi
	Use of ejective	ẽnek → ẽnek'
	Error on aspirated consonant	pʰʊl → pʊl
	Error of manner	pãɳi → mãɳi
3;0–3;5	Use of ejective	ɑk → ɑk'
	Affrication	sɑːf → tʃɑːk
	Use of lateral fricative	ʃer → ɬer
	r error	ɾona → bona
	Use of glottal stop	fɛɾɪʃ → fɛʔɪʃ
3;6–3;11	nasal to liquid	næk → læk
	Metathesis	ṭopi → boti
	r error	ʃeːɾ → ʃeːb
	Metathesis	kʌpəɾ̥ẽ → pʌkəre
4;0–4;5	Error on aspirated consonant	ɑtʰi → ɑθi
5;6–5;11	Aspirated consonant → retroflex	ɑtʰi → ɑṭi

mother tongue and therefore were more reluctant to attempt items about which they were unsure.

Consonants attempted and percentage of consonants correct

The mean number of consonants attempted shows an essentially upward trend until the age of 4;11 when it plateaus for 12 months before showing a slight downward trend from the age of 6;0. The percentage of consonants correct shows an upward trend until the age of 7;5, thereafter showing a slight decline. Again these figures may well reflect the impact of exposure to English and the increased demand from education staff for expression in English from the age of 5;0.

Age of acquisition of consonants

The data presented suggests a relatively late establishment of consonants in this speech community. In fact this should be viewed as a refection of the relative difficulty of eliciting speech samples rather than an overall delay per se. Broadly speaking the data presented here reflect the findings of Khan (1984) with regard to order of acquisition of consonants *viz.* plosives followed by fricatives. Nasals are also among the first sounds to be firmly established. The unexpectedly early appearance of a dentalized alveolar plosive relative to other consonants is explained by the use of the word /d̪ʊd̪/ (milk) to elicit this sound. The prolonged role played by milk in the diet of children in the target community (where it is commonplace for children still to have bottles of milk at the age of five) ensures that this remains a high frequency word.

Phonological processes
The phonological processes identified in the data are broadly in line with those identified by Holm *et al.* (1999). Interestingly there was a high incidence of fronting observed here which is not reported in the earlier data. The incidence of reduplication is explained by the use of the target word /d̪ʊd̪/ (milk) which adults tend to realise in an immature, reduplicated style as /d̪ʊd̪ʊ/ when talking to young children.

Application of Data to Clinical Cases

Two examples of clinical findings are outlined below. In both cases application of the data presented here facilitates a differential diagnosis of delayed versus disordered phonological development.

Case study of disordered phonological development

S.M. was assessed at the age of 6:0 years. He has an unremarkable developmental history with no medical problems. He attends an English-language school in the United Kingdom. He was exposed to Mirpuri from birth and English on school entry. Parents and school have no concerns about S.M.'s non-verbal abilities. Formal assessment by an Educational Psychologist has shown S.M. to have high average non-verbal skills.

Summary of speech and language skills

Comprehension skills are age appropriate in both Mirpuri and English. His expressive language in both languages is delayed. S.M.'s spontaneous speech is almost completely unintelligible and his own immediate family have difficulty understanding him. S.M.'s speech exhibits simplification processes that are observed in younger children's speech (phonological delay) and also unusual sound substitutions which suggest a disordered phonological system.

Example of language skills in Mirpuri

Mirpuri target sentence	dʒənani	ʈaɾi	maɾni	pi
Mirpuri to English literal translation	Lady	clap	doing + female	is + female
S.M.'s sentence	ʌmi	aʈʰ		
Mirpuri to English literal translation	Mum	hand		

Example of language skills in English

English target	She's cuddling the teddy bear
S.M.'s utterance	With the teddy bear

English target	She's picked up the baby to post the letter
S.M.'s utterance	Big girl baby letter

Phonological assessment: Features of delay

Process	*Mirpuri*	*English*
Assimilation	naʰk – *nose* → [dæt]	red → [ded]
Fronting	kan – *ear* → [tæn] pʰəkana – *balloon* → [bəutana] naʰk – *nose* → [dæt] ga – *cow* → [da] ʔag – *fire* → [aʈʰ]	cars → [tɑʰ] smoke → [bəut] girl → [dɜl] sugar → [dudə] bag → [bæd]
Stopping of fricatives	saʰp – *snake* → [dæpʰ] dʒaz – *aeroplane* → [dæd] ʃeɾ – *lion* → [dɜ] ɦuʃ – *happy* → [ʌt] dʒɛnda – *flag* → [dena] ɾitʃ – *bear* → [dɪtʰ]	knife → [naɪt] sun → [dʊn] dress → [det] sugar → [dudə] pushing → [pʊtɪn] crash → [twæd] zip → [dɪp] nose → [dɒd] chair → [tɛə] watch → [dɒt]

Continued

(*Continued*)

Process	Mirpuri	English
Initial consonant deletion	tʌsvir – *picture* → [ədije] kʌɽi – *watch* → [edi] ɦaṯ – *letter* → [ætʰa] lefafa – *envelope* → [Ifata]	Not present
Cluster reduction	Initial clusters not frequent in Mirpuri inventory	smoke → [bəʊt] snake → [deɪd] swimming' → [wɪdɪ] sleeping → [dipɪn] spider → [paɪd] or [faɪd] stamp → [dæm] sky → [aɪ] blue → [bu] crown → [daʊn] clown → [dæn] grass → [dæt]

Phonological assessment: Unusual sound substitutions

Target	Mirpuri	English
/b/	bɪli – *cat* → [mɪni] bʌkɾi – *goat* → [wædi] baɾɪʃ – *rain* → [fadi]	On target
/m/	muɽgi – *chicken* → [fʌdi] mʌkʰi – *spider* → [bʌdʒi] or on target.	On target
/l/	bɪli – *cat* → [mɪni]	On target
/r/	rɪtʃ – *bear* → [dɪtʰ]	Phoneme not present in English inventory
/ʈ/	ʈoʈi – *chapatti* → [doɖi]	Phoneme not present in English inventory
/w/	Not sampled	web → [fed] flower → [fadə]

Case Study of Phonological Delay

H.A. was assessed at the age of 3;11 years. He was exposed to Punjabi from birth and English since school entry (eight months prior to assessment). H.A. has delayed comprehension and expression in Punjabi.

Expressive language skills

Punjabi target sentence	kʊɾi	d̪ʊd̪	pind̪i	je
Punjabi to English literal translation	girl	milk	drink – ing + female	is + female
H.A.'s sentence	d̪ʊd̪u	kʰand̪i		
Punjabi to English literal translation	milk	eating + female		

Phonological assessment: Features of delay

Process	*Mirpuri*	*English*
Reduplication	d̪ʊd̪ – *milk* → [d̪ʊd̪u]	
Gliding	kʊkəɾi – *chicken* → [kʊkəli]	bridge → [bwɪ]
Stopping of fricatives	sɑːf – *clean* → [tɑ]	fishing → [wɪtɪŋ]
Cluster reduction	mʊnd̪a – *boy* → [mʊd̪a]	gloves → [gəlʌb]
Initial consonant deletion	kela – *banana* → [ela]	
Final consonant deletion	fɛɾɪʃ - *floor* → [fɛlɪ]	watch → [wɒ]

Conclusion

The Pakistani heritage community is a significant minority ethnic population in the United Kingdom, but one about which surprisingly little data has been previously reported. Given the inevitably heterogeneous nature of any bilingual population some degree of caution should be exercised when extrapolating these findings and applying them to other children from a Pakistani heritage background. In particular the clinician should take into account the level of deprivation encountered in the community reported here. Nevertheless, it is believed that the data presented above will give clinicians valuable guidelines concerning the developmental patterns of phoneme acquisition and patterns of disordered phonology within the Pakistani heritage community in the United Kingdom.

Acknowledgements

The authors wish to thank the children and parents who participated in this study. Our particular thanks go to the staff at South Street Nursery,

Belfield, Deeplish, Marland Hill, Sparrow Hill and St John's schools in Rochdale who tolerated our intrusion into their busy routines with such good humour. Shazye Iqbal, Zahida Warriach, Nazmeen Kausar, Tahira Mahmood, Rosie Chamberlain and Claire Hannay assisted with data collection.

Chapter 14
Phonological Development and Disorder of Bilingual Children Acquiring Welsh and English

M.J. BALL, N. MÜLLER and S. MUNRO

Introduction

Welsh is a member of the Brythonic branch of the Celtic group of the Indo-European language family. According to the 2001 census, Welsh is spoken by 575,168 in Wales, representing 20.5% of the population over the age of three (National Statistics Online, 2003b). This percentage is an increase of around 2% since the 1991 census and is, in fact, the first increase in speakers (both percentage and in real terms) since figures started to be collected in the late 19th century. In the capital city, Cardiff, the number of Welsh speakers has increased from 5.67% of the city's population in 1981 to 10.86% today.

The long history of decline of the language reached a turning point in the 1960s and 1970s when there was a major increase in direct action (including civil disobedience) by Welsh speakers concerned with collapsing numbers of speakers and the erosion of traditionally Welsh-speaking society. These campaigns persuaded generally reluctant British governments to instigate legal and educational changes to raise the status of the language. Coupled with increased media usage of Welsh (including Welsh-language radio and television channels), and with self-funded and run Welsh immersion nursery schooling (often supported by parents who were not Welsh speaking), these developments have helped turn around the pattern of decline. It should be noted, however, that increases in Welsh speakers are mostly centred in the main cities and urban areas, with a new Welsh-speaking middle class elite. Traditionally Welsh-speaking rural communities are still seeing losses of speakers, as Welsh speakers move out to seek work, to be replaced by second-home buyers and retirees from England. A fuller examination of the social context of the language is available in Ball (in press).

The section following on Welsh phonology follows closely Ball (in press), and that work also includes information on other aspects of the grammar of the language.

The Phonology of Welsh

Phonology

Northern standard pronunciation of Welsh will form the basis of this section as the phonological system is fuller than in southern varieties. Where these differ, this will be noted in the relevant places.

Consonants

The consonant system consists of contrastive units in the plosive, nasal, fricative, affricate, trill and approximant categories. There are six plosive phonemes: /p, b, t, d, k, g/, where the fortis plosives are normally realised as strongly aspirated, and the lenis subject to varying degrees of devoicing (even in intervocalic position). The apical plosives are normally dental in northern varieties, but alveolar in southern (this distinction also applies to the apical nasal and lateral).

Some authorities posit six contrastive nasal stops as well: /m̥, m, n̥, n, ŋ̥, ŋ/. However, as the so-called 'voiceless' nasals (which are usually realised as voiced or partially voiced nasals with heavy aspiration) only occur in certain morphosyntactic contexts as reflexes of fortis plosives (see *mutations* below), it is normal to exclude them from the phonological system, and assume they are clusters of nasal plus /h/.

Welsh has eight contrastive fricatives: fortis-lenis pairs at the labiodental and dental positions, and voiceless fricatives at the alveolar, postalveolar, velar/uvular and glottal places: /f, v, θ, ð, s, ʃ, χ, h/. A voiced alveolar fricative may be used in some loan words from English, especially by southern speakers (e.g. *sŵ*/su/~/zu/, 'zoo'). The point of articulation of the dorsal fricative does appear to vary between velar and uvular (see Ball & Williams, 2001). This may be dialectal (northern varieties seem to use a uvular articulation more often), or an idiosyncratic feature. The lenis fricatives are usually subject to considerable devoicing, with duration and intensity being the main acoustic cues to the fortis-lenis contrast. The glottal fricative is often omitted in casual speech in southern varieties.

Affricates at the postalveolar position (/tʃ, dʒ/) are found in the language, but are the result of borrowings from English or are speech rate variants of clusters of /t/+/j/ or /d/+/j/.

Welsh has a series of four liquids: a voiced and a voiceless trill, a voiced lateral approximant and a voiceless lateral fricative (for the sake of symmetry we class the lateral fricative here with the lateral approximant; this is supported by morphosyntactic alternations between the two): /r, r̥, l, ɬ/.

The trills are alveolar and normally consist of two or three contacts (tapped articulations may also occur); the voiceless trill is normally followed by aspiration, but this sound may be missing from southern varieties who merge it with its voiced counterpart. In /tr-/ and /dr-/ clusters, an approximant or fricative postalveolar realisation is usual: [t̥ɹ̥], [dɹ]. The lateral approximant is dark in northern varieties, but clear in southern. The phonological evidence for full contrastivity between the fortis and lenis trills is not strong. Apart from in loan words, the lenis is restricted to medial and final syllable position, while the fortis occurs only syllable initially. However, the morphosyntactic alternations known as 'soft mutation' (see below) do produce word-initial lenis trills, so in these circumstances a contrast occurs. Similarly, the voiced lateral approximant only occurs in loans word-initially (though both laterals can occur elsewhere), and again mutation can bring about initial contrastivity.

Finally, the language has two central approximants, the labio-velar /w/ and the palatal /j/. Both approximants have fortis variants in certain morphosyntactic contexts (e.g. *iaith* [jaɪθ] 'language' ~ *ei hiaith* [i hjaɪθ] 'her language'; *wats* [watʃ] 'watch' ~ *ei hwats* [i hwatʃ] 'her watch'), but these are normally considered to be clusters of /h/ plus the approximant.

Vowels

The vowel system is large in northern varieties, with 13 monophthongs and 13 diphthongs. Southern varieties have smaller systems, however, with a formal register probably distinguishing 11 monophthongs and eight diphthongs. Monophthongs are normally paired in descriptions of the language into phonologically long and short vowels; northern varieties have smaller qualitative differences between the members of each pair than southern. In the following transcriptions we will not show vowel length, adopting instead a different symbol for each vowel to show the kind of quality distinctions that are heard.

The short vowels are /ɪ, ɛ, a, ɔ, ʊ, ɨ/ and the long vowels /i, e, ɑ, o, u, ɨ/. There is also an unpaired mid-central vowel /ə/ which, unlike schwa in English, can appear in stressed syllables and also enters into morphophonological alternations with the high central vowels /ɨ, ɨ/ (though only with those written 'y', e.g. *mynydd* ~ *mynyddoedd* ['mənɨð] ~ [məˈnəðoɨð], 'mountain' ~ 'mountains'). It should be noted that generally only northern varieties of Welsh retain the high central vowels, in southern varieties they are merged with the short and long high front vowels. Then, the morphophonological alternations just described take place between schwa and /ɪ, i/, but only those instances of these vowels derived from northern /ɨ, ɨ/.

The northern diphthong system has three subsystems: three glides moving towards the high front position, five glides moving towards a high back position, and five moving towards a high central position.

This gives us /aɪ, ɔɪ, əɪ/, /iʊ, ɛʊ, aʊ, əʊ, ɨʊ/ and /aɨ, ɑɨ, oɨ, ʊɨ, əɨ/. The main distinction between the diphthongs /aɨ/ and /ɑɨ/ is that the later has a longer first element than the former; likewise with /ɔɪ/ and /oɨ/ where the latter has a longer first element, though here the final elements are different as well.

In southern varieties, the diphthongs with a close central element are replaced by those with a close front one. This gives us two subsystems: four glides to a high front position and four to a high back position: /aɪ, ɔɪ, ʊɪ, əɪ/ and /iʊ, ɛʊ, aʊ, əʊ/. It should be noted, however, that in non-formal registers the northern /ɑɨ/ diphthong may be realised as /ɑ/, while the northern /aɪ/ diphthong may be realised as /ɔɪ/.

Phonotactics

One final aspect of segmental phonology we can consider is phonotactics. We do not have the space to go into this in any great detail (see Awbery, 1984 for a thorough treatment). We do include in Table 14.1 possible syllable shapes and consonant clusters adapted from Ball and Williams (2001).

Table 14.1 Phonotactic patterns of Welsh

Syllable type	Consonant type	Examples
CV*	Obstruents Sonorants	p t k b d g f v θ s ʃ χ ɬ tʃ dʒ m n l r̥ j w h
VCV	Obstruents Sonorants	p t k b d g f v θ ð s ʃ χ ɬ tʃ dʒ m n ɬ r̥ j w h
VC	Obstruents Sonorants	p t k b d g f v θ ð s ʃ χ ɬ tʃ dʒ m n ŋ l r
CCV*	Obstruents + obstruent Obstruent + sonorant	e.g. sb, sd, sg e.g. kn, tr, dr, tl, fr, gl
VCCV	Obstruents + obstruent Sonorant + sonorant Sonorant + obstruent Obstruent + sonorant	e.g. gv, χg, ɬd e.g. rm, rl, mn e.g. ŋg, mð, rd, rθ e.g. dn, br, vn, vl
VCC	Obstruents + obstruent Sonorant + sonorant Sonorant + obstruent Obstruent + sonorant†	e.g. sg, ɬd e.g. rn, rm e.g. mp, rd, rð, lχ e.g. dr, br, vn
CCCV	/s/ + stop + liquid	e.g. sdr, sgl
VCCCV	/s/ + stop + liquid Nasal + stop + liquid	e.g. sgr, sbr e.g. ndl, ntr

*Excluding mutation reflexes (see below).
†Except in very formal speech these clusters are normally separated by a copy epenthetic vowel in southern varieties.

There are also constraints on phonologically long and short vowels and coda consonants, some of which differ between varieties (see Awbery, 1984). Minimal pairs with these vowels are only possible in syllables closed with /m, n, ŋ, l, r/.

Prosody

Suprasegmental aspects of Welsh phonology have not been studied to such an extent as segmental (though see Ball & Williams, 2001 and references cited within). Word stress in Welsh is regularly on the penult with a very small number of exceptions (mostly borrowings, or the result of syllabic contraction). Interestingly, however, major pitch movements of the intonation system take place on the final syllable of accented words and so pitch and stress are separated (this phenomenon is also reported for Welsh English, see Walters, 1999). Nuclear tones (or major pitches) have been described by several authors (Ball & Williams, 2001; Pilch, 1975; Rhys, 1984; Thomas, 1967). The consensus view is that the language has four broad categories of pitch movement: fall, rise, rise-fall and level, but that high and low versions of these exist, at least at the level of phonetic difference. Thomas (1967) posits a variety of prenuclear patterns in intonation (both 'pre-heads' and 'heads'), and Williams (1985) found some support for these. They are normal, high rising, high level and low level preheads, and saw-toothed, rising and level heads.

Mutations

Mutations are phonological changes to word-initial consonants that are triggered by a range of morphosyntactic contexts. Initial consonant mutations are common to all the Celtic languages and are historical remnants of processes once triggered by phonological context, which have subsequently been lost during various sound changes. A full account of mutations and the environments that trigger them is given in Ball and Müller (1992), but we can give a brief description of them here. There are three main sets of consonants changes: soft mutation (SM) or lenition, nasal mutation (NM) or nasalisation, and aspirate mutations (AM) or spirantisation. Table 14.2 shows the changes in orthography and phonology.

Common triggering environments for these mutations are as follows:

SM: feminine singular noun after the article, after the numeral *un*; adjective following feminine singular noun; word following *ei* 'his', *dy* 'your' sing.; words following a range of common prepositions; verbs following a range of preverbal particles (e.g. marking questions, statements, negatives); items following a range of numeral forms (e.g. *dau/dwy* 'two', *ail* 'second'); adjectives following the complementiser *yn* (but not verbs); direct object of an inflected verb (but not of a periphrastic construction), and adverbials of time, among numerous others.

NM: words following *fy* 'my'; nouns following the preposition *yn* 'in'; various set expressions with numerals and time expressions.

Table 14.2 Initial consonant mutations

Radical		SM		NM		AM	
p	p	b	b	mh	m^h	ph	f
t	t	d	d	nh	n^h	th	θ
c	k	g	g	ngh	ŋ^h	ch	χ
b	b	f	v	m	m		
d	d	dd	ð	n	n		
g	g	deleted	–	ng	ŋ		
m	m	f	v				
ll	ɬ	l	l				
rh	r̥	r	r				

Note: Unfilled boxes mean that the mutation does not changes the radical in these cases.

AM: words following *ei* 'her'; words following a range of prepositions (*â*, *gyda* 'with', *tua* 'towards'); words following various negative particles; words following the numerals *tri* 'three' masc., *chwe* 'six', and the adverb *tra* 'very'.

A feature called pre-vocalic aspiration by Ball and Müller (1992) can also occur in some contexts, and here an /h/ is added to vowel-initial words, for example, following *ei, ein, eu* 'her, our, their'.

Orthography

The grapheme–phoneme correspondence in Welsh is fairly close, especially for the northern accents. Generally, each phoneme described above has only one written form, and each grapheme only one pronunciation. There is some departure from this ideal, but often this is predictable. For consonants, /p, t, k, b, d, g/ are written *p, t, c, b, d, g*; /m, n, ŋ/ are written *m, n, ng* (though *ng* can occasionally represent /ŋg/); /f, v, θ, ð, s, ʃ, χ, h/, are written *ff, f, th, dd, s, si/sh, ch, h*; /ɬ, l, r̥, r/ are written *ll, l, rh, r*; and /j, w/ written *i, w*. The borrowed affricates /tʃ, dʒ/ are written *tsi/tsh, j*.

The written symbol *i* represents the vowels /ɪ, i/ with a circumflex occasionally being used to show the long vowels in the few contexts where this is not predictable (the same is the case with all the long-short vowel pairs). Similarly, *e* represents /ɛ, e/; *a* represents /a, ɑ/; *o* represents /ɔ, o/; *w* represents /ʊ, u/; and *u* represents /ɨ, ɨ/. The unpaired central vowel /ə/ is written with the letter *y*, though this letter is another way of representing /ɨ, ɨ/ when in final syllables (except for a handful of function words when it stands for the schwa in their final open syllables). Diphthongs are written with the relevant vowel symbols that represent the first and last parts of the diphthong.

Speech Therapy Practice in Wales: The Use of Welsh and English

Currently only 259 speech and language therapists work in Wales. Only a small proportion of these are Welsh speaking and by no means all of these work with Welsh/English bilingual children. The number of therapists who have the ability to assess the children in both languages, who have knowledge of the phonological structures concerned, and who have access to relevant data, is therefore small.

This is no doubt the reason why Welsh-language assessments for disordered speech and language are so scarce. Ball and Munro (1981) describe a picture elicitation procedure designed to provide input for an assessment of Welsh phonology, and developments of this early work were employed in Munro (1985) and in Munro *et al.* (2005) (these last two covering studies on normal and disordered phonology described later in this chapter). Ball (1989) describes some suggestions for the transcription of suprasegmentals in Welsh, although this does not constitute an assessment protocol. Finally, we can note that Ball (1988) is an adaptation of the LARSP grammatical screening and assessment procedure for English originally designed by Crystal *et al.* (1989).

Previous Studies on the Acquisition of Welsh Phonology

Very little information exists on the normal development of Welsh phonology in previously published research. An early work was the research report of Harrison and Thomas (1975), but this work was mainly concerned with investigating the factors that maximised the likelihood of familial transmission of Welsh compared to those which favoured monolingual English transmission. Bellin (1984, 1988) provides the first attempt to provide data on the phonological acquisition of Welsh. Unfortunately, Bellin's data is derived from the study of only four children, though he uses a broader base of speakers in some studies of the acquisition of the mutation system (although this area is outside our scope of phonological acquisition). He devotes quite a lot of space to the discussion of patterns of babbling, and to early syllable structure. Of more interest, perhaps, are the patterns of substitutions he notes in the children once word combinations begin and vocabulary starts to expand. He finds, for example, typical patterns of cluster reduction, velar fronting, fricative simplification and consonant harmony. His data also show difficulties with target /ɬ/ with cluster realisations such as [sl], [θl], [xl] and [fl] gradually giving way to singleton [x]. Welsh /r/ was also subject to gliding with some subjects ([l]) and to spirantisation with others ([v]).

Siencyn (1985) and Hatton (1988) both studied language acquisition in the school situation. However, Hatton's work was on the mutation system which we will not consider here, and Siencyn makes only very limited reference to phonology. She does comment that one child she studied showed difficulties with Welsh /ɬ/, /r/ and /x/ but little data is provided.

The Study of Normal Phonological Acquisition

The study was conducted in southeast Wales, specifically in Cardiff and surrounding areas. It was felt that the acquisition patterns of children in the south east would be broadly representative of patterns in Wales generally. Although data on vowel patterns were collected, the primary focus of the study was the consonantal systems of the children. There are, of course, a number of Welsh and English dialects in Wales which display a range of consonantal variation, but at a phonemic level the similarities are sufficient to allow for broad generalisations to be made.

Furthermore, and with specific reference to Welsh, children in Wales learn the language within diverse linguistic, educational and familial contexts, so that children in the southeast represent those contexts likely to be found in other parts of Wales.

Method

Subjects

In order to fully reflect the formative years of phonological development subjects ranged in age from 2;6 to 5;0. Children younger than 2;6 would have posed a particular challenge in the elicitation of speech samples which could reasonably be compared with those obtained from the older subjects. The upper age limit was derived from the investigations of monolingual children summarised in Grunwell (1985, 1987) which suggest that the main stages of development in normal children have been mastered by 5;0, although some difficulties may persist for a number of years.

Subjects were divided into five age cohorts, each six months apart (2;6–3;0, 3;0–3;6, etc.). It was originally intended that there be 20 subjects in each cohort, with equal distribution of males and females, but as will be seen later, issues related to bilingualism militated significantly against the acquisition of 20 subjects for Group A (the youngest group). Children were included in the study if they had used Welsh and English for listening or speaking at any level.

Despite this, it was not possible to obtain more than six subjects for the youngest cohort, all of whom were first language Welsh. This reflects the tendency in south Wales for children reared in predominantly Welsh homes to be automatically exposed to the wider, dominant English environment. On the other hand, children from English speaking homes are not usually exposed to Welsh until their parents elect to place them in Welsh medium playgroups and nurseries.

Given the potential for diversity, it was considered necessary to use an initial classification of speakers. Various methods of classifying bilinguals are available although Baker (1988) argues that they are usually a priori procedures and frequently fail to take into account the fact that children's languages exist on a variety of dimensions. These classifications may not therefore be sensitive to types and (sub)groups of bilingual speakers as they exist in reality.

While the problems in rigidly adhering to an a priori means of classifying were recognised, it was nevertheless felt that some means of identifying subjects was required. This was in order to ensure that subjects were at least likely to contain some first language Welsh and some first language English speakers within each age group. In order to do this, language background questionnaires were given to parents and nursery leaders for completion (see Munro et al., 2005).

Language background was selected because it could provide profiles on a variety of dimensions which could, at least to some extent, lead to clustering of subjects. However, it has to be recognised that language background measures a child's use of two languages with a variety of people in various contexts and does not address issues of skill and ability in the languages. The term 'language dominant' as a classification guide is therefore mainly utilised to indicate, loosely, frequency of usage.

Following the above method, the cohort numbers were as presented in Table 14.3.

Analysis

The type and depth of analysis required, to an extent, determined the nature of the data. Two methods of analysing child phonology were employed in the project. The first was based upon a description of the child's speech as an independent phonological system. This approach

Table 14.3 Age-distributed cohorts

Group	Age range	*Language dominant*				
		Welsh		*English*		
		Male	*Female*	*Male*	*Female*	*Totals*
A	2;6–3;0	3	3	0	0	6
B	3:0–3:6	4	5	5	3	17
C	3:6–4;0	3	7	5	4	19
D	4;0–4;6	5	5	7	4	21
E	4;6–5.0	5	4	5	6	20
Totals		**20**	**24**	**22**	**17**	**83**

was originated by Bloomfield (1933) and his followers and was applied later to atypical speech in monolingual children by Grunwell (1981b, 1985, 1987) and Ingram (1989b).

The analysis of a child's phonological system highlights the function of the sound patterns found in the child's speech. In order to render themselves intelligible children must develop the distinctive differences in sounds which characterise the adult's spoken language. A contrastive analysis of child speech describes the extent to which a child's speech is communicatively effective.

The advantage of such an analysis for bilingual children is that it is based on formal, universal properties of phonological systems. These include, for example, stipulations that:

(1) there be hierarchical organisation of features, phonemes and syllables forming words;
(2) there be rules for their combination;
(3) there be sets of contrastive units established for the child's phonological system *in toto* or for different positions in (word or syllable) structure.

There is an argument here for a level of processing common to both languages. However, the analyses must also allow for detection of language-specific characteristics, but application of general principles need not preclude such specificity. Indeed, one of the advantages of using this method for bilingual phonology is that it can disclose the existence of 'asymmetry', when a child fails to exploit the contrastive resources of the system so that speech sounds which are normally contrastive for both adult target languages are contrastive in only one of the languages in the child's system.

The second aspect of the analysis of data was a description of the children's phonological simplifying processes, and these are discussed later.

Data collection

A minimum of 50 words per language at the single word level were elicited via picture naming. In order to explore syntagmatic and paradigmatic aspects of the phonologies of both languages as economically as possible two 50-word lists were drawn up (see Appendix 3). These lists were compiled according to the following criteria:

(1) able to be elicited via pictorial representation;
(2) likely to be familiar to young children;
(3) contained a variety of consonant vowel sequences so that the effects of phonotactic complexity could be analysed;
(4) included multisyllabic words;

(5) some of the words were bimorphemic;
(6) the multisyllabic words contained examples of different stress patterns;
(7) there was a representative sample of vowels;
(8) there were examples of word classes other than nouns.

Thus, derivation of normative data from a preponderance of monosyllabic words with CVC shape was avoided (as subsequently recommended by James, 2001).

A further consideration in word selection was the frequency of occurrence of particular sounds/sound sequences. However, in some cases it was difficult to reflect the frequency because the type of word in which it was found (e.g. function words) could not be easily represented pictorially.

In Welsh, sounds such as [tʃ] and [dʒ] which were historically regarded as not belonging to Welsh are now found so commonly in south Wales that they were considered by the authors to be part of the phonology of the accent and therefore incorporated into the target words. [z], also not considered to be part of Welsh phonology, occurs much less frequently and has limited distribution. It was consequently excluded as a target. However, where children spontaneously uttered (modified) loan words, these were included in the Welsh analyses where appropriate.

Also excluded were the voiceless nasals [m̥], [n̥] and [ŋ̊] because, as stated earlier, they are the result of nasal mutation (see Ball & Müller, 1992 for a description of consonant mutation in Welsh). It was not the purpose of the study to deliberately elicit mutated forms as this introduced another element of language acquisition.

A few loan words from English were included in the Welsh word list as they were totally integrated in the Welsh language. The entire list is given in Munro *et al.* (2005).

In both languages target speech sounds were allocated according to position in the word i.e. initial, medial, final. Not all possible places were chosen for each contrastive speech sound as some have restricted distribution.

A further consideration was that children do not develop contrasts on an all-or-nothing basis and so procedures which elicit sounds in only one context are limited in their potential to examine the development of phonology. Children may show phonological errors in connected speech which are not evident in the production of single words. In order to take this into account children were systematically encouraged to comment on the pictures and any multi-word utterances were transcribed and subsequently included in the analyses.

The children were audio-tape recorded by the research assistant (RA) attached to the project, using a Marantz CP230 cassette tape recorder. The RA made preliminary transcriptions of the subjects while they were speaking. All data were transcribed using the International Phonetic Alphabet and, where needed, the extensions to the IPA (Duckworth *et al.* 1990).

Whole-word transcription was adopted in order to allow for analysis of phonological simplifying processes and for maximum use of the data, avoiding, whenever possible, single evaluations of phonemes.

In order to verify the reliability of the transcriptions an experienced phonetician (who was also a qualified speech and language therapist) was asked independently to transcribe a randomly selected sample of the total recorded corpus. Interscorer reliability measures exceeded 90% in virtually all cases.

Words which could not be spontaneously elicited from the children were provided by the RA. Imitated words were allocated a specific code in case of the need for future, separate analysis. However, elicitation by imitation was not considered to be an issue of concern given that a number of authors (e.g. Siegel *et al.*, 1963) had not found a difference in error patterns between imitated and spontaneous responses.

Results

Full results are given in Munro *et al.* (2005). Figures 14.1 to 14.4 show the stages of acquisition of the speech sounds according to target language and language dominance. As the aim of these figures is to indicate broad patterns, information for the different sexes is not presented separately as the statistical analysis showed that, while there were a few interaction effects related to sex, there were very few main effects.

Acquisition was defined as the developmental sequence of phonological contrasts. This raised the issue of how to reflect which sounds in the children's phonetic inventories were used contrastively. Frequency

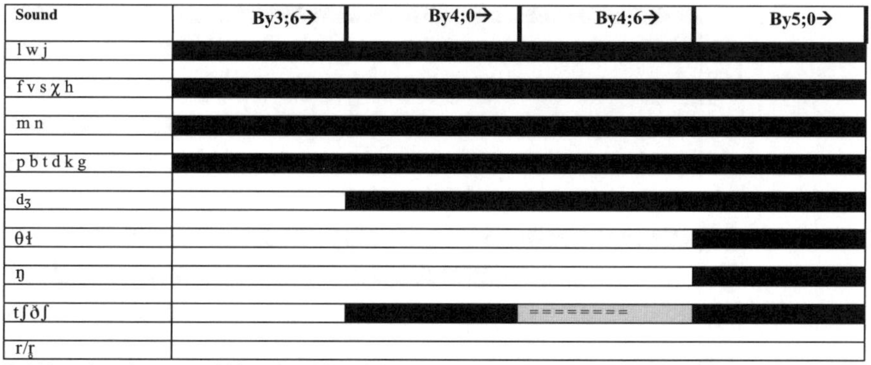

Sound	By3;6→	By4;0→	By4;6→	By5;0→
l w j				
f v s χ h				
m n				
p b t d k g				
dʒ				
θ ɬ				
ŋ				
tʃ ð ʃ			-------	
r/r̥				

Bold insertions denote acquisition, dotted lines indicate where acquisition is not maintained.

Figure 14.1 Welsh acquisition stages: Welsh dominant subjects

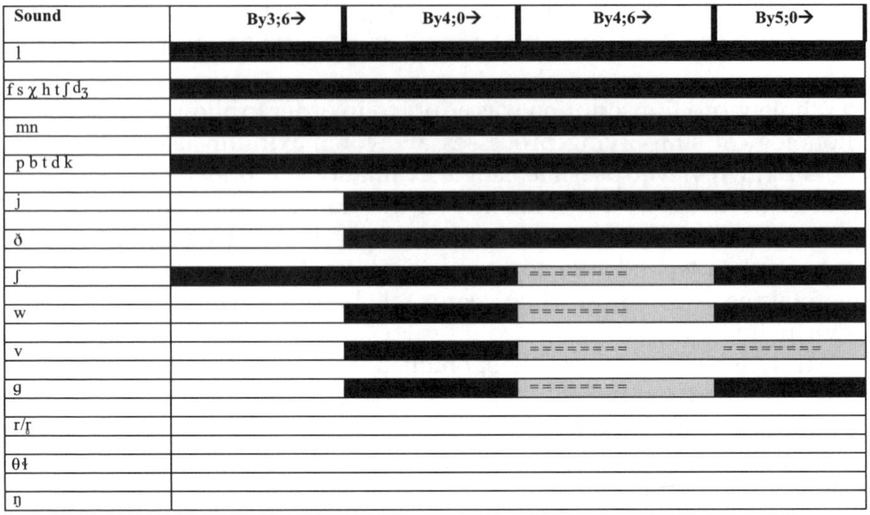

Sound	By3;6→	By4;0→	By4;6→	By5;0→
l				
f s χ h t ʃ dʒ				
m n				
p b t d k				
j				
ð				
ʃ			========	
w			========	
v			========	========
g			========	
r/ɾ				
θɬ				
ŋ				

Bold insertions denote acquisition, dotted lines indicate where acquisition is not maintained.

Figure 14.2 Welsh acquisition stages: English dominant subjects

definitions are crude but are convenient for analysis of data from large numbers of children. Although the use of age groups allowed for a longitudinal dimension, it was not possible to capture diachronic change for individual subjects. Rather, the aim was a synchronic analysis of groups of subjects. With the group aspect in mind, the frequency formula adopted was that a speech sound was deemed to be acquired for each cohort if at least 75% of the children in that cohort achieved at least 75% accuracy for each sound in question.

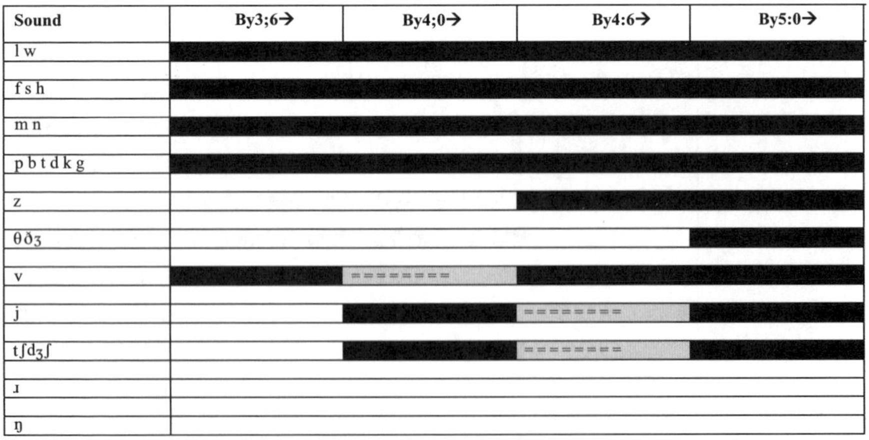

Sound	By3;6→	By4;0→	By4:6→	By5:0→
l w				
f s h				
m n				
p b t d k g				
z				
θ ð ʒ				
v		========		
j			========	
tʃ dʒ ʃ			========	
ɹ				
ŋ				

Bold insertions denote acquisition, dotted lines indicate where acquisition is not maintained.

Figure 14.3 English acquisition data: Welsh dominant subjects

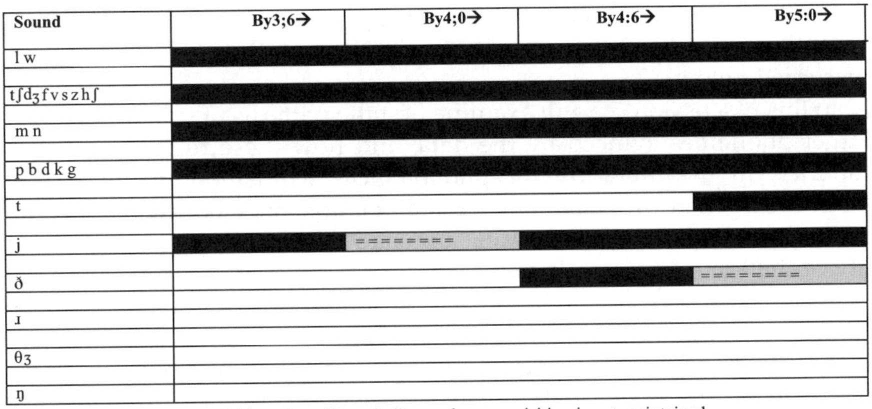

Sound	By3;6→	By4;0→	By4;6→	By5;0→
l w	███████	███████	███████	███████
tʃ dʒ f v s z h ʃ	███████	███████	███████	███████
m n	███████	███████	███████	███████
p b d k g	███████	███████	███████	███████
t				███████
j	███████	=======	███████	███████
ð			███████	=======
ɹ				
θ ʒ				
ŋ				

Bold insertions denote acquisition, dotted lines indicate where acquisition is not maintained.

Figure 14.4 English acquisition data: English dominant subjects

Some phonemes were 'permanently' acquired before 3;6 (i.e. the pattern of acquisition did not change for older children). These were the plosives /p b d k/, nasals /m n/, fricatives /f s h/ and approximant /l/. English /z/ was acquired by 4;0. Welsh /r/r̥/ and English /ɹ/ were still not acquired by 5;0.

Welsh /t/ was acquired before 3;6 regardless of dominance, but English /t/ only by the Welsh dominant children. English /t/ was not acquired until 4;6 by the English dominant subjects. English /g/ and /w/ were acquired before 3;6 as were Welsh /g/ and /w/ by the Welsh dominant children, but once again the English dominant subjects differed, showing uneven patterns (in Welsh).

Other phonemes are shown to be acquired after 3;6 in some of the figures but not at all in corresponding figures. Welsh /ŋ/ was acquired by 4;6 for the Welsh dominant group but did not reach the acquisition criterion elsewhere. For the language-specific English /ʒ/ and Welsh /ɬ/, it is the dominance which appears to mark the difference. English and Welsh /θ/ are acquired by 4;6 on the figures for Welsh dominance but /θ/ does not reach criterion on the other two figures.

For the remaining phonemes there is variability characterised by:

(1) different acquisition ages across figures;
(2) uneven patterns of acquisition within figures, where there is apparent acquisition by younger children which is not maintained by older children.

Various combinations of (1) and (2) are evidenced for /tʃ dʒ j v ð ʃ/.

Discussion

To examine the effects of the three factors (age, sex and language dominance) and any interactions between them, the data were analysed using three-way unrelated analyses of variance. Full results of the statistical analysis are given in Munro *et al.* (2005), but the broad trends are discussed below.

In this discussion we will examine first the patterns of substitutions for target phonemes evinced by the data, and how these relate to patterns reported in the literature for phonological acquisition in a range of languages. Then we will look at the relationships between the non-linguistic factors of age, sex and language dominance and the patterns of acquisition described above.

Patterns of substitution

As we have seen in the results, the children of both language-dominance groups gradually increased their accuracy of production of the consonants of both languages across the age ranges. It is interesting to compare the patterns of substitutions used for Welsh and for English for those sounds that were not already mastered at age 3;0–3;6 (the age of our Group B subjects: the first group with both Welsh and English dominant speakers).

As we can see from Figures 14.1 and 14.2, a large range of Welsh phonemes are acquired at the 75% accuracy rate or better by this group: /l, f, v, s, χ, h, m, n, p, b, t, d, k/, while the Welsh dominant subjects have also acquired /g, w, j/, and the English dominant /tʃ, ʤ, ʃ/. As we might expect from developmental studies of other languages (see Grunwell, 1987, 1997), velar fronting is the commonest substitution pattern for /g/ with the English dominant subjects, and for /ŋ/ with both dominance groups. Gibbon (e.g. 1990) has explained the prevalence for velar fronting in phonological acquisition as related to slow development of the ability to separate front and back tongue gestures, and her electropalatographic evidence suggests that fronted velars have different tongue-palate contact patterns than intended alveolars, but the timing of articulatory release produces an identical acoustic impression.

A range of fricative simplifications are seen with the unacquired fricatives (including devoicing with /v/), and both stopping and various stop-fricative clusters are seen with the affricates. The voiced dental fricative /ð/ still manifests some fricative stopping substitution patterns. Again, these patterns are similar to those reported for other languages.

Substitutions for the approximants are few and too varied to discern any pattern. The particular cases of the lateral fricative and the two rhotic consonants have been dealt with elsewhere (Ball *et al.*, 2001a, b, c), but we can briefly summarise their findings here. With the lateral fricative, a large number of substitutions were used though the tendency among English-dominant subjects was to use a voiceless velar/uvular fricative, or that fricative together with the voiced alveolar lateral approximant ([χ], [χl]). Even with Group E speakers substitutions were still common. With the Welsh dominant subjects the lateral fricative was less often substituted, and was totally correct for all Group E speakers. Patterns of [s] and [χ] usage were noted, but the use of fricative plus lateral clusters was less common than with the English dominant group.

The Welsh trill was the sound that showed the most varied substitution patterns of all (46), though many of these occurred only once or twice. As we might expect, the English dominant subjects demonstrated a considerable usage of the approximant-r ([ɹ]), as found in English, and this was a common substitution for the Welsh dominant speakers as well (though they used a larger number of target forms in all the age groups). Interestingly, there was also a considerable use of voiced fricatives (especially [ð]) by all subjects. Ball *et al.* (2001c) speculate that this choice was due to the acoustic similarity between this fricative and the target trill.

The English approximant-r showed many fewer substitutions: most commonly used were [ʋ] and [w], with other glides and liquids also occurring. Such a pattern of 'liquid gliding' has often been reported in the literature (see Grunwell, 1987, 1997). Interestingly, some speakers used [ɹ] for target Welsh /r/r̥/ while at the same time using [ʋ] or some other substitution for English target /ɹ/.

Turning to the substitution patterns with the other English target phonemes, we see that English dominant subjects had acquired all the consonant phonemes of English by 3;6 except: /t, ð, θ, ʒ, ŋ, r/ (this last we have already discussed). /t/ in syllable final position was often substituted by [ʔ] which is a dialect feature of Cardiff English (though, interestingly, not of Welsh in this area). It could be argued, therefore, that substitutions of [ʔ] for /t/ in relevant syllable positions should be counted as regionally correct; in which case, /t/ would be acquired earlier by the English dominant group. The fact that the English dominant children have different behaviours as regards the acquisition of /t/ in English and in Welsh supports the idea that they have already begun, at least, to treat the phonologies of the two languages separately. On the other hand, the fact that Welsh dominant subjects do not demonstrate glottaling or tapping behaviours with English /t/ could mean that they still have a single representation for /t/ in both languages, but is probably just a reflection of the Cardiff Welsh-speaking community's norm for this sound.

The three fricatives showed simplification patterns, though while /θ/ normally simplified to [f], /ð/ and /ʒ/ showed a variety of patterns including some stops. The velar nasal showed mostly fronting to alveolar position, consistent with the velar fronting process we noted above for Welsh.

The Welsh dominant subjects acquiring English showed similar trends in terms of substitution patterns. However, they did not demonstrate the glottal replacement of syllable final /t/ (as noted above, this was not part of their dialect of Welsh, so this is a clear example of influence from the dominant language). They did, though, show problems with English /z/ (we noted earlier the peripheral nature of /z/ in the phonemic system of Welsh). Deletions, and substitutions by a variety of other fricatives and affricates were found for /z/, but no clear pattern emerged. Simplifications of the postalveolar fricatives and affricates were also seen in these subjects, with alveolar substitutions the commonest pattern. Finally, we can note the substitution of [l] for /j/ for some subjects accounted for a later acquisition stage for this phoneme with the Welsh dominant subjects than the English, despite the fact that Welsh dominant speakers had no problems with Welsh /j/, while English dominant subjects did. This suggests that there is possibly some subtle phonetic (or indeed phonological) difference between /j/ in the two languages which has yet to be described.

Relationships with sex of speaker

The only statistically significant effect of sex was with the Welsh fricatives /χ/ and /ɫ/, though it is difficult to suggest reasons for these effects. The effect of sex and dominance with the plosive /t/ in English was interesting, as it supports the finding of sociolinguistic studies showing females more likely to use standard variants of phonological variables than males (see discussion in, e.g. Chambers, 2003).

Relationships with age of speaker

Clearly, only those sounds that were not already acquired at age 3;0 will be subject to any age effects so, broadly speaking, we expect to find possible effects with velars, fricatives and approximants. What is of particular interest is the occurrence of fluctuating acquisition of certain sounds over the age ranges. For example, English-dominant subjects of age range 3;6–4;0 acquire Welsh /ʃ, w, v, g/, but these sounds drop below the 75% threshold for age range 4;0–4;6 (and in the case of /v/, for age range 4;6–5;0 also). What is surprising about these results is that the same group of subjects have no such problems with these sounds when we look at English (though they display fluctuating acquisition of /j/ and /ð/ which is not the case with these sounds in Welsh). Welsh dominant speakers show fluctuating patterns with English /v, j, dʒ/, Welsh /ð/ and with both Welsh and English /ʃ, tʃ/.

The reasons for these patterns may well be found in the numbers of subjects and tokens involved, but there is also the tendency for advances in phonological acquisition to be followed by short periods of increased variability in usage, perhaps because the system needs time to fully integrate new forms (see Ingram, 1986b, 1989a). This is supported from our data if we consider that most of the sounds involved are intermediate or later acquired sounds, such as velars, fricatives and affricates. It must be assumed that such periods of increased variability are more likely in the less dominant language in bilingual acquisition. Further, the fact that these periods are mainly manifested for sounds in one language only, supports the notion that the children already have separate phonologies for English and for Welsh.

Relationships with language dominance of speaker

The results show that dominance effects are mainly manifested on sounds within the velar, fricative, trill, and approximant groups. Language dominance may be related to performance in both languages or one.

In Welsh words dominance effects are found with the velars /g/ and /ŋ/, where the Welsh dominant subjects perform significantly better than the English dominant ones. Likewise, with the fricatives /v, θ, ʃ, ɬ/ Welsh dominant subjects outperform English dominant ones. This was clearly to be expected for the Welsh-only fricative /ɬ/, and a greater frequency of occurrence might explain the effect with /v, θ/. As we would expect, Welsh dominance significantly aids the acquisition of the Welsh trill, but surprisingly Welsh target /w/ and /j/ also demonstrate this dominance effect (perhaps relating to a greater functional load for /w/ at least in Welsh).

In English words there are also a number of effects with language dominance. Above we noted a correlation between age and /t/, and this reoccurs with language dominance. Interestingly, the pattern here shows that Welsh dominant subjects perform better than English dominant ones on English target /t/. This may be due to the lack of glottalising tendencies in Cardiff Welsh that we have discussed previously, and if such realisations had been marked as dialectally correct, this effect would not be present. The other English target sounds showing a dominance effect were the fricatives /s, ʃ/ and the affricates /tʃ, dʒ/, where English dominant subjects outperformed Welsh ones. For the two affricates this is understandable given the greater frequency of these in English; however, the two fricatives are more problematic (especially as the opposite effect was demonstrated with Welsh /ʃ/). Whether subtle realisational differences or distributional patterns might account for these results needs to be investigated further, but at any rate these effects give added support to the notion that the subjects have separate phonological representations for similar consonants in Welsh and English.

A final interesting interaction is with English target /h/: here again the Welsh dominant subjects outperform the English. While both south Walian English and Welsh are subject to /h/-dropping, it appears that the models of Welsh presented to the children may have stressed /h/ retention. Certainly all subjects use /h/ with very high frequency in their Welsh, and only the English dominant subjects display any marked degree of /h/-dropping in their English (though, interestingly, the Group E speakers do not display this dropping tendency). It may well be, then, that /h/ retention in the Welsh dominant subjects is an interzlanguage feature, rather than a more native-like acquisition pattern.

Language performance interactions

The statistical analysis also examined overall performance on different sounds between the two languages: that is, whether percentage correctness in one language correlated with percentage correctness in the other. In all instances where such correlations occurred, the direction was always that the higher percentage correctness was in English, the higher it was in Welsh too. At the 0.01 degree of confidence such correlations existed for /b, k, g, θ, ʃ, tʃ, dʒ, l/, while at the lower 0.05 degree they existed for /p, ŋ, h/.

This result suggests the strong effect of English on all subjects irrespective of language background. For, while performance in English may enhance performance in Welsh, it would appear that the converse is seldom the case.

The Study of Disordered Phonology

Little published work exists which investigates the error patterns of Welsh/English bilingual children diagnosed with speech disorder. If one is to attempt to compare these patterns with normal phoneme acquisition and phonological processes, there are further limitations. It is possible to use what is available to begin the process of comparing with data on monolingual English speaking children. However, comparisons with monolingual Welsh speakers would be more problematic. As the majority of Welsh speaking children are bilingual, information on monolingual Welsh phonological acquisition is scarce. There are studies of normal bilingual Welsh/English acquisition (see above) but these are limited in number and, in some cases, only quite recently published.

Although published information on bilingual phonological difficulties is not readily available, there is much untapped potential in the speech and language therapy clinics in Wales. However, there have been no recent studies which use clinical data to systematically compare with normal (monolingual and bilingual) development, to compare across two languages in the same child or to use findings to inform phonological theory. In addition to the limitations mentioned above, one also needs to consider that, as noted earlier, only small proportion of Speech-Language therapists in Wales are Welsh speaking and have the opportunity to work with Welsh/English bilingual children.

One piece of work, that did study phonological difficulties in Welsh/English bilingual children, was by Munro (1985). Although not recent, it is used as the basis to the following discussion as it attempted to address a number of issues embedded in questions subsequently posed by Holm and Dodd (1999b) (see below). Where issues more recently raised in the literature were not addressed it is possible to revisit the original Welsh/English study in order to consider the significance of its data.

Case study 1: Nigel

At the time of the study Nigel was eight years and nine months old. He had mild general learning difficulties and his hearing was reported to be within normal limits. Nigel's parents and grandmother (who lived in the family home) were fluent speakers of Welsh and English; Nigel had been exposed to both languages from birth. He attended a school where both Welsh and English were used informally but English was the medium of education. At the time of the study his dominant language was English.

Research conducted since this study has indicated that there are four subgroups of children with speech disorder. Using the groupings suggested by Bradford and Dodd (1994), it is not easy to classify Nigel's speech. There was evidence of 'articulation impairment' as he was unable to produce acceptable versions of a range of phonemes. There was also evidence of 'inconsistent speech disorder', with variable production of words and phonemes and a history of difficulty in planning motor sequences.

Significantly, his phonetic inventories for Welsh and English were similar, with the range of audible units being largely restricted to liquids, glides and nasals. The two languages were also similar with regard to correspondence between (adult) target phonemes and Nigel's realisations of them. The most striking similarities were the large number of correct realisations for target /m/ and /n/ but a weighting towards [ʔ] and nil realisations. In both languages there was variability in realisations, homonymy and unintelligibility.

Therefore, in reply to one of the questions posed by Holm and Dodd (1999b) which asks if speech errors are characteristic of a particular subgroup of speech disorder, the data suggest that Nigel's error patterns were identified with the same subgroup(s) in both of his languages.

Case study 2: Rhodri

Rhodri was five years and eight months old when studied. He had a history of slight delay in speech and language development but at the time of the study only his speech was problematic, this being frequently unintelligible. He was considered to be of above average intellectual ability and his hearing was normal.

Like Nigel, he had been raised in a home where his parents spoke Welsh and English fluently, Welsh being the dominant language. Rhodri attended a Welsh medium school. Literacy skills were developing normally.

Although there was some evidence of 'articulation impairment' (e.g. absence of /s/ and /z/ in the phonetic inventories of both languages), the predominant picture was that of 'inconsistent speech disorder'. Rhodri had developed a larger number of contrastive phonemes than Nigel but there was overlapping of these at all places in word structure with consequent inconsistency and unpredictability. There were also non-contrastive variants, which contributed further to the unpredictability. These patterns were characteristic of both languages. Therefore, despite there being some differences between Rhodri's Welsh and English phonological systems (see below), the predominant characteristics placed his speech in the same subgroup for both languages.

Another important question to ask is whether children's speech errors indicate the same underlying deficit for both languages. This raises the issue of the nature of 'underlying deficit' and it may be argued that there is a need to move beyond surface phenomena and focus attention on the organisation principles of the children's phonologies.

This was the approach taken by Munro (1985) in a study that suggested that separate descriptions of the phonologies of bilingual children with phonological impairment did not provide an explanation of how children arrived at these phonologies. One method of attempting such an explanation was argued to be the application of a procedure that would look at the strategies adopted by the children that would be sufficiently fundamental to serve both languages. The original study debated the nature of 'strategies' but the details of that debate are not repeated here.

Although the original work measured the degree of correspondence between (adult) target phonemes and subjects' realisations of them, correspondence analyses did not take into account the number of words distinguished by any particular phonemic contrast and thus the pattern-forming aspects of the child's phonology. The 1985 study therefore concluded that an insightful method would be the analysis of a child's speech as an independent phonological system. Consequently, the analyses were based on the work of Grunwell (1977) who had argued that analyses of phonological systems highlighted the function of sound patterns and thus the communicative implications of any abnormal patterns.

The approach was based on universal principles and argued that the child's independent phonological system was his/her pattern of organisation. Munro (1985) suggested that this organisational capacity, being fundamental, could be activated by either of the bilingual child's languages and would serve them both. This implied a general plane of functioning common to both languages, but as these principles of organisation might have differing effects in each language, a specific plane could be postulated for each.

The universal aspects were implicit in the analyses by the nature of the properties selected *viz*. phonetic inventories, consonant vowel sequencing, contrastivity and feature composition (some of which are included below).

Also included in the analyses were the subjects' phonological (simplifying) processes as these were regarded by Grunwell as inextricably linked to the phonological systems. These too were related to universality as they had been attested in a substantial number of languages. It was not suggested that all children of all languages demonstrated the same processes but rather that this means of organising was universally available, its manifestations varying between languages and individuals.

The additional advantages of the two approaches were that they could be used to analyse clinical phonological data as well as data from normally developing children. In the original study, complete phonetic inventories were presented followed by basic inventories which excluded infrequent phonetic variations and phonetic units for which there were only a few tokens. It is evident from Tables 14.1 and 14.2 that the basic inventories were virtually identical and were highly restricted in the same way.

The basic inventories for Rhodri (Tables 14.3 and 14.4), while not as restricted as Nigel's, were nevertheless marked by similarity across Welsh and English, showing the same inadequacies. The [ɬ] and [x] in the Welsh inventory reflect the nature of the target phonology.

Contrastive phonemes were analysed according to word position. To avoid confusion with target language phonemes, the contrastive phonemes of the two speech disordered children described here are put into vertical brackets, as suggested by Grunwell (1985). Word initially for both languages |m|, |n|, |l|, |ʋ|, |j|, |ʔ|, |m⁻| were contrastive. Overlapping was a characteristic of both languages.

Word medially the contrastive phonemes in both languages were |m|, |n|, |l|, |ʔ|, |m⁻|, and the degree of overlapping was less in both. However, some language specificity was evident in that |j| and |w| were contrastive only in his Welsh system.

Table 14.4 Basic phonetic inventory for S1: Nigel – Welsh

				ʔ
m		n		
				h
w	ʋ	l	j	
m⁻*				

*[m⁻] denotes non-audible release.

Nil realisations were not included when contrastivity was calculated which, word finally, left very few tokens with a result that contrastivity could not be established with confidence except in the case of |m|, |n| and |l|. These were contrastive for both languages with no language-specific patterns. In all word positions there was non-contrastive variability in both languages.

In Rhodri's case, the contrastive phonemes in his word initial system were |p|, |b|, |t|, |d|, |m|, |n|, |f|, |v|, |l|, |w| and |ʔ|. They were contrastive for both Welsh and English. There were quite a number of non-contrastive variants and some overlapping although the latter was not as widespread as for Nigel. Again, these characteristics were noted across languages.

Additionally, there were two interesting patterns. Both [ɬ] and [f] occurred with equal frequency for Welsh-specific target /ɬ/; and [ʊ] and [v] occurred equally for Welsh /r/ or English /ɹ/. As each pair appeared to operate contrastively, each was regarded as a unit composed of two items.

Word medially, [ʊ] and [v] once again appeared to operate as a unit and were therefore included as such in the list of contrastive phonemes. These were |p|, |b|, |t|, |d|, |m|, |n|, |l|, |f|, |v| and |v~ʊ| in both Welsh and English. There was one language-specific feature which was the appearance of |k| as contrastive only in Rhodri's English system. There was overlapping in both languages.

Although Rhodri's word final system was surprisingly well developed within the context of clinical phonology, it was still susceptible to overlapping. The contrastive phonemes across languages were |p|, |b|, |t|, |d|, |k|, |g|, |m|, |n|, |f| and |l|. The appearance of |v|, |x| and |v~ʊ| were reflections of the target language (see below).

To summarise, underlying the phonologies of both languages for both subjects were

- restricted phonetic inventories;
- restricted use of contrastive phonemes at all places in word structure;
- overlapping and homonymy;
- non-contrastive variants.

With regard to phonological processes the two subjects simplified in very similar ways in their two languages. Not only did the same processes appear but also they were of approximately similar proportions. The only exception was that Rhodri demonstrated what appeared to be Final Consonant Deletion only in his Welsh. However, the number of examples was very small and there was a possibility that it was not a process as such (see later).

Major processes in Nigel's data were

- Cluster reduction
- Final consonant deletion
- Favourite articulation

Minor processes for the same subject were

- Consonant harmony
- Metathesis
- Gliding
- Fronting

Major processes in Rhodri's data were

- Cluster reduction
- Consonant harmony
- Favourite articulation

The only minor process operating in both of his languages was metathesis.

Similarities existed also in terms of how the processes were used. For example, in word initial Cluster Reduction of /s/ + stop, it was the fricative that was omitted in both languages and Nigel's version of the stop which was retained. It was also the fricative that was omitted in /s/ + nasal clusters. In Rhodri's case the type of cluster reduction was more unusual as it was his version of the fricative which was maintained and the stop or nasal omitted. However, the pattern was consistent across languages. It should be noted that the little research that exists on processes in phonologically normal Welsh/English bilingual children indicates that maintenance of the fricative is unusual in Welsh as it is in English.

The above similarities and the fact that both subjects' error patterns could be allocated to the same subgroup(s) of speech disorder in both languages 'validates the hypothesis that a single deficit underlies disorder in the two phonological systems of each child' (Holm & Dodd, 1999b: 127).

Despite the commonality described there was evidence of the language specificity implied in the third question posed by Holm and Dodd which concerned itself with differentiation of a bilingual child's phonological systems.

As stated above, the major difference in processes between the two languages (and the two subjects) was Rhodri's possible use of Final Consonant Deletion. However, a possible explanation was that it was not a process but the result of a 'mechanical' event. All of the omissions occurred during spontaneous conversation and might have been due to Rhodri's speed of utterance; his approach to the less familiar English conversational context was more cautious.

In Nigel's case, there were a few subtle language-specific patterns. For instance, variations between Welsh and English existed for him in that realisations of target English consonant +/ɹ/ clusters showed attempts to signal the /ɹ/ in both word initial and word medial positions whereas in Welsh consonant +/r/ clusters, the second element appeared almost exclusively word initially. The reason for the increased incidence of this word medial Cluster Reduction in Welsh was unclear particularly as the clusters in question are well defined in the Welsh target phonology.

More convincing evidence of a differentiation between languages existed in the analyses of the children's phonological systems, in particular the analysis of their contrastive phonemes. Contrastivity was linked explicitly to the target phonemes in Tables 14.5–14.9 where targets above the dotted line apply to both languages and those below the dotted line apply only to one.

It was possible to track where patterns in the child's system related directly to the target phonology and where they were reflections of the child's independent organisation.

The phonemes marked with * reflected the adult systems. The /ɬ/ was specific to Welsh. Although /v/ and /θ/ can occur word initially in Welsh, their use is largely triggered by particular syntactic environments, a result of the Welsh initial consonant mutation system (see Table 14.8).

The appearance of |ʊ| as contrastive for the Welsh trilled /r/ was interesting. The English target /ɹ/ maybe articulated differently but it does, nevertheless, have a place in the word initial system of adult English.

Other instances of differentiation were found in the use of the already established |mˀ| as contrastive for /p/, /b/ and /f/ only in his Welsh system.

With the exclusion of |w| and |j| the phonemes were contrastive for both languages albeit with marked language-specific distribution. The

Table 14.5 Basic phonetic inventory for S1: Nigel – English

mˀʔ				ʔ
m		n		
				h
w	ʊ	l	j	
mˀ				

Table 14.6 Basic phonetic inventory for S2: Rhodri – Welsh

p b		t d	k g		ʔ
m		n			
		l			
	f v			x	
		ɬ			
	ʊ				

Table 14.7 Basic phonetic inventory for S2: Rhodri – English

p b		t d	k g		ʔ
m		n			
		l			
	f v				
		tʃ			
	ʋ				
w					

specificity demonstrated in the rows marked with * tended to parallel the pattern in the target languages concerned for the phonemes specified are either exclusive to or far more common word medially in that language.

However, the use of contrastive equivalents for targets /n/ and /b/ in English only appeared to be peculiar to Nigel's own system.

As stated above, Nigel's word final contrastive system could not be established with confidence and therefore no table is provided at this point.

Language differentiation in Table 14.10 was related to specific characteristics of the target languages.

Like the |w| and |j| of Table 14.6, the |k| in Table 14.11 did not appear as contrastive at all in one language. Unlike the glides, the [k] was absent in Welsh and this absence was not related in any way to the target Welsh phonology. This type of asymmetry, i.e. a failure to exploit contrastive resources, was not referred to by Grunwell (1977) as it relates particularly to the bilingual context.

Table 14.8 Contrastive phonemes word initially for S1: Nigel

Contrastive phoneme	Target(s) for which phoneme is contrastive		
m	m		
n	n		
l	l		
j	j		
ʔ	t d k g tʃ dʒ s z ʃ		
	ɬ* h		
ʋ	r		v
m̚	p b f		θ*
	Welsh only		English only

Table 14.9 Contrastive phonemes word medially for S1: Nigel

Contrastive phoneme	Target(s) for which phoneme is contrastive	
m	m	
n	ŋ	
l	l	
ʔ	t d k g s ʃ	
m̚	f	
n		n
ʔ	*θ x ɬ	tʃ dʒ z ʒ*
m̚		b
	Welsh only	English only
w	w*	
j	j*	

Language differentiation word finally (Table 14.12) was related to the nature of the respective adult phonologies.

Moving on to the fourth of Holm and Dodd's questions (1999b: 117), 'Were the error patterns typical of monolingual children in each

Table 14.10 Contrastive phonemes word initially for S2: Rhodri

Contrastive phoneme	Target(s) for which phoneme is contrastive	
p	p	
b	b	
t	t	
d	d	
m	m	
n	n	
l	l	
w	w	
ʔ	h	
f	f s ʃ	
v	v	
v~ʋ	r	ɹ
f		θ
f~ɬ	ɬ	
	Welsh only	English only

Table 14.11 Contrastive phonemes word medially for S2: Rhodri

Contrastive phoneme	Target(s) for which phoneme is contrastive	
p	p	
b	b	
t	t	
d	d	
m	m	
n	n	
l	l	
f	f s ʃ θ	
v	v	
v~ʋ	r	ɹ
	Welsh only	English only
k		k

language?', it is very clear that both subjects had English speech systems which did not compare with their monolingual English counterparts. In addition to restrictions in the number of phonemes acquired, both subjects used non-English sounds.

Comparison of the subjects' processes in the English data with normal developmental English patterns indicates that both Nigel and Rhodri used delayed as well as atypical processes.

Delayed (similar to younger normally developing children)
Nigel: Cluster reduction; Consonant harmony; Final consonant deletion; Gliding; Fronting
Rhodri: Cluster reduction; Consonant harmony

Atypical (absent or very infrequent in normal developmental data)
Nigel: Metathesis; Favourite articulation
Rhodri: Metathesis; Favourite articulation

It is not possible to compare the subjects' phonological systems and processes with monolingual Welsh children for the reasons given previously.

Future directions

A useful next step would be to compare the data for Nigel and Rhodri with that provided for normally developing bilingual children. A degree of comparison could be achieved by using the normal bilingual data

Table 14.12 Contrastive phonemes word finally for S2: Rhodri

Contrastive phoneme	Target(s) for which phoneme is contrastive		
p	p		
b	b		
t	t		
d	d		
k	k		
g	g		
m	m		
n	n		
f	f s θ		
l	l		
n			ŋ
ɬ	ɬ		
v	ð		z
v~ʊ	r		
	Welsh only		English only
x	x		

covered at the start of this chapter. However, it should be noted that Nigel and Rhodri were simultaneous bilinguals whereas a proportion of the children providing the normal data were successive bilinguals. Furthermore, both the normally developing children and the speech disordered subjects varied in language dominance patterns.

Therapy

Limited research exists on generalisation of therapy across a bilingual child's languages. Holm *et al.* (1997) argued that effects of articulation therapy in one language generalised to the other language. However, they did not find evidence of generalisation as a result of phonological therapy.

Rhodri had received speech therapy in Welsh for approximately one year but when he was almost five years old the therapist left. Therapy then terminated as Rhodri's parents refused to take him to a monolingual English speaking speech and language therapist. The concentration had been on articulatory placement and a little improvement had been noted. Unfortunately, no information was available on the actual therapy targets and no indication as to whether improvement applied only to his Welsh.

Nigel had been seen by various speech and language therapists for a number of years but input had been irregular and progress very limited. There were no reports of bilingual therapy. Just after initial data collection Nigel received intensive speech therapy for two weeks in English which concentrated on articulation of [f].

An analysis of post intensive therapy data (post data) revealed some interesting patterns. These can be exemplified by using the data relating to Nigel's word initial phonological system.

Prior to intensive speech therapy (pre data) Nigel correctly and consistently realised targets /m/, /n/ and /l/ in both languages. This pattern was maintained in the post data. In both sets of data, for both languages, |ʔ| was used contrastively by Nigel for targets /t/, /d/, /k/, /g/, /tʃ/, /dʒ/, /s/, /z/ and /ʃ/. Maintenance of contrastive |ʔ| was also evidenced across pre and post data with regard to Welsh-specific target /ɬ/. In the pre data, a type of asymmetry had existed because |ʔ| had been the major realisation for Welsh target /h/ but this was not the case in English. However, the post data indicated that |ʔ| was being used contrastively for /h/ in English also.

|ʊ| appeared contrastively for English-specific target /v/ in the pre data but this was not maintained in post data although there were more instances of correct realisations in the post data. In the post data |ʊ| was contrastive for English target /ɹ/ but this had not been the case in the pre data. This pattern was the reverse to the pattern for target /v/. Maintenance across data was seen in the contrastive use of |ʊ| for Welsh target /r/.

A significant development was the appearance of |f¬| as contrastive for /f/ in the English post data. The disappearance of |m¬| as the major realisation for target /f/ was also evident in the Welsh post data but there was no replacement of |m¬| by |f¬| in Welsh. Instead, the Welsh realisations became more variable.

There were also other patterns relating to contrastive use of |m¬| across data sets:

English-specific target /θ/:	pre data, |m¬| contrastive
	post data, [m¬] not contrastive
English target /p/, /b/:	pre data, [m¬] not contrastive
	post data, [m¬] not contrastive
Welsh target /p/, /b/:	pre data, |m¬| contrastive for /p/ and /b/
	post data, |m¬| contrastive for /b/ only

Finally, |j| was consistently correct in the pre data for both languages but lost its status as a contrastive phoneme in the post data, again in both languages.

In the pre data all of the contrastive phonemes in Nigel's system were contrastive in Welsh and English although there were language-specific differences in the targets with which they were associated. Following intensive therapy, the |fˀ| became the one phoneme to be contrastive within Nigel's own system in one language only (English). The loss of the previously contrastive |mˀ| for word initial /f/ in Welsh without replacement by |fˀ| may be evidence of inter-language generalisation. Nigel may be 'reappraising' his Welsh phonological system. Although the effect is not obviously positive, the resulting variability may perhaps be regarded as a precursor to a pattern nearer to the adult phonology.

Intra-language generalisation may be an explanation for the loss in English of |mˀ| as contrastive for /θ/, and |ʋ| for /v/ with an increase in variability. Both changes relate to target fricatives although the latter change may be the more positive as it is associated with increased instances of the correct [v]. The examples of |fˀ| for /θ/ appear to indicate an inappropriate generalisation of the labio-dental contact established for English target /f/.

Increase in variability in the English post data was not evidenced for targets /h/ and /ɹ/, in fact the reverse was true with |ʔ| and |ʋ| respectively becoming more consistently used for those targets. This might have been due to Nigel's increasing awareness of the requirements of the English target system as an effect of therapy but it is not clear why some effects would involve decrease in variability an other effects an increase in variability. Also puzzling are the changes in |j| and Welsh |p| described above.

Conclusion

This chapter has demonstrated some of the drawbacks of working with minority languages: there are never enough speakers, and there is never enough research available. Nevertheless, both the study of normal phonological development and the study of the disordered speakers have demonstrated cross-linguistic similarities with other languages (including those investigated in this collection), as well as language specific characteristics. It is our hope that this account may stimulate further research into Welsh phonology – both normal and disordered – and the provision of more assessment materials in the language that may lead to a greater use of Welsh in intervention in the speech clinic.

Appendix 1: Consonant Chart

	Bilabial	Labiodental	Dental	Alveolar	Postalveolar	Palatal	Velar	Uvular	Glottal
Plosive	p b			t d			k g		
Nasal	m			n			ŋ		
Affricate					tʃ dʒ				
Fricative		f v	θ ð	s (z)	ʃ			χ	h
Lateral fricative				ɬ					
Approximant	w					j			
Lateral approximant				l					
Trill				r					

Note: Northern varieties have dental rather than alveolar /t, d, n/. /χ/ may be realised as [x] by some speakers. /z/ is marginal, found in borrowings in southern varieties where northern varieties replace it with /s/. /l/ is clear in southern varieties, and dark in northern.

Appendix 2: Vowel Charts

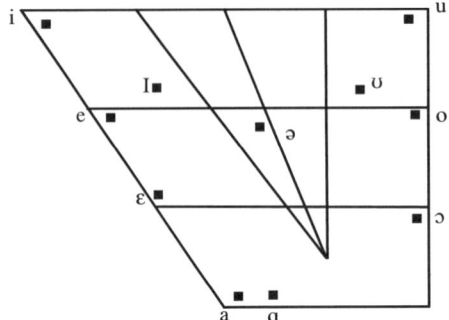

Vowel Chart 1 Main variants of the monophthong vowel phonemes of southern Welsh

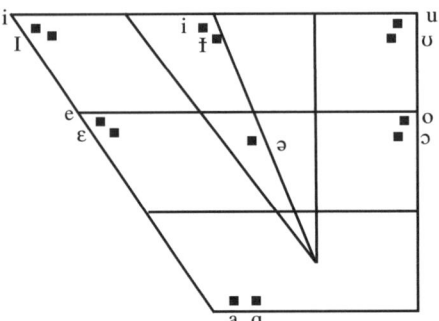

Vowel Chart 2 Main variants of the monophthong vowel phonemes of northern Welsh

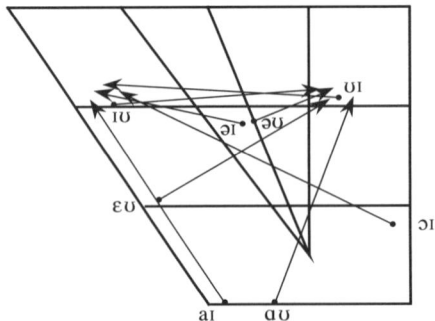

Vowel Chart 3 The diphthongs of southern Welsh

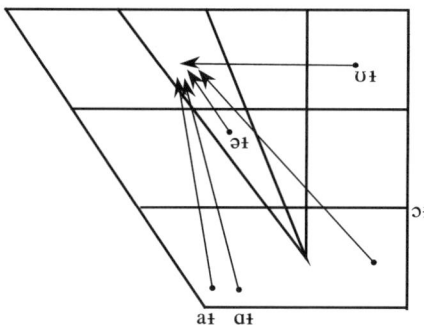

Vowel Chart 4 The centring diphthongs of northern Welsh

Appendix 3: Differences from English

	Welsh	British English
Syllable initial consonants	p t k b d g f v θ s ʃ χ ɬ m n l r̥ j w h tʃ dʒ	p t k b d g f v θ ð s z ʃ m n l ɹ j w h tʃ dʒ
Syllable initial clusters	p b t d k g f+l r ʃ+r k+n s+b d g m n l s+b d g+r s+g+l	p b t d k g f θ ʃ+l ɹ j w s+p t k m n l w s+p t k+l ɹ w j
Syllable final consonants	p t k b d g f v θ ð s ʃ χ ɬ tʃ dʒ m n ŋ l r	p t k b d g f v θ ð s z ʃ ʒ m n l (ɹ) tʃ dʒ
Vowels	i ɪ e ɛ a ɑ ɔ o ʊ u ə *northern, also* ɨ ɨ̞ aɪ ɔɪ ʊɪ əɪ ɪʊ ɛʊ aʊ əʊ *northern* aɨ ɔɨ əɨ ɪʊ ɛʊ aʊ əʊ ɨʊ aɨ ɑɨ ɔɨ ʊɨ ɪə	i ɪ ɛ æ ʌ ɑ ɒ ɔ ʊ u ɜ ɪ ə aɪ aʊ ɔɪ ɪə ɛə (ɔə) ʊə (eɪə əʊə aʊə ɔɪə)
Word-initial consonant mutation	Soft mutation (voiceless plosives change to voiced; voiced plosives change to voiced fricatives, though /g/ deletes; /m/ changes to /v/; /r̥/ changes to /r/; /ɬ/ changes to /l/) Nasal mutation (plosives change to homorganic nasals) Aspirate mutation (voiceless plosives change to voiceless fricatives)	None
Stress	Fixed: penultimate	Variable
Syllable structure	C_{0-3} V C_{0-2}	C_{0-3} V C_{0-4}

Note: Based on south Welsh varieties except where noted.

Appendix 4: Map showing one or more skills in the Welsh language (2001 census) by unitary authority areas

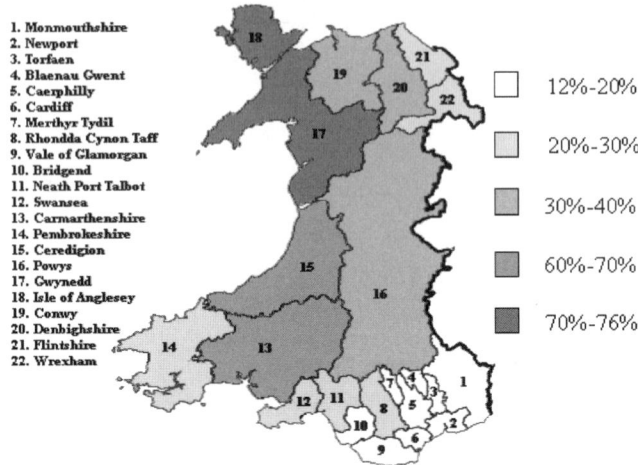

Local authority	Percentage	Ranking	Local authority	Percentage	Ranking
Gwynedd/ Gwynedd	76.1	1	Flintshire/Sir y Fflint	21.4	12
Isle of Anglesey/ Ynys Môn	70.4	2	Rhondda Cynon Taff/Rhondda Cynon Taf	21.1	13
Carmarthenshire/ Sir Gaerfyrddin	63.6	3	Bridgend/Pen-y-bont ar Ogwr	19.9	14
Ceredigion/ Ceredigion	61.2	4	Merthyr Tydfil/ Merthyr Tudful	17.7	15
Conwy/Conwy	39.7	5	Vale of Glamorgan/Bro Morgannwg	16.9	16
Denbighshire/Sir Ddinbych	36.0	6	Caerphilly/ Caerffili	16.7	17
Powys/Powys	30.1	7	Cardiff/ Caerdydd	16.3	18
Pembrokeshire/ Sir Benfro	29.4	8	Torfaen/Tor-faen	14.5	19
Neath Port Talbot/ Castell-nedd Port Talbot	28.8	9	Newport/ Casnewydd	13.4	20
Wrexham/ Wrecsam	22.9	10	Blaenau Gwent/ Blaenau Gwent	13.3	21
Swansea/ Abertawe	22.5	11	Monmouthshire/ Sir Fynwy	12.9	22

Appendix 5: Age Ranges for Segments

Age range	Dominant Welsh: Welsh	Dominant Welsh: English	Dominant English: Welsh	Dominant English: English
3;0–3;6	p t k b d g m n f v s χ h l w j	p t k b d g m n f v s h l w	p t k b d m n f s ʃ χ h tʃ dʒ l	p k b d g m n f v s z ʃ h tʃ dʒ l w j
3;6–4;0	ð ʃ tʃ dʒ	ʃ tʃ dʒ j	g v ð w j	
4;0–4;6		z		ð
4;6–5;0	ŋ θ ɬ	θ ð ʒ		t
Unacquired by 5;0	r/r̥	ŋ ɹ	ŋ θ ɬ r r̥	ŋ θ ʒ ɹ

Comparison of age emergence of Welsh and English phonemes: dominant Welsh and dominant English bilinguals (75% criterion).

Appendix 6: Age Ranges for Process

	Age ranges			
	3;0–3;6	3;6–4;0	4;0–4;6	4;6–5;0
Final consonant deletion	– – – – –			
Cluster reduction	———	– – – – –		
Stopping	– – – – –			
Fricative simplification (mostly θ)	– – – – –	– – – – –	– – – – –	– – – – –
Velar fronting (mostly ŋ)	– – – – –	– – – – –	– – – – –	– – – – –
Trill fricativisation/ approximantisation	———	———	———	———
Lateral fricative simplification/ decoupling	———	———	———	– – – – –

Note: Earlier processes are not found due to the age ranges of the children studied.

Appendix 7: Chronology of Phonological Processes for Welsh

Simplification process	Welsh–English bilinguals: Welsh		Welsh–English bilinguals: English	
	N	PD	N	PD
Cluster reduction	X	X	X	X
Final consonant deletion	X	X	X	X
Final cons devoicing	–	–	–	–
Fricative stopping/ simplification	X	X	X	X
Fronting	X	X	X	X
Liquid gliding	–	X	X	X
Assimilation	–	X	–	X
Weak syllable deletion	–	–	–	–
Trill fricativisation/ approximantisation	X	X	NA	NA
Lateral fricative simplification/ decoupling	X	X	NA	NA

Key: N = normally developing; PD = phonologically disordered; X = phonological process exhibited; NA = not applicable.
Note: The lack of some processes in the normally developing children may be due to the age range of the youngest cohort in the study being already 2;6–3;0. The results for the phonologically disordered children are based on the two children described in the chapter.

Chapter 15
Phonological Acquisition by Arabic-English Bilingual Children

G. KHATTAB

Introduction

This chapter differs from most contributions to this book in four main ways. First, most of the studies were conducted using a large number of subjects, allowing the presentation of normative data. This chapter concentrates on three bilingual subjects, but includes English and Arabic monolingual children and adult controls who were chosen from the bilinguals' immediate environment. This original approach allows a more reliable assessment of the behaviour of the bilingual subjects. The case study approach emphasises the importance of individual differences in phonological acquisition. It also allows a detailed analysis of bilingual speech using instrumental techniques that until recently have rarely been used in bilingual research. Second, while other chapters have focused on children aged between two and five, this study looks at older subjects (ages five, seven, and 10), showing that children's phonologies continue to develop after the age of five. Third, this study provides a detailed phonetic description of aspects of phonological acquisition that are important not only for understanding phonemic contrast, but that also play a role in native-like acquisition of each language and in the acquisition of sociolinguistic competence. Finally, this is one of the very few studies that have taken the language mode (Grosjean, 1998), or context, into consideration when analysing bilingual speech. Phonological and phonetic aspects of code-switches have been analysed separately from single-language utterances. This study indicates that the bilingual's production differs depending on certain contextual aspects such as the identity of their interlocutor and the base language. These factors need to be taken into consideration when interpreting bilingual phonological behaviour.

Background to the Study

This chapter presents data on consonant production by three English–Arabic bilingual children aged five, seven, and 10, who were born and raised in Yorkshire, England. These two languages have rarely been studied in combination in bilingual phonological acquisition. Several aspects of sound production by bilinguals are examined in order to contribute to existing debates on bilingual phonological acquisition (e.g. De Houwer, 1995; Genesee, 1989), in particular the issue of whether a bilingual child starts with one phonological system or two at the onset of language development. This question has produced mixed results, in part due to differences in the methodologies used in studying bilinguals, but also due to a problem that is inherent in the question itself.

It is difficult to define a system even in monolingual acquisition, due to the debate over what a phonological system looks like and at what age it emerges (Docherty et al., 2005). While in simple terms we might talk about the 'system' of English and the 'system' of Arabic, it is clear that each system is only identifiable in an abstract sense. If we focus on an aspect of the phonological system of English such as /t/, it is hard to define exactly what evidence we need to look for to decide whether a child has successfully acquired it. For example, in English, /t/ varies in its phonetic realisation according to word position. It is often aspirated in stressed syllable-initial position, unaspirated in unstressed position, and unreleased in final position (Cruttenden, 2001: 162–65). Moreover, it varies across dialects, and even systematically within its dialects. For instance, /t/ glottalling and glottalisation are frequent in many British dialects and have been shown to vary in frequency and realisation according to linguistic context but also according to social factors such as age, gender and social class (Docherty & Foulkes, 2004).

Insights from sociolinguistic studies of monolingual acquisition have argued that different types of dialectal, individual and stylistic variability are learned by children via the input they receive. Such aspects of variability constitute part of the 'system' acquired by children. Foulkes et al. (1999), Docherty and Foulkes (2000), Local (1983), Roberts (1997), Roberts and Labov (1995), and Scobbie (2005) show that there is often no stable target model for the child to acquire, and that children acquire the range of sociophonetic variation that is acceptable in their speech community and the systematic distribution of conditioned variants from a very early age. Results from these studies have important implications for bilingual as well as monolingual studies of phonological acquisition, and suggest that it is not enough to look for the acquisition of sound features that are lexically contrastive for evidence that the child has acquired a given phonological system. Therefore, when approaching the phonological aspects of both bilingual and monolingual acquisition, it is important that a thorough assessment be made of variable targets a child must aim for in order to speak like a mature member of its immediate community.

The bilingual child faces an added degree of variability by being exposed to input that may vary between standard, non-standard, and non-native varieties for either language. Studies of bilingual development, however, have mainly concentrated on a monolithic view of the two languages under investigation and have mainly taken the child's acquisition of contrastive sounds in either language as evidence for phonological differentiation. Even when comparing two standard varieties, a phoneme like /t/ might be judged as the 'same' in two languages, despite important differences that may govern its production in each language. These include subtle differences in articulatory coordination, phonotactic distribution, as well as systematic social and stylistic differences. For instance, English and Arabic /t/ may vary in place of articulation, with Lebanese Arabic /t/ being produced as a dental stop (Nasr, 1966) and British English /t/ as an alveolar one (Cruttenden, 2001). Moreover, /t/ is unaspirated in stressed syllable-initial position in Arabic (Yeni-Komshian *et al.*, 1977) but aspirated in English. It is therefore important to look for signs of acquisition of these subtle differences in /t/ realisation between the two languages when trying to establish evidence for language differentiation.

In order to take variability into account, the present study adopts a different methodology in that it does not only rely on published accounts of consonant production patterns in either language. Since it is expected that the bilinguals' social network has an influence on their linguistic choices, monolingual English friends of the bilingual children were also taped for the project, along with monolingual Arabic controls and the parents of all bilinguals and monolinguals (see section The Subjects). The study also addresses the issue of interaction (code-switching and code-mixing) between the bilingual's languages. Research has shown that interaction is inevitable, even when bilinguals acquire their languages simultaneously and show clear evidence of differentiation. This has led to the more recently adopted view that bilinguals have separate but non-autonomous phonological systems, as summarised by Grosjean (1995). However, language interaction has often been interpreted as evidence for grammatical interference (deviation from the language being spoken due to the influence of the other language), without regard to the context or the language mode in which the so-called 'interference' took place (Grosjean, 1998). This study will offer evidence for different phonological modes in the bilingual by showing that each language mode has a different impact on the bilingual's production.

Chapter Outline

This chapter will concentrate on five interrelated issues in phonological acquisition. First, a brief description of Lebanese consonants in the next section highlights some relevant phonetic and phonological differences between English and Arabic consonant production, while the Methodology section describes the methodology that was followed in the current investigation. Next, complex phonetic features are examined, in this case emphasis and voicing lead in Arabic, and the impact they have on phonological acquisition is observed. This will highlight the importance of looking at data from monolingual controls (children and adults) when studying bilinguals, as it is an essential step towards a better understanding and interpretation of results obtained from bilinguals. The examination of complex features will also show that the bilinguals' phonological systems undergo change even after the age of five. The outcome of that change is influenced by both input and age. Next, the study outlines the importance of looking at detailed sociophonetic features. A look at sociolinguistic competence in bilinguals shows how they may deploy acquired features to suit certain communicative contexts but also how their speech undergoes parental, societal, and language mode influence.

Lebanese Consonants

Aspects of Egyptian Arabic phonology (phonemic inventory, syllable structure, phonotactics) are covered by Ammar and Morsi (this volume). Consonants are discussed here (Table 15.1) in more detail due to differences in the sound inventories of Lebanese and Egyptian Arabic and because this chapter will mainly concentrate on consonantal aspects in the bilinguals' production.

Notes on sounds in brackets: In Arabic, no native /p/ exists. However, proper names and loan words, principally from French (*piscine, pyjama*), are frequent in the Lebanese dialect and are usually produced with [p] by the majority of people, especially if they are highly educated. [b] and [ḅ] can also be heard as realisations for [p], especially among the uneducated. Similarly, no native /g/ exists in Lebanese Arabic, but people usually produce it accurately in loan words (e.g. *garage, gateau*). /g/ is also familiar to the Lebanese due to its use in nearby Arabic dialects such as Palestinian and Egyptian (e.g. Al-Shareef, 2002; Ammar and Morsi, this volume). However, [k] is sometimes heard as a realisation for /g/ in loan words. As for /q/, it is mainly realised as [ʔ] in Lebanese Arabic, although a handful of lexical items that are borrowed from classical Arabic have kept the original [q] pronunciation (e.g. [quṭḅ] 'pole'). /θ/ and /ð/ are restricted to standard Arabic usage (e.g. news reading, sermons, etc.) and are normally realised as [t] (or [s]) and [d] (e.g.

Table 15.1 Lebanese–Arabic consonants

	Bilabial	Labio-dental	Dental	Alveolar	Post-alveolar	Palatal	Velar	Pharyngeal	Glottal
	(p) b		t d tˤ dˤ				k (g) (q)		ʔ
		f	(θ) (ð)	s z sˤ dˤ	ʃ ʒ		x ɣ (χ) (ʁ)	ħ ʕ	h
					(tʃ) (dʒ)				
	m			n					
				ɾ r					
	w			l lˤ		j			

[tleːte] for /θalaːθa/ 'three'; [sawɾa] for /θawɾa/; [danab] for /ðanab/ 'tail'). Finally, [χ] and [ʁ] are in free variation with [x] and [ɣ], while /tʃ/ and /dʒ/ are either produced in loan words (e.g. *Chernobyl*; *jeans*) or are realisation of CVC syllables with reduced vowels (e.g. [tʃamːas] for /taʃamːasa/ 'he sun-bathed').

Methodology

The subjects

A total of 23 subjects were recorded for this study, including three English–Arabic bilingual children and three monolingual children from each language, along with both parents of all children (Table 15.2). With respect to the children, there are three age groups (5, 7 and 10) and all subjects in a given group are of the same sex. Two of the monolingual children (A5 and A7) and two of the bilinguals (B7 and B10) are siblings, so there are only four parents in each of the bilingual and monolingual Arabic groups.

The monolingual English subjects are close friends of the bilinguals. Although the monolinguals were born and raised in Yorkshire, their parents come from different areas in Britain. The bilingual subjects are children of Lebanese families who have lived in Yorkshire for over 10 years. All the bilinguals' parents are native speakers of Lebanese Arabic and mainly use Arabic with their children at home, but code-switching is a common feature in the speech of parents and children alike. All three children started attending English nurseries from around age 1;0 and all are English-dominant. The only contact that the children have with Arabic is from their parents and a couple of other Lebanese families living in other cities. The families are keen on bringing up the children as bilinguals and have positive attitudes towards both languages. The monolingual Arabic subjects were chosen from the same district as the bilinguals' parents in the Lebanon.

Procedure

Tape-recording sessions took place in the subjects' homes and were designed around picture-naming activities, story-telling and free-play sessions for the children, and word lists, story-telling and interviews for the adults. A Tascam DA-P1 DAT recorder was used during all sessions, with Trantec external microphones clipped to the subjects' clothes. For the picture-naming activities, the bilingual children were recorded twice, following a one-language-per-session format in order to control for the language context. While I conducted the sessions with the children in English, the mothers were asked to conduct the Arabic sessions on the basis that the children would be more likely to use Arabic with their parents than with anybody else in their

Table 15.2 Details of subjects and their parents

Subject	Age	Sex	Mother	Father
Monolingual English				
E5	5;5	F	EF5	EM5
E7	7;5	M	EF7	EM7
E10	10;3	M	EF10	EM10
Bilingual				
B5	5;6	F	BF5	BM5
B7	7;1	M	BF7	BM7
B10	10;2	M		
Monolingual Arabic				
A5	5;4	F	AF5	AM5
A7	7;4	M		
A10	10;3	M	AF10	AM10
Total = 23		9	7	7

environment. However, while the children used only English in the English sessions, they frequently reverted to code-switching during the Arabic sessions or responded in English even when the mothers were asking them questions in Arabic.

The code-switched utterances were analysed and interpreted separately from the single-language utterances and proved significant in the overall interpretation of the results. The consonants or consonantal features that were analysed in both languages include: (1) Voice Onset Time (VOT) patterns in voiced and voiceless stops (mainly /p t k/ and /b d g/), (2) /r/ production and phonotactic rules governing its realisation in each language, and (3) /l/ production and the social and phonetic factors governing its realisation in different syllable positions. Detailed results for all the consonants examined in this study can be found in Khattab (1998, 2002a, b, c). The next five sections present the most salient findings in terms of the discussion of the main issues that were outlined previously.

The Acquisition of Complex Phonetic Features

Developmental features in phonological acquisition often appear in a child's production when a given phonetic feature that is being acquired is complex and requires mature articulatory ability before adult-like production can be attained. Immature productions appear in the speech of monolingual and bilingual children alike, and it is therefore important to be aware of the developmental patterns that are expected for a given language when looking at bilingual production. Otherwise the child's bilingual background tends to be used as an explanation that is often based on the concept of 'interference' (e.g. Weinreich, 1953) from the bilingual's other language. Two examples will be used to illustrate this point, emphasis and voice onset time (VOT) acquisition in Arabic.

Emphatic /l/ in Arabic

Arabic /l/ is clear in all word positions (e.g. [liːfe] 'sponge' and [fiːl] 'elephant'), apart from when it is found in limited emphatic environments. These include (1) an emphatic context e.g. [lˤabatˤ] 'he kicked', (2) words involving the name of God e.g. [alˤlˤa], and (3) unpredictable words, sometimes loan words e.g. [ˈlˤambˤa] 'lamp' (Anani, 1985: 130). In terms of articulatory properties, clear [l] in Arabic embodies a back cavity shape of a wide unobstructed pharynx and a gradual narrowing of the mouth cavity towards the region of articulatory constriction, while dark [lˤ] has another place of articulation dividing the back cavity behind the alveolar point of articulation (Anani, 1985: 130).

/l/ production normally emerges earlier in Arabic than in English (around the age of 2;0–2;6), reaches an acceptable performance around the age of 3;6, and is fully mastered around the age of six (Amayreh & Dyson, 1998, 2000; Dyson & Amayreh; 2000; Omar, 1973). Developmental processes include cluster reduction e.g. [keːb̥] 'dogs' for adult [kleːb], assimilation, e.g. [ˈħiwwe] 'pretty' for adult [ˈħilwe], and gliding, which is less frequent in Arabic than in English and tends to be restricted to [j] (e.g. [ˈʔajam] 'pen' for adult [ˈʔalam]; [ħajiːb] 'milk' for adult [ħaliːb]). Another rare substitution for /l/ in Arabic is [n] (Dyson & Amayreh, 2000: 109).

As for emphatic [lˤ], the difficulty in its production is related to the general difficulty experienced by Arab children in acquiring emphatics due to the articulatory complexity of these sounds. Emphatics involve simultaneous articulatory postures, one for the primary place of articulation of the consonant and another one in the velo-pharyngeal area of the mouth (Ferguson, 1956). Emphasis is therefore one of the sound features that are acquired very late in children and often remain only partially developed until the age of 14 (Dyson & Amayreh, 2000: 84; Omar, 1973: 55). The usual pattern that appears in the production of emphatics by children is de-emphasis, i.e. the loss of the secondary articulation and therefore producing the plain counterpart of the emphatic sound in question, e.g. [latiːf] for adult [lˤatˤiːf]. Though the incidence of de-emphasis gradually declines with age, it does not easily disappear and sometimes persists even after the age of six due to the infrequency and low functional load of emphatics in Arabic (Dyson & Amayreh, 2000: 100).

In the current study, the /l/ tokens that were produced by the subjects in an emphatic environment were smaller in number than those for initial and final environments. For this reason, results below are presented in tokens rather than percentages. Figures 15.1 and 15.2 show the patterns for /l/ production in emphatic environments by both adults and children.

Starting with the adults, it is interesting to note that none of the speakers produces categorical dark [lˤ]'s in all the target tokens. There are various reasons for this finding. First, emphasis did not always spread to the next syllable ([e.g. [ʕadˤaˈleːt] 'muscles'; [ˈtˤɑːwle] 'table') or to the preceding one (e.g. [maxˈluːtˤa] 'mixed nuts'; [lˈʔarədˤ] 'the earth'; [ˈjɪlbʊtˤ] 'he shoots'). Even when /l/ occurred in the same syllable as the emphatic sound, it tended to be de-emphasised if it occurred in word final position (e.g. [basˤal] 'onions'; [batˤel] 'hero'). Apart from contextual differences, there were individual differences among the speakers in that some of them produced plain rather than emphatic consonants in some of the tokens, which ruled out the possibility of a dark [lˤ] since the emphatic context that is needed to trigger it was lost. There was a slight tendency for males to produce more emphatics than females, which is a pattern reported for other dialects as well (Kahn, 1975). But the major

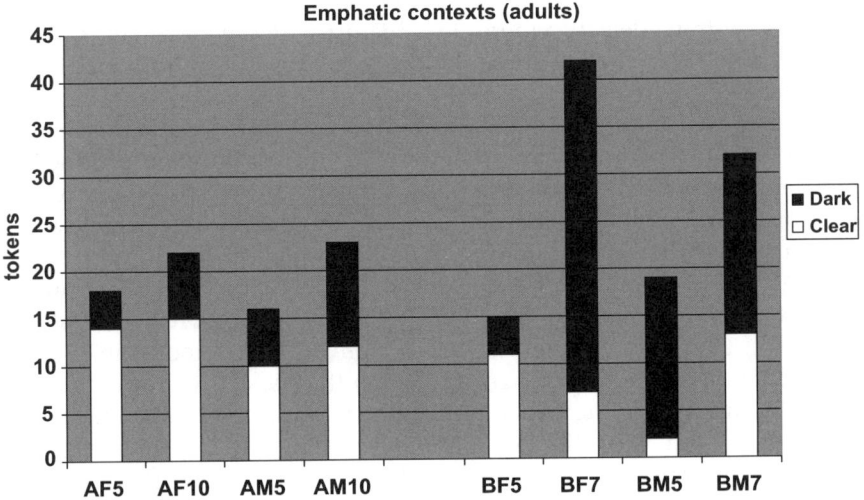

Figure 15.1 Results for /l/ in emphatic contexts in Arabic by the monolinguals' parents (left) and the bilinguals' parents (right) [*n* (tokens) = 187]

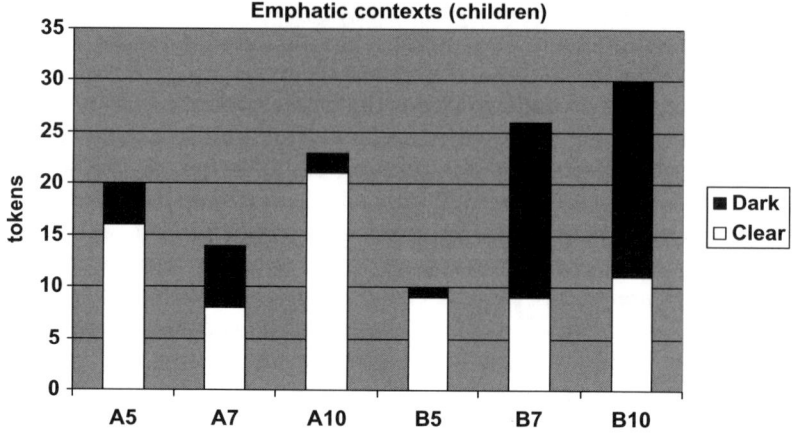

Figure 15.2 Results for /l/ in emphatic contexts in Arabic by the monolingual Arabic and the bilingual children ($n = 123$)

difference between the speakers was not due to gender. It emerged that the two speakers who produced emphatic tokens the most belong to the same family (BF7 and BM7) and produce emphatic glottal stops that are otherwise plain in the other speakers' productions (e.g. [ħalˤaʔˤ] as opposed to [ħalaʔ] 'earrings'; [ʔˤlˤeːm]as opposed to [ʔleːm] 'pens'). Such behaviour appears to be particular to the accent of certain localities within Beirut, where the historic uvular plosive [q] that changed into [ʔ] in the Lebanese dialect is still produced with emphasis, therefore [ʔˤ].

The contextual, accentual and individual variability in the production of the adults seems to be reflected in the children's production (Figure 15.2). Many of the emphatic consonants in the target words were produced as their plain counterparts by all children, which ruled out the possibility of examining /l/'s (e.g. [dalːit] for [dˤalˤːit] 'she stayed'). Even when emphatic consonants were produced, emphasis did not always spread to the /l/'s (e.g. [basˤɐl] 'onions'; [ʕadˤɐˈleːt] 'muscles'). There did not seem to be any noticeable differences in emphasis production depending on age or whether the subjects were bilingual or monolingual. Rather, the two subjects who produce emphatic tokens the most are B7 and B10, BF7 and BM7's children. The two brothers also produce emphatic glottal stops (e.g. [ˈʔˤalˤʕa] 'fortress'; [ˈlˤaʔˤɪt] 'she found'; [ˈʔˤaːlˤɪt] 'she found'). This might be interpreted as evidence for the importance of input in the acquisition of complex and accent-specific features. Variability in the input seems to be attended to rather than ignored during the process of acquisition (Foulkes *et al.*, 2005).

In sum, /l/ realisations in emphatic contexts proved to be highly variable in their production due to developmental, contextual, social, and accentual factors (e.g. Kahn, 1975; Lehn, 1963; Mitchell, 1993). Such variability points to the difficulty in assessing whether any child has acquired its production and it is therefore not surprising that both the monolingual and the bilingual children produced a great number of clear [l]'s. What is interesting though is that two of the bilinguals actually produced more emphatic [lˤ]'s than the monolingual controls. This may be due to an accent feature that was revealed in the speech of the bilinguals' parents (emphatic glottal stops [ʔˤ]) and that is not well-documented in the literature.

Voice Onset Time (VOT)

While the contrast in homorganic stops in English is mainly one of aspiration, Arabic follows a binary system of presence or absence of glottal pulsing during the closure period of the stop (e.g. Flege & Port, 1981: 126; Yeni-Komshian et al., 1977: 35) (Figure 15.3).

VOT acquisition studies in English suggest that usual development for all stops is to be initially produced in the short lag range during the early acquisition stages (e.g. Foulkes et al., 1999; Gilbert, 1977; Kewley-Port & Preston, 1974; Macken & Barton, 1980a; Simon, 1976, 1978a,b; Snow, 1997; Stoel-Gammon & Buder, 1999; Zlatin & Koenigsknecht, 1976). By 24 months, VOT distinctions usually start to emerge, and the production is extended to the long lag and long lead ranges. Children are also known to produce VOT with longer duration and more variability than adults do. Adult-like consistency is usually achieved around 10–12 years of age, after reductions in the duration of speech sounds and in variability gradually have taken place. Still, there are important individual differences in

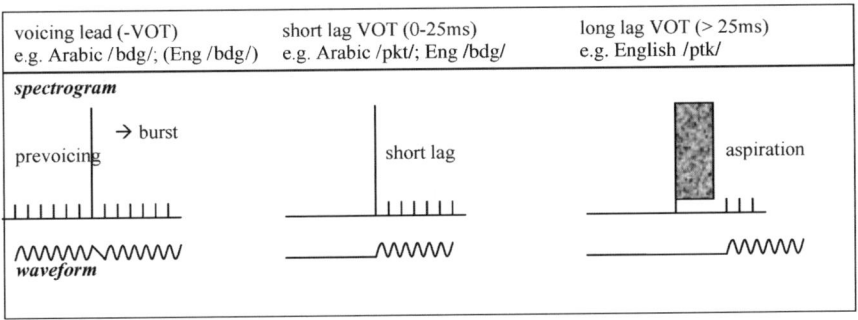

Figure 15.3 Schematic representation of the VOT continuum which shows the relationship between English and Arabic stops

the developmental patterns of children, and gradual decrease in the duration of sounds is not always the norm (cf. Smith & Kenny, 1999).

Acquisition of voicing lead

A number of studies have shown that voicing lead develops late (e.g. Allen, 1985; Konefal & Fokes, 1981; Macken & Barton, 1980b). In physiological terms, the difficulty in producing voicing lead is due to the fact that, when the pressure increase behind the stop closure reaches the level of subglottal pressure, transglottal airflow ceases and voicing is difficult (Docherty, 1992: 62; Ohala, 1997: 687). Children, with shorter vocal tracts, will be unable to sustain voicing in this condition for as long as adults, which may prompt them to seek compensatory strategies if they are attempting to match the values of adult speech. Some of these strategies include spirantisation of voiced stops, which was observed by Macken and Barton (1980b) for Spanish-speaking children. They found that Spanish children first produced predominantly short lag stops as monolingual English children did, but that the Spanish lead/lag voicing contrast did not develop as early as the English contrast (Macken & Barton, 1980a). Few tokens of voicing lead stops were found in the data for their two-year-old subjects, and even the four-year-olds had not fully developed the lead/lag contrast. Most of their tokens fell in the short lag range, and the evidence of voicing contrast that they used was often based on short lag for VOICELESS versus continuants for VOICED. Similar results were found from other studies on Spanish and French (Allen, 1985; Konefal & Fokes, 1981). Allen (1985) reported prenasalisation and prevocalisation with an oral or nasalised vowel by 1;9–2;8 aged French speakers, while Heselwood and McChrystal (2000) reported all of the above features in their 10-year-old Punjabi–English bilinguals, with different subjects choosing different strategies.

There are hardly any studies on the acquisition of VOT by Arabic children, let alone Lebanese ones. One exception is the study by Preston *et al.* (1967), who attempted a cross-cultural comparison of apical stop production by one Lebanese and one American infant who were both 12 months old. The authors' findings were similar to those of the French and Spanish data, as both infants produced their stops in the short lag region with VOT values ranging between 0 and 30 ms. Preston *et al.* (1967) concluded that short VOT intervals may be the easiest for infants to accomplish as opposed to voicing lead and long lag which require careful timing between supraglottal and glottal articulators.

VOT in bilingual studies

Several investigations into the phonological acquisition of bilingual children have compared the production and/or perception of VOT in their subjects' languages, especially where the two languages differ in their use of the VOT continuum, as in English and French (e.g. Caramazza *et al.*, 1973; Elman *et al.*, 1977), English and Spanish (e.g. Bond *et al.*, 1980; Deuchar & Clark, 1995), English and Portuguese (e.g. Sancier & Fowler, 1997; Rocca & Marcelino, 1999) or English and Punjabi (e.g. Heselwood & McChrystal, 2000). In all cases, the languages being examined are described as having similar phonological contrasts in terms of the binary opposition between VOICED and VOICELESS stops (except for Punjabi, which has a three-way contrast), but as differing in their phonetic realisation of the voicing contrast in that English follows the short lag – long lag distinction, whereas French, Spanish and Portuguese follow the voicing lead – short lag distinction.

Overall, studies suggest that bilinguals behave in ways that are at once distinct from monolinguals but also very similar to them. During the early stages of production, it is often difficult to look for signs of differentiation between the VOT systems of two languages since (1) the little amount of data produced by the child at this stage does not allow for any firm conclusions to be drawn (Deuchar & Clark, 1995) and (2) the production of certain phonetic categories (e.g. voicing lead) is at the mercy of articulatory maturation and therefore affects both bilingual and monolingual production (e.g. Macken & Barton, 1980a, b). At a later stage, some studies have found that bilinguals do develop monolingual-like VOT production patterns for each language (e.g. Bond *et al.*, 1980), whereas others note that there might still be subtle acoustic differences that are imperceptible to the listener (e.g. Watson, 1991). In the case of late and/or less proficient bilinguals, on the other hand, noticeable signs of interference from the VOT patterns of the first and/or dominant language have been documented (Rocca & Marcelino, 1999).

VOT results for VOICED stops from the current study

Looking at the bilinguals' results first (Figure 15.4), it seems that two of the subjects (B5 and B10) have not acquired voicing lead for Arabic. Instead, they are applying the short lag pattern for the production of their VOICED stops in both languages. While this can be interpreted as interference from English, results from the monolingual Arabic controls (Figure 15.5) show that all three subjects also produce short lag for some of their VOICED stop productions. In this case, however, there are signs of gradual approximation towards adult-like figures according to age (the percentage of prevoiced tokens increases with age). Possible reasons for why bilinguals do not show similar progression towards adult values for their VOICED stops are discussed in the following two sections. What is important at this stage is to highlight the role of including controls in the design of bilingual studies. Results from monolingual data in this study show signs of incomplete acquisition of the voicing lead

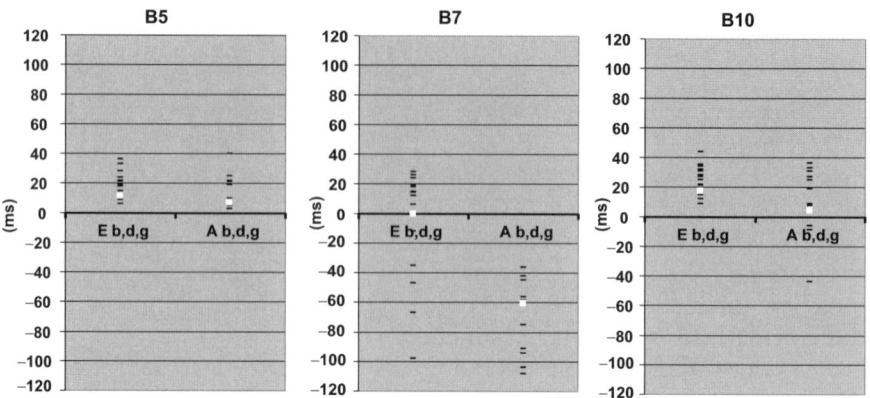

Figure 15.4 Mean VOT values (white squares) and distributions (in ms) for English and Arabic /b d g/ as produced by the three bilingual subjects ($n = 190$)

even up to the age of 10. These results are similar to the ones reported for Spanish and French children (see Acquisition of Voicing Lead section). They suggest that the lack of prevoiced tokens in the bilinguals' data is not only due to influence from English, but may also be due to developmental factors.

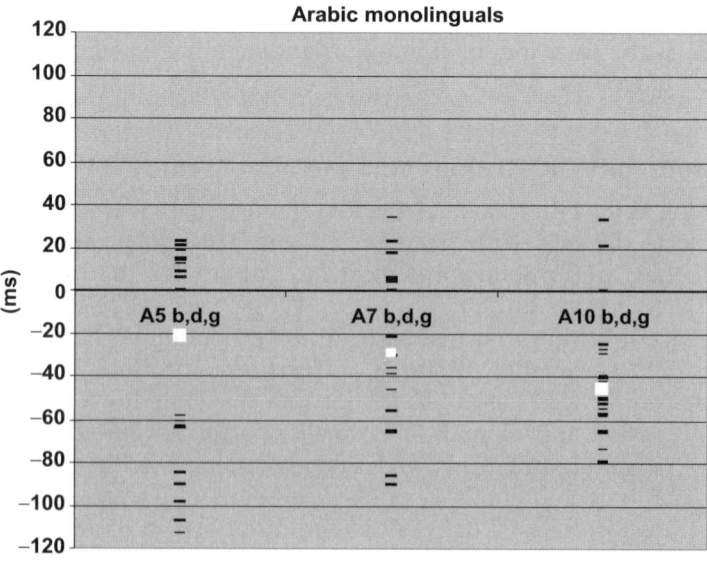

Figure 15.5 Mean VOT values (white squares) and distributions (in ms) for Arabic /b d g/ as produced by the three monolingual Arabic subjects ($n = 86$)

The Role of Input

As noted earlier, not all studies have taken adult input into consideration. One exception is Deuchar and Clark's (1995) study, which shows how the child's adoption of a given VOT pattern (in this case voicing lag instead of voicing lead for Spanish VOICED stops) might actually be traced to the input that she receives (in this case that of her native-English mother who also spoke Spanish to the child). Watson's (1991) study shows that both bilingual and monolingual adults exhibit a lot of variability in their productions, which might in turn be displayed in the children's productions.

In the current study, B7 seems to be the only bilingual who uses prevoicing for his VOICED stops in both English and Arabic. What is particular about B7's prevoiced stops in both languages is that in the majority of his prevoiced tokens (six out of nine tokens in English and 11 out of 24 in Arabic), the auditory impression was that of a homorganic nasal preceding the stop (e.g. [əm'bɛd³ɹʉm] 'bedroom'; ['mbaʔrɐ] for /'baʔra/ 'cow'), or of an implosive (e.g. ['ɓʌtʰə] for 'butter'). Spectrographic analysis revealed that the laryngeal voicing preceding these stops was accompanied by energy above the F0 level and traces of formant structure (Figure 15.6), thus confirming the auditory impression. B7's use of a nasal-like sound can be seen as a strategy that is not dissimilar to that of Allen's (1985) monolingual French subjects who preceded French VOICED targets with a nasal or a vowel segment that permitted continuous voicing, Macken and Barton's (1980b) monolingual Spanish subjects who spirantised their Spanish VOICED stops, or Heselwood and McChrystal's (2000) Punjabi–English subjects who showed both features. In all four cases (Arabic, French, Spanish and Punjabi), the subjects are choosing an articulation that does not involve a complete obstruction of

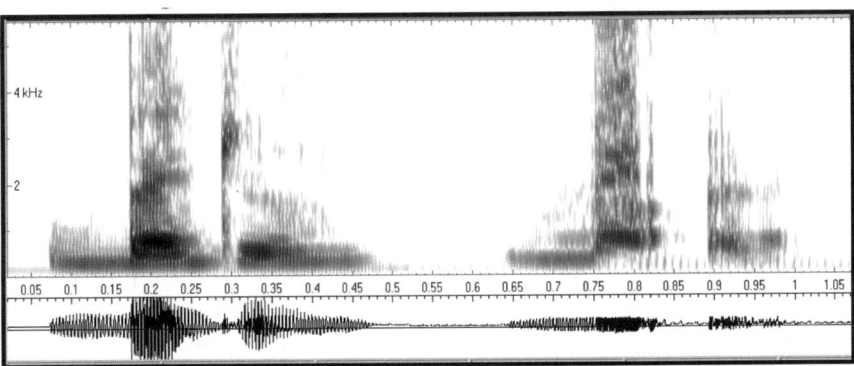

Figure 15.6 Spectrogram of the words 'bedroom' (left) and /'baʔra/ 'cow' (right) as produced by B7 as [əm'bɛd³ɹʉm] and ['mbaʔrɐ], respectively

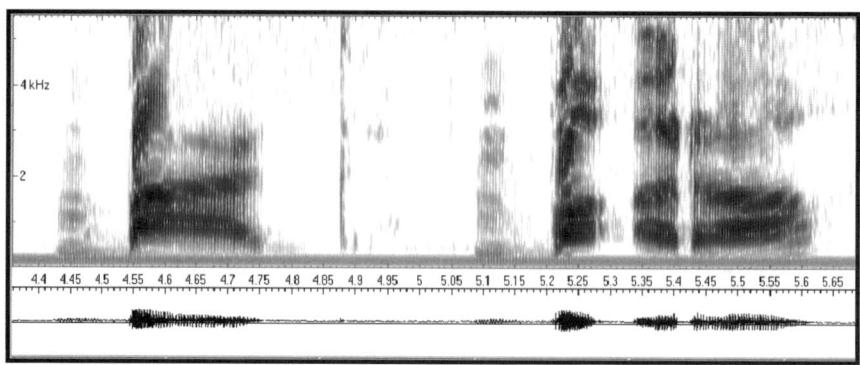

Figure 15.7 Spectrogram of the words 'bag' (left) and /'baʔra/ 'cow' (right) as produced by BF7 as [ᵊmbag] and [ᵊm'baʔra], respectively

the airstream in order for them to prolong the voicing articulation. B7's production of implosives can also be considered as another strategy used to maintain glottal vibration (Heselwood, 1998).

However, nasals and implosives may not only be showing signs of developmental features by B7, as closer analysis of his mother's prevoiced tokens (BF7) revealed very similar patterns. BF7 frequently produced audible and acoustically detectable nasals before her VOICED stops in English and Arabic (Figure 15.7). The nasals were homorganic with the stops, e.g. [mbɛːr] 'bear', [ndoːr] 'door' and were sometimes preceded by what sounded like a schwa, e.g. [ᵊm'baʔra] for 'cow'. Note that these tokens did not sound like pause-fillers as might be expected, and only occurred with voiced tokens, never with voiceless ones.

The Interaction Between Input and Age in Phonological Development

The VOT results that were presented in Figure 15.4 suggested that B7 was the only bilingual subject to have acquired the voicing lead associated with Arabic VOICED stops while B5 and B10 produce their VOICED stops with short lag. A further examination of the differences in the production of Arabic VOICED stops by the two bilingual brothers B7 and B10 was conducted. The aim was to investigate how each of the patterns emerged in the production of each child and what factors affected their acquisition in such a way that only B7 acquired voicing lead in Arabic. Results from an earlier study conducted with B7 and B10 only (Khattab, 1998) show that 18 months prior to the current study, neither of the two brothers had acquired voicing lead in Arabic yet. Only /b/, /d/, /t/ and /k/ tokens were collected for Arabic in the 1998 study, but the VOT patterns obtained then offer the opportunity to trace the development of VOT patterns in the two subjects over a period of 18 months. At the time of the recording for the later study (Khattab, 2002a), the brothers had been attending a weekend Arabic school for 15 months. The outcome of these changes was an increased input in Arabic for the two brothers. At the time of the first recording the parents were the only source of Arabic to the children. One can safely assume that such an increase in Arabic input would increase their exposure to prevoiced stops from a variety of Arabic speakers.

Looking at B7's developmental changes in Arabic (Figure 15.8), one can notice a major change in VOT patterns for his VOICED stops. While in 1998 B7's /b d/ production in Arabic fell mainly in the short lag region, his production markedly changed by the time of the second recording. Most of his VOICED stops are now produced with voicing lead. The differences between the 1998 and 2000 values are significant for both /b/ and /d/ (t-test, $p < 0.001$). B10, on the other hand, shows no significant difference in his VOT production patterns between 1998 and 2000.

Knowing that the two brothers experienced the same changes in Arabic input, the uneven change in their behaviour may be attributed to their age. B7 was still five years old when he experienced the increased Arabic input and showed faster and greater development than his brother. B10 was eight and had developed more stable patterns that may have been more difficult to change despite the new increase in Arabic input. As in monolingual situations, the acquisition of certain complex features that require early and extensive exposure might therefore be delayed or not acquired if these features are lacking in the input. B10 was probably past the 'critical' age required for the acquisition of voicing lead (Flege, 1995).

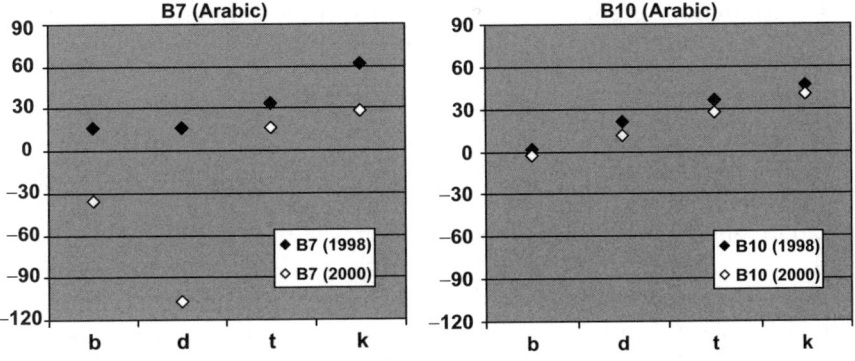

Figure 15.8 Mean VOT values for Arabic /b, d, t, k/ as produced by B7 and B10 in 1998 and 2000 ($n = 176$)

Acquisition of Socio-Phonetic Features

In this section, the bilinguals' production of sounds that are known to vary in their production in the two languages according to sociolinguistic factors such as age, dialect and style are investigated. The aim is to examine whether the bilinguals have acquired sociolinguistically appropriate realisations for these sounds. This issue has not been the main focus of research on bilingualism due to the predominant interest in looking for evidence for the acquisition of sounds that are important for lexical contrast in the respective languages. But as mentioned in the background to this chapter, this study adopts the view that variability in the speech input that a child is exposed to constitutes part of the 'system' acquired by children and is acquired at a very early age as part of the development of their sociolinguistic competence. Data from (l) and (r) production are presented here to illustrate this issue.

(l) Patterns

In many varieties of English, clear [l] occurs mainly in syllable-initial position ('lip' [lɪp]; 'sailor' ['seɪlə]; 'blow' [bləʊ]), whereas dark [ɫ] tends to occur in syllable-final and syllabic position ('peel' [piːɫ]; 'bulb' [bʌɫb]; 'table' [teɪbɫ̩]/) (e.g. Cruttenden, 2001: 201). However, this allophonic difference does not hold for all dialects. For instance, in Yorkshire, there is little phonetic distinction between syllable-initial and syllable finals /l/'s. Wells (1982: 371) describes initial /l/ as 'dark-ish'. Moreover, some dialects of English permit vocalisation of syllable-final /l/ with a range of back vocoids used as the reflex of [ɫ] e.g. 'milk' [miʊk], 'fill' [fɪʏ]. It is well known that vocalisation is spreading rapidly through the urban dialects of England (Wells, 1982).

In this study /l/ was analysed in order to find out whether the bilinguals show any signs of initial dark /l/'s and/or vocalised final /l/'s in their production. Figures 15.9 and 15.10 show the English /l/ patterns that were found for the bilinguals and monolinguals from this study. Results are presented as raw tokens.

Both monolingual and bilingual groups produce few initial dark [ɫ]'s. Although it was expected that Yorkshire /l/'s would be dark in all positions (Wells, 1982), it emerged that some but not all of the monolingual English parents recorded for this study produced dark initial [ɫ]'s (Khattab, 2002b). What is important though is that results for the bilinguals (who also produce initial clear [l]'s) turned out to be similar to those of the monolinguals of the same age. Therefore the bilinguals' behaviour should not necessarily be interpreted as a failure to acquire sociolinguistic features that are present in their environment, or as an influence from their parents' L2 productions. In coda position, on the

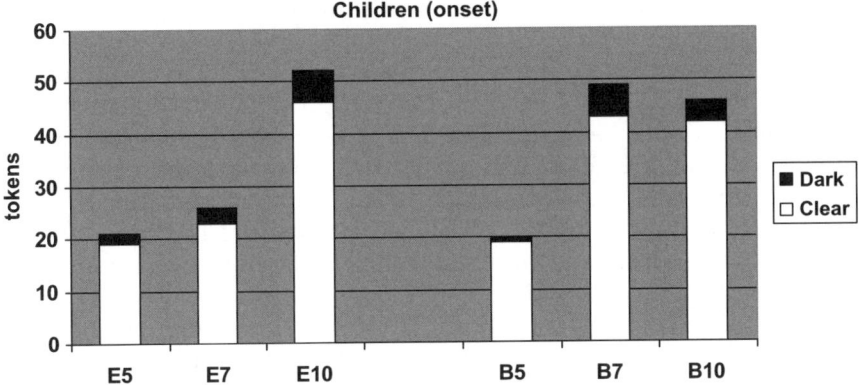

Figure 15.9 Results for /l/ in onset position in English for the monolingual and bilingual children ($n = 214$)

other hand, both groups of children seem to follow the monolingual adult patterns in terms of the production of dark [ɫ]'s, despite the fact that the bilinguals' parents mainly produce clear [l]'s in this position (Khattab, 2002b). The bilingual children also produce a small number of clear [l]'s, but these seem to decrease in number with age. Clear [l]'s also appeared in the production of the monolingual English five-year-old, and may be part of developmental features, as clear [l] is normally

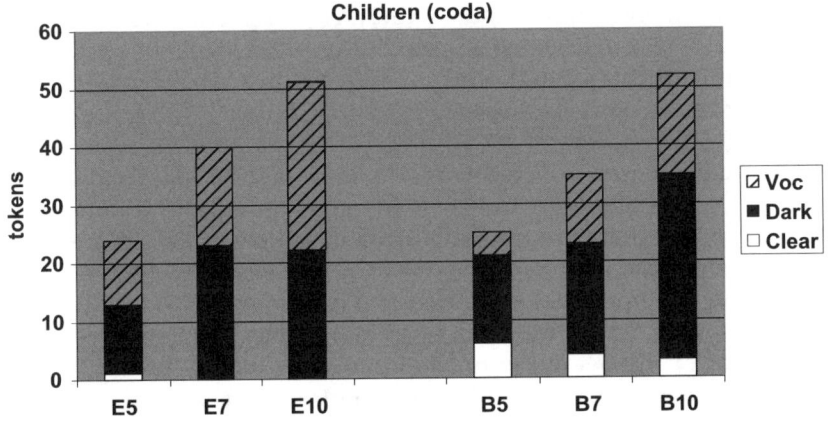

Figure 15.10 Results for syllable-final /l/ in English by the monolingual and bilingual children (E = English; B = Bilingual) ($n = 229$)

acquired before dark [ɫ], the latter being prone to gliding and vocalic substitutions (Cruttenden, 2001: 204). What's more interesting is that vocalised /l/'s seem to gradually increase with age for both groups of children (Figure 15.10). This rules out the possible interpretation that vocalisation is only being produced here as a developmental feature, since we would predict that it would gradually disappear with age. Here, /l/ vocalisation is maintained by the children and, since it was also found in the monolingual English parents' production (Khattab, 2002b), it can be considered an accent feature in the children's community. Therefore, the bilingual children not only show evidence of having acquired the expected dark variant (despite a small number of clear [l]'s), but also show possible signs of sensitivity to local sociolinguistic norms by producing a considerable amount of /l/ vocalisation.

(r) Patterns

In most English accents, /r/ is produced as a voiced alveolar or post-alveolar approximant [ɹ] (Hughes & Trudgill, 1996: 90; Wells, 1982: 368) while the Arabic /r/ is mainly realised as a tap or a trill, depending on free and allophonic variation (Anani, 1985: 132; Nasr, 1966: 5; Shaheen, 1979: 142). Moreover, most urban Yorkshire accents are non-rhotic, i.e. post-vocalic /r/ is absent before a consonant or in absolute final position, e.g. *farm* [fɑːm]; *far* [fɑː] (Cruttenden, 1994: 268; Hughes & Trudgill, 1996: 33; Wells, 1982: 368). Arabic /r/, on the other hand, is produced in all contexts.

The production of [ɹ] is known to involve physically complex articulations and usually emerges late in children's speech, commonly around the age of 4;5 in English (Cruttenden, 2001: 209; Edwards, 1973: 9; Vihman, 1996: 219, 239), and 5;6 in Arabic (Amayreh & Dyson, 1998: 646; Omar, 1973: 48–56). In English, [ɹ] is frequently replaced by [w] and [ʋ] in initial position, e.g. 'rabbit' [wæbɪʔ]; 'red' [ʋɛd]. In Arabic, developmental features normally include deletion e.g. [naː] 'fire' for adult [naːɾ], assimilation, e.g. [ʔikkab] 'I ride' for adult [ˈʔirkab] and substitution, which is more frequent and mainly involves lateralisation, e.g. [ˈlasam] 'he drew' for adult [ˈrasam]. Another occasional type of /r/ substitution is gliding of /r/ to [j], but there are normally no occurrences of [w] for either /r/ or /l/. This pattern is quite different from English where /r/ gliding to [w] is frequent whereas lateralisation is uncommon.

Acquisition of /r/ by bilinguals has mainly been looked at as part of case studies of the overall phonological development of a given child. While early views argue for an initial single system for the acquisition of /r/'s by bilinguals (e.g. Leopold, 1970), later studies offer evidence for the bilinguals' ability to distinguish between the patterns of /r/ production in each of their languages from an early age (e.g. Ball *et al.*, 2001c; Ingram, 1982). In this study /r/ tokens were collected from words produced in isolation during the picture-naming and story-telling activities for the children. All the words that had 'r's in the spelling as well as in the pronunciation were examined in both languages in order to compare the occurrence of post-vocalic /r/'s by different subjects and in different languages. Figures 15.11 and 15.12 show the /r/ results for the bilingual and monolingual children from this study.

The patterns produced by the bilinguals were on the whole similar to those of the monolinguals. In English, both groups of children mainly produced the alveolar approximant [ɹ], while [ʊ] showed a gradual decrease across age groups. In Arabic, both groups of children produced mainly taps and trills, and sporadic productions of the approximant [ɹ]. Within tap production, there was a weak variant [ɾ] that was also found in the adults' production and that showed possible gender correlation that was being picked up by the children (see discussion of this variant in Khattab, 2002c).

Developmental features such as omissions, assimilations and substitutions appeared in the productions of all three groups of children. However, there were two differences between the bilinguals and the monolinguals in Arabic. First, developmental features in the monolingual group decreased with age whereas in the bilingual group, B7 had more omissions and other realisations of /r/ than B5. Still, B10 had the lowest number of omissions and other realisations. Second, other realisations by the monolingual Arabic children included variants normally reported in the literature for children acquiring Arabic, e.g. [l], [j] and [n] and assimilation to a following obstruent (Dyson & Amayreh, 2000). The bilinguals, on the other hand, produced these and other realisations

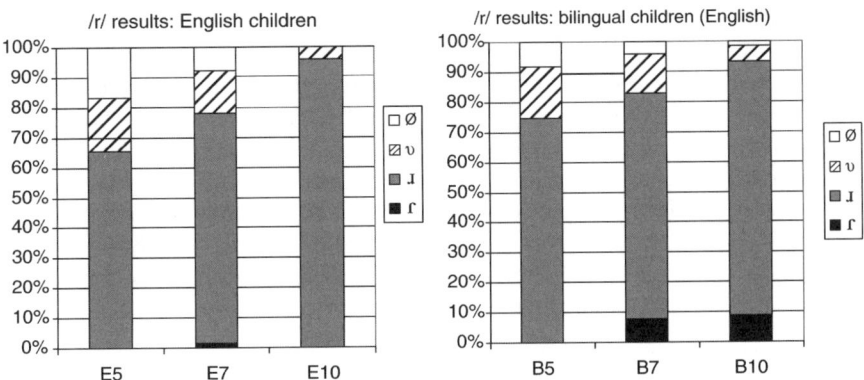

Figure 15.11 Results for the English /r/ variants produced by the monolingual and bilingual children during the English sessions. 'Ø' includes deletions and other realisations ($n = 440$)

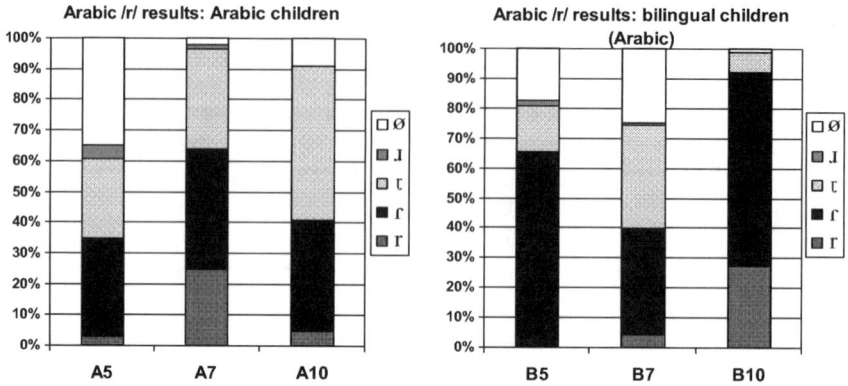

Figure 15.12 Results for the different Arabic /r/ variants produced by the monolingual and bilingual children. 'Ø' includes deletions and other realisations ($n = 726$)

not normally reported for monolingual Arabic children, including retroflex taps, retroflex approximants and rhoticised vowels e.g. [ɚ], [ɪ˞] and [a˞]. These realisations suggest that the bilinguals have a wider repertoire of /r/ sounds than that of the monolinguals and the interaction between Arabic, native-English, and other non-native varieties of English that the children are exposed to. The bilinguals' /r/ patterns in Arabic were still significantly different from the ones found for English.

Role of Language Mode

So far, the data presented in this chapter have been taken from the English-only or Arabic-only sessions that were conducted with the bilingual subjects. But as mentioned previously, the bilinguals frequently reverted to code-switching during the Arabic sessions or responded in English even when the mothers were asking them questions in Arabic. The English code-switches that were produced by the children during the Arabic sessions displayed phonetic patterns that were different from the patterns observed during the English-only sessions. While most tokens were taken from isolated words (Example 1), others were part of an utterance (Example 2).

1   **Mother** (pointing at a kettle):   [ʃu haɪda]?
                                                   What that (masc.)?
                                                   'What is that?'
    Child: ['kɛtəl]
                                                     KETTLE

2 **Child** (describing an action):   [natˤtˤo bɪl puːl]
jump-past-3rd pers.pl. in <u>POOL</u>
'they jumped in the pool'

The code-switched tokens that were found for each of the phonetic features being studied were not numerous. Still, they needed to be examined separately from the data presented so far in order to test the difference in patterns that the children exhibited depending on the language context. As most of the code-switches to English contained lexical items that the bilinguals had also produced in the English sessions, this allowed direct comparison of two productions of the 'same' word. Data from VOT, /l/ and /r/ will now be presented to illustrate the difference in the bilinguals' phonetic realisations of English utterances depending on the language session.

Code-switching and VOT

Table 15.3 shows a small selection of words that were produced by the bilinguals in both the English and the Arabic sessions (see Khattab, 2002b for full data and discussion). Two major patterns emerged. First, English words with initial VOICELESS stops almost invariably had shorter VOT

Table 15.3 VOT measurements of English target words produced by the bilinguals during each of the Arabic and the English sessions

			Arabic sessions		*English sessions*	
		Gloss	IPA	VOT (ms)	IPA	VOT (ms)
p		pool	puːəl	28	pʰʉɤ	84
		Po	pʰoᵘ	56	pʰoʊ	92
t		tummy	ˈtʌmiː	12	ˈtʰʊmɪ	42
		teapot	ˈtiˑ pɔt̚	19	ˈtʰiːpɔtʰ	76
k		kettle	ˈkɛtəl	37	ˈkʰɛtəɫ	70
		carrot	ˈkɐɾˑət	25	ˈkʰaɹət	57
b		bottle	ˈbɔtəl	0	ˈbɒtɐ	12
		beer	biɐ̯ɾ	− 165	ˈbɪə	0
d		deer	diːɾ	13	dɪə	31
		duck	d̪ɜk	12	dʊk	21
g		guitar	g̊iˈtɑˑɾ̥	13	gɪˈtʰɑː	34
		goat	goːt	25	gəʊt	21

when produced during the Arabic sessions. This pattern applied mainly to B7 and B10, while B5's production tended to follow the English pattern regardless of the language session. As for VOICED stops, there was no significant difference in VOT production of the 'same' words depending on the language session. This may be due to the fact that two of the bilinguals did not produce any prevoicing for their Arabic stops anyway. There was, however, a tendency to produce longer VOT in the English sessions than in the Arabic ones. More importantly, VOT was not the only feature that changed depending on the language session. As can be seen from Table 15.3, a whole set of language- and dialect-specific phonetic and phonological features appeared to vary in the production of the 'same' words depending on the language context. This included clear versus dark variants of /l/, rhoticity, vowel quality, etc. This suggests that the bilinguals can manipulate VOT features in the same way that they manipulate other vocalic and consonantal features to make the words sound more Arab- or English-like. More evidence can be provided from /l/ and /r/ patterns (see next subsection).

Similar evidence for VOT code-switching has been found at the perceptual level. For instance, Elman *et al.* (1977) tested Spanish–English bilinguals on voice onset time (VOT) continua (/ba-pa/; /da-ta/; /ga-ka/) and obtained different identification curves in English and in Spanish. The language sets were obtained by changing experimenters (one English, one Spanish), the settings, and the language instructions. The bilinguals behaved like English listeners when in an English mode and like Spanish listeners when in a Spanish mode (i.e. they showed a perceptual boundary shift).

Code-switching and the production of liquids

Tables 15.4 and 15.5 show a selection of /l/ and /r/ tokens words that were produced by the bilinguals in both the English and the Arabic sessions (see Khattab, 2002a for full data and discussion). As with the results found for VOT, the bilinguals' productions display different consonantal and vocalic features depending on the language of the session. Since the code-switched tokens with target /r/'s were frequent enough to allow for comparison with the English pattern, Figure 15.13 combines the results for /r/ patterns by the bilinguals from the English sessions, the Arabic sessions, and the English code-switches produced during the Arabic sessions. The differences across results from the three contexts suggest that different language modes were operating during each context, with some overlap. This issue will be discussed further in the next section.

Table 15.4 English /l/ tokens produced by the bilinguals in Arabic sessions compared with productions of the same tokens in English sessions

Gloss	Produced in Arabic sessions	Produced in English sessions
castle	ˈkʰa̰səl	ˈkʰasɫ
kettle	ˈkɛtəl	ˈkʰɛtəɫ
purple	ˈpɜːpəl	ˈpɜːpɵ
muscle	ˈmʌsˤl̩	ˈmʌsɫ̥
football	fətˈboːl	ˈfʊʔbəʊ
bottle	ˈbɔtəl	ˈbɒtɐ
elbow	ˈɛlbɔ	ˈɛɫbɔᵊ
nails	neɪəɫz̥	neɪɫz̥
castle	ˈkasl̩	ˈkʰasɵ
pool	puːl	pʰᵾɤ
football	fotˈboːl	fʊʔbɔʊ

Table 15.5 English /r/ tokens produced by the bilinguals in Arabic sessions compared with productions of the same tokens in English sessions

	Gloss	Produced in Arabic sessions	Produced in English sessions
Pre-V	present (noun)	ˈpʰɾ̥ɛzẽnt	ˈpʰɹ̝̊zɔ̃nʔs
	microphone	ˈmaɪkɾəfõ	ˈmaɪkʰəfə̃ʊn
	umbrella	ʔʌmˈbrɛllə	ṹmˈbɹˑɛlə
Post-V	beer	biɾ̝	bɪə
	circus	sɜɾˈkʰas	ˈsɜːkəs
	star	staˑɾ	staːz̥
	waiter	ˈweɪtɐɾ	ˈweɪtə
	cartoons	kʰa̰ˈtʰɜːn	ˈkʰɑːtʰᵾːnz
	fireman	fɛjɛɾˈmãn	ˈfaɪəmən
	guitar	giˈtɑ̰ɾ	gɪˈtʰɑː
	deer	diːɾ	dɪə
	scarf	skɑ̰ɾf	skɑˑf

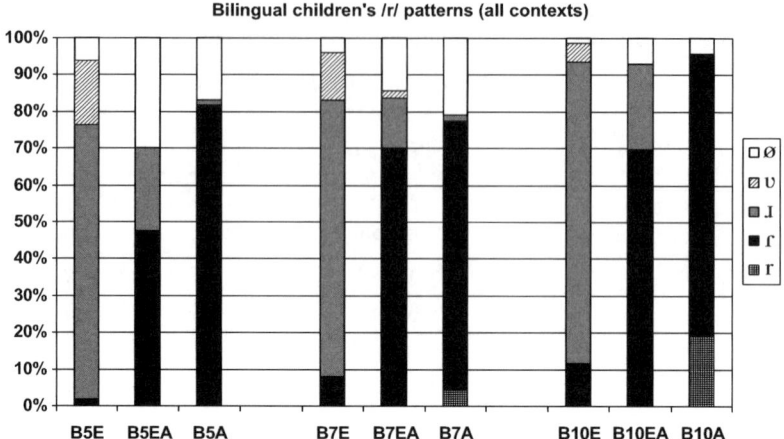

Figure 15.13 Summary of the /r/ patterns found for the bilinguals in the three different language contexts (E = English; EA = English in Arabic context; A = Arabic)

Discussion

The results obtained from this chapter offer important observations related to methodological issues in the study of bilingual and monolingual phonological acquisition. Although there are three bilingual children at the heart of the study, the inclusion of their parents along with monolingual children and adults from each language has offered a substantial contribution to the analysis of the bilinguals' production in the two languages. Moreover, if the bilinguals' language modes had not been taken into account, some misinterpretations of their linguistic behaviour might have been reached.

The description of the bilingual children's acquisition of complex features was able to distinguish between features that the bilingual subjects had not acquired because of their bilingual background and those that were missing due to continuing language development. For example, although the three bilinguals produced some clear [l]'s in emphatic contexts, the results indicated that the monolingual children were also producing clear [l]'s. Emphatic [lˤ] in Arabic develops very late and may not be mastered till the early teenage years. Moreover, the contextual and dialectal factors showed that even the adults were producing some clear [l]'s in emphatic contexts. This again underlines the importance of looking at the input that both bilingual and monolingual children receive.

Similarly, although B5 and B10's VOICED stops in Arabic are produced with short lag rather than long lead, such patterns cannot be solely attributed to English dominance. The monolingual Arabic controls also showed evidence of incomplete acquisition of this complex phonetic feature. The VOT patterns that were found for VOICED Arabic stops in this study are similar to results obtained in monolingual (Allen, 1985; Macken & Burton, 1980b) and bilingual studies (Deuchar & Clark, 1995; Heselwood & McChrystal, 2000; Konefal & Fokes, 1981). They show that some adult patterns develop later than others. In this case, the complexity of the articulatory gestures involved in the production of voicing lead and the difficulty of co-ordination of laryngeal control with a particular supra-laryngeal articulatory gesture may delay the children's acquisition of voicing lead (Kewley-Port & Preston, 1974; Zlatin & Koenigsknecht, 1976). Therefore, while adult-like VOT patterns in English normally start appearing around the age of two, it must be kept in mind that children who acquire languages that contrast voicing lead with voicing lag might develop those patterns at a later age.

B7's later acquisition of voicing lead suggests that, when the two conditions of input and age are met, bilinguals will follow similar acquisitional patterns to those of monolinguals, or even 'catch up' with them. In the process of doing so, bilinguals will exhibit developmental patterns that are similar to monolingual ones, such as the use of short lag instead of voicing lead, or the use of continuants preceding the prevoiced stops (Allen, 1985; Macken & Barton, 1980a). Similarly, B7's use of strategies that are similar to those used by monolinguals points to the necessity of looking for normal developmental processes in order to explain the speech patterns observed in bilinguals before resorting to explanations based on language interference. Such processes may be due to the articulatory difficulty associated with some gestures (in this case consonantal ones) that can delay children's acquisition of speech timing, regardless of whether they are monolingual or bilingual. Moreover, B10's use of short lag is not necessarily caused by an influence from English, but may be due to the fact that he did not receive enough Arabic input at an early age to master the complex articulatory features required for the production of voicing lead. What is considered a developmental feature or an error may also turn out to be part of adult speech, such as the production of nasals and vowels before prevoiced stops by BF7.

The /l/ and /r/ patterns that were acquired for each language by the bilinguals show evidence of acquisition of dialect-specific features that were similar to those observed in their immediate input. Therefore, contrary to what is assumed in many accounts of phonological learning, children do not only acquire the full inventory of adult phonological oppositions, but may also preserve fine phonetic details of the speech input (e.g. Docherty & Foulkes, 2000; Foulkes *et al.*, 1999; Local, 1983; Roberts & Labov, 1995; Williams & Kerswill, 1999). This allows them to imitate and reproduce speech patterns heard in their surrounding environment, and therefore provides them with a huge benefit in acquiring the phonology of the local dialect from speakers they are exposed to early in life (Pisoni, 1997: 28; Pisoni & Lively, 1995: 439). Yet the tradition in most bilingual research has been to treat the two languages that the bilingual seeks to acquire as homogeneous sets of well-defined phonological representations (often consisting of a set of abstract phonemes some of which are exclusive to one language while others are 'shared' between the two languages). The child's productions are therefore judged against these targets, and 'unexpected' patterns in one language are often attributed to influence from the other, imperfect learning, or developmental problems. The present study shows that these 'unexpected' patterns may be actually due to the input that the children receive and to possible variability in the input. These patterns should not be discarded or considered as problematic. They may provide evidence for the child's attention to relevant social-indexical features in the input that he/she receives.

The language and social context(s) from which the bilingual's utterances are extracted and analysed also constitutes an important factor that affects bilingual production but that has not always been factored in as part of the methodology in bilingual studies. For instance, questions such as whether the bilingual was communicating with a monolingual or with a bilingual interviewer and in the latter case, whether two languages were used or whether the researcher followed a one-language-per session approach all have a bearing on the interpretation of the data. The effect of the interlocutor on the bilingual's linguistic choices is often discussed in terms of the bilingual's decision to use one language or two during a conversation, and, in the latter case, how much code-switching to engage in. What this study suggests is that similar decisions might apply on a more subtle and detailed level, for instance, with regards to the phonetic patterns produced for a given language depending on the interlocutor and on whether one or both languages are activated.

Grosjean (2001: 8) notes that even though language mode has been alluded to by several researchers over the years, it has not been the object of systematic study until quite recently. Accounting for the language mode can partly account for problematic ambiguous findings relating to interference, code-switching, and language mixing in bilingual children. For instance, researchers who have examined bilingual language production have often reported instances of interference. Schnitzer and Krasinski (1994: 616) give examples of interferences by their son Fernando that include dark [ɫ] for clear [l] in Spanish from age 3;3 to 3;4, and Spanish [r] for English [ɾ] (allophone of /t/) at age 3;8. These are considered errors in judgement as to which phonological system is appropriate; however, there was no mention of the language context in which they were produced. When interferences occur in a bilingual or intermediate mode, they are very difficult to separate from other forms of language mixing, especially borrowings. What might appear to be interference could be a guest element or structure produced by the speaker who is aware that his or her interlocutor can understand mixed language. In other words, language interference can only be identified correctly if deviations from the language being spoken (due to influences from the other language) took place in a near-monolingual mode.

In this study, the English tokens that were produced in the Arabic sessions contained a mixture of features that belong to both languages. Moreover, many of the patterns that were found in the children's code-switches resembled the patterns that were found in their parents' productions of the English targets. This suggests that the children have learned their parents' foreign-accented pronunciations of particular words rather than filtering out the foreign accent features that they are exposed to. However, the children seem to limit these productions to interactions with their parents. Informal observations of mother–child interactions also suggested that the children were accommodating to their mothers' productions in English. This was part of an overall tendency for the children to explain English expressions to their mothers and to repeat utterances slowly when they detect misunderstanding on the part of their mother. Accommodation is often reported as being part of the bilingual's behaviour and is a sign of communicative competence (Fantini, 1985: 116; Hamers & Blanc, 2000: 253; Hoffmann, 1991: 180).

If the patterns found for the English words produced during the Arabic sessions were to be included with the rest of the data that were analysed in previous sections, one might have reached the erroneous conclusion that the bilinguals have not acquired separate patterns for each of their languages. However, by taking the language mode into account, one can see that the bilinguals may actually be showing signs of highly sophisticated sociolinguistic competence by manipulating vocalic, consonantal and prosodic features in their speech to enhance communication in their weaker language.

Finally, any examination of bilingual speech needs to take account of the difficulty in specifying the phonological targets that are available to the bilingual for each language. Bilinguals are exposed to input that normally ranges between standard, non-standard, and non-native varieties; these varieties consist of overlapping phonological systems that create fuzzy boundaries for a given phonological target. Variability is also recognised as one of the most obvious characteristics of children's speech, so this issue needs to be taken into consideration when interpreting bilingual children's production. Developmental factors are exerted on all phonological representations as children enlarge their knowledge of language and its structure, expand their resources for using language and communicating effectively and mature in their social interactions. Similarly, bilingual children draw on their multiple representations that pertain to knowing and using language as they continue to develop more complete representations for each language they are learning (Bialystok, 2001: 120). Like monolingual children, they make do with whatever linguistic resources they have available to express themselves. The only difference is that, unlike monolingual children who are limited to the resources of one language, bilingual children can draw on two (Genesee *et al.*, 1995: 629).

Chapter 16
Phonological Development of Cantonese-Putonghua Bilingual Children

L.K.H. SO and C.S.S. LEUNG

Introduction

Bilingual children start to separate the phonological systems of their two languages at around two years of age. Watson (1991) suggests that there are three possible outcomes in the phonological systems of balanced bilinguals. The bilinguals may have:

(1) two independent phonological systems that are the same as those of the monolinguals,
(2) some integration of the two systems, or
(3) two systems that differ from those of monolinguals.

In successive bilinguals, the influence of one language over the other is more than that in balanced bilinguals. Research has focused on the relationship between age of learning and native-like phonological competence (Scovel, 1988; Patkowski, 1994; Yavaş, 1998), and on phonological interference between the two languages acquired. Weinreich (1953) reported four interference patterns in bilinguals: under-differentiation of phonemes, over-differentiation of phonemes, reinterpretation of distinction and phone substitution.

Although there have been studies on different aspects of phonological development e.g. phoneme mastery order (Ingram, 1989a); underlying cognitive processes in phonological acquisition (Macken & Ferguson, 1983); relationship between metalinguistic awareness and phonological acquisition (Magnusson, 1991), there is a lack of solid empirical data for the phonological development of monolingual English-speaking children (Holm & Dodd, 1999a). Data on the phonological development in bilingual children are rare. Since information on the phonological acquisition of normally developing bilingual children is essential for diagnosis and treatment of bilingual phonological disorder, it is important to investigate the phonological development of typical bilingual children.

There have been some studies on the phonological development of bilingual children who acquired English and another language e.g. English–Spanish (Yavaş & Goldstein, 1998), English–Welsh (Ball *et al.*, this volume) and English–Cantonese (Dodd *et al.*, 1997). Little work, however, has focused on the phonological development of bilingual children who are acquiring two languages, one of which is not English. This chapter reports a study of the phonological development of Putonghua–Cantonese bilingual children. There appears to be no previous data on the phonological development of children acquiring two tonal languages.

The Chinese context

Putonghua is the standardised variety of language promoted by the Chinese government. Surveys report that over 90% of the population in mainland China understands Putonghua while about 50% are able to communicate in Putonghua (Wu & Yin, 1984). Chinese children are often exposed to both Putonghua, since it is taught in schools, and their own native dialect/language. Dialects are often used at home and in the community. Shenzhen is an immigrant city and many people speak their own dialects as well as Putonghua. Shenzhen is therefore an ideal place to collect data on Putonghua–Cantonese bilingual children's speech development. The findings would provide evidence concerning the effect of phonological interference between two tonal languages on phonological development of bilingual children and clarify our understanding of universal patterns that may occur in phonological acquisition. It was predicted that:

- the bilingual children's phonological development will be similar and/or generally delayed in comparison with monolingual children;
- the bilingual children's phonological error patterns will be different for Putonghua and Cantonese;
- patterns of bilingual phonological development will be characterised by some speech error patterns that are similar to those of monolingual counterparts but delayed, and atypical patterns will also be found.

Contrast between Putonghua and Cantonese phonology

Despite the fact that both Putonghua and Cantonese belong to the same family of Chinese languages, they have quite different phonologies. A speaker of Putonghua cannot understand a speaker of Cantonese and vice versa. Some linguists describe Cantonese as a different language from Putonghua, since they are mutually unintelligible. As descriptions of Putonghua and Cantonese are provided in previous chapters by Zhu (Chapter 5) and So (Chapter 6), we will only highlight the major contrasts between the two languages or dialects.

Syllable structure

In the syllable structure of both Putonghua and Cantonese, the onset and the coda can be optional but the vowel nucleus is compulsory. The syllable structure in Putonghua is (C) V (C); and of Cantonese is (C) (G) V (C/G).

Onset and coda

The onset in Putonghua can be one of 21 consonants (except /ŋ/), whereas the onset in Cantonese can be one of 17 consonants (except /ŋ/). Putonghua has no consonant clusters, whereas in Cantonese, /kw/ and /kʰw/ are sometimes described as consonant clusters. The coda in Putonghua can only be one of two consonants, /n/ and /ŋ/. In Cantonese the coda can be either a stop (/p/, /t/, /k/), a nasal (/m/, /n/ or /ŋ/) or a glide.

Nucleus

The nucleus in a Putonghua syllable is the vowel. It may have a prenuclear glide (medial vowel). In Cantonese, the nucleus is made up solely of vowels.

Segments

There are 22 consonants in Putonghua and 17 contrastive consonants and two consonant clusters[1] in Cantonese. In both languages, aspiration is a distinctive feature. All aspirated and unaspirated consonants are voiceless.

Vowels

There are 22 vowels in Putonghua, i.e. nine simple vowels, nine diphthongs and four triphthongs. There are eight vowel phonemes in Cantonese, namely, /i, y, e, a, œ, ɐ, ɔ, u/.[2]

Tones

Both Putonghua and Cantonese are tonal languages. There are four tones in Putonghua, i.e. one level tone (high level) and three contour tones (rising, fall-rising, high falling). There is also a neutral tone. In Cantonese, six contrastive tones have been identified (i.e. high level, high-rise, mid-level, low-fall, low-rise, low-level). In traditional Cantonese phonology, the tones ending with /−p/, /−t/, /−k/ are called entering tones, thus making nine tones in total.

Method

Subjects

Forty bilingual (Cantonese and Putonghua) children aged from 2;6 to 5;6 who attended kindergartens in China were recruited. Putonghua was the primary language spoken at school for all children. Either Cantonese or Putonghua was spoken at home but the language used in the community is mainly Putonghua, e.g. in the school playground. The subjects were divided into six age cohorts, of six monthly bands. There were four to nine subjects in each age group. All children were recruited from nurseries and kindergartens in Shenzhen. Teachers and childcare workers were asked to exclude children who had oro-motor structural abnormalities, hearing or cognitive problems. None of the subjects had any history of language disorders. Parental consent for their children's participation in the study was obtained prior to data collection. All parents were asked to fill in a questionnaire to collect background information on language use by the child and family (see Appendix).

Procedure

Children were assessed in a room on two occasions with two different data collectors. The data collector for the Putonghua speech sample only spoke Putonghua to the children while the data collector for Cantonese speech sample only spoke Cantonese. This encouraged the children to speak the targeted language. The first 10 minutes of each session were spent establishing rapport with the children through free play. Once the children were happy to co-operate, they took either the 80-word research version of the Putonghua Segmental Phonology Test (So & Zhou, 1997) or the 57-word research version of the Cantonese Segmental Phonology Test (So, 1992). These picture-naming tests sampled all initial and final Putonghua or Cantonese consonants, vowels and tones. Consonants were also tested in the medial position. Spontaneous speech samples, as well as picture naming, were obtained from all the children, except for the youngest age group. It was difficult to obtain spontaneous speech from the youngest children and the data was derived from the picture naming tasks. The children's speech sample was audiotaped with a Sony MD recorder (MZ-R50).

Analyses

Both data collectors, who had good phonetic training, phonetically transcribed the speech samples. Intra-rater and inter-rater reliability were conducted on 10% of the data. The intra-rater reliability for Cantonese was 98.5% and the inter-rater reliability for Cantonese was 97.5%. For Putonghua, intra-rater reliability was 97.6% and inter-rater reliability was 96.5%. The rating calculated included comparison of all segments: consonant, vowels and tones.

The transcriptions of the children's speech samples were inspected to establish the children's mastery of Putonghua and Cantonese consonants, vowels and tones. A phoneme was considered to be part of a child's phonemic inventory if it was used three times correctly in different lexical items. Patterns of phonological errors were identified. A phonological rule was judged to be used if there were at least two examples of its application in different lexical items and no counter examples of another error type occurred. These phonological measures were derived from single word responses and from the continuous speech samples.

Results

Bilingual subjects' performance in Cantonese

Age of emergence of syllable-initial and -final consonant phonemes

Bilingual children completed their Cantonese phoneme repertoire later than the monolingual children. Seventy-five percent of Cantonese monolingual children completed their acquisition by 3;5 (So, 1992) whereas 75% of bilingual children completed their phoneme acquisition only by the age of four (see Table 16.1).

The children's acquisition of Cantonese initial and final consonants was compared to that of monolingual children. For the syllable initial consonants, both the bilingual and monolingual children acquired bilabial plosives, unaspirated alveolar plosives, fricatives, nasals and glides before the aspirated velar plosives and aspirated affricates. The bilingual children acquired the clusters much later than the monolingual children while they acquired the aspirated alveolar plosives earlier than the monolingual children. As for syllable-final consonants the bilingual children acquired the plosives and bilabial and alveolar nasals earlier than the velar nasals. The patterns and rate of the acquisition was similar to that of monolingual children.

Age of emergence of vowel phonemes

A vowel phoneme was judged to be acquired if 75% of the children in an age-group produced the phoneme correctly in at least three words. The bilingual children acquired vowels by the age of two and diphthongs by the age of 2;6. Their acquisition rate of Cantonese vowels is the same as Cantonese monolingual children. Table 16.2 shows the order of acquisition of Cantonese bilingual children and Cantonese monolingual children.

Tone acquisition

Only 5% of the subjects made any tonal errors, i.e. changed tone two (high rise) into tone five (low rise) or vice versa.

Table 16.1 Comparison of bilingual children's acquisition of Cantonese consonants with Cantonese monolingual children ($n = 40$) (75% criterion)

		p	pʰ	t	k	f	s	h	m	n	ŋ	l	w	j	ts	-p	-t	-k	-m	-n	tʰ	kʰ	tsʰ	-ŋ	kʰw	kw
2;6–2;11	Bilingual	■	■	■	■	■	■	■	■	■	■	■	■	■	■	■	■	■	■	■	■	■	■	■	■	■
	Cantonese monolingual	■	■	■	■	■	■	■	■	■	■	■	■	■	■	■	■	■	■	■	■	■	□	■	■	■
3–3;5	Bilingual	■	■	■	■	■	■	■	■	■	■	■	■	■	■	■	■	■	■	■	■	■	■	■	□	■
	Cantonese monolingual	■	■	■	■	■	■	■	■	■	■	■	■	■	■	■	■	■	■	■	■	■	■	■	■	■
3;6–3;11	Bilingual	■	■	■	■	■	■	■	■	■	■	■	■	■	■	■	■	■	■	■	■	■	■	■	■	■
	Cantonese monolingual	■	■	■	■	■	■	■	■	■	■	■	■	■	■	■	■	■	■	■	■	■	■	■	■	■

Note: Shared phonemes between Cantonese and Putonghua are shaded in bold types.

Table 16.2 Comparison of age of emergence of Cantonese vowels: bilingual and Cantonese monolingual children (75% criterion)

Age	Bilingual children	Cantonese monolingual children
Before 2;0	a, i, ɛ, u, œ, y, ɐ, ɔ	a, i, ɛ, u, œ, y, ɐ, ɔ ai, ui, ei, ɐi, ɔi, au, ɐu, ou, iu, ɵy
After 2;0	ai, ui, ei, ɐi, ɔi, au, ɐu, ou, iu, ɵy	

Comparison of Cantonese phonological rules

Table 16.3 shows the percentage of bilingual children producing different error patterns affecting syllable-initial, syllable-final consonants and vowels. Bilingual children showed both delayed and disordered patterns of Cantonese phonological development when compared with Cantonese monolingual children. Altogether 12 error patterns were observed in the bilingual children's speech: cluster reduction, stopping, fronting, deaspiration, deaffrication, final consonant deletion, initial consonant deletion, frication, aspiration, gliding, backing and vowel errors.

Cluster reduction persisted in the bilingual children even by the age of five. Fronting, final consonant deletion and vowel errors disappeared by the age of five. Deaspiration, aspiration, gliding, backing, frication still occur at the age of 4;5 while stopping, deaffrication, and initial consonant deletion disappeared by the age of four.

Bilingual subjects' performance in Putonghua

Age of emergence of syllable-initial and -final consonant phonemes

When 75% of the children in the same age-group produced the phoneme correctly in at least three words, the phoneme was considered to be acquired by children of that age group. The bilingual children acquired the bilabial and alveolar plosives, the unaspirated velar plosive /k/, the labio-dental fricative /f/ and the nasals by the age of three. They acquired the palatal and alveolar fricatives and affricates /ɕ, tɕ, tɕʰ, s, ts, tsʰ/ and the lateral /l/ by the age of 3;6. By five years of age, they had acquired the retroflex fricative and affricatives /ʂ, tʂ, tʂʰ/ and /ʐ/. Table 16.4 shows the acquisition of Putonghua phonemes by bilingual children and the comparison with Putonghua monolingual children.

Both the bilingual and Putonghua monolingual children acquired the bilabial and alveolar plosives, the unaspirated velar plosive, the labio-dental fricative and the nasals before the other phonemes. The lateral /l/ was acquired by the bilingual children (at about 2;6–2;11) earlier

Table 16.3 Percentage of bilingual children using error patterns affecting Cantonese consonants and vowels

	Percentage of children using error patterns						Examples of error
Age	2;6–2;11	3;0–3;5	3;6–3;11	4;0–4;5	4;6–4;11	5;0+	
No. of subjects	n = 4	n = 9	n = 6	n = 9	n = 7	n = 5	
No. of errors	–	11	16	–	–	80	
Cluster reduction	50	11	16	22	43	20	kw: [k]
Stopping	25	11	16	–	–	–	s: [t]
Fronting	–	–	–	–	14	–	k: [t]
Deaspiration	50	44	16	22	–	–	$p^h\,t^h\,k^h\,ts^h\,k^hw$: [p, t, k, ts, kw]
Deaffrication	50	44	16	–	14	–	ts, ts^h: [s]
Final consonant deletion	50	56	–	22	–	–	mit: [mi]
Initial consonant deletion	25	–	16	–	–	–	lap: [ap]
Frication	50	56	–	17	–	–	t, t^h: [s]
Aspiration	–	11	–	22	–	–	p, t, k, ts, kw: [p^h, t^h, k^h, t^hs, k^hw]
Gliding	–	56	16	22	–	–	l: [j]
Backing	50	–	16	22	–	–	t, t^h: [k, k^h]
Change vowels	50	56	20	22	29	–	e:[a]

Table 16.4 Age of emergence of Putonghua syllable-initial and -final consonants of bilingual children compared with Putonghua monolingual children (75% criterion)

Phonemes / Age		p	pʰ	t	tʰ	k	kʰ	m	n	ŋ	kʰ	ɕ	tɕ	tɕʰ	l	s	tsʰ	ʂ	tʂ	tʂʰ	z
2;6–2;11	Bilingual																				
	Putonghua monolingual																				
3;0–3;5	Bilingual																				
	Putonghua monolingual																				
3;6–3;11	Bilingual																				
	Putonghua monolingual																				
4;0–4;5	Bilingual																				
	Putonghua monolingual																				
4;6–4;11	Bilingual																				
	Putonghua monolingual																				
5;0+	Bilingual																				
	Putonghua monolingual																				

Note: Shared phonemes between Cantonese and Putonghua are shaded in bold types.

than the Putonghua monolingual children (at about 3;6–3;11). Affricates /ɕ, tɕ, tɕʰ/ were acquired by both groups of children at 3;0–3;5. The alveolar fricative and affricates were acquired earlier by bilingual children than by Putonghua monolingual children. As for the retroflex fricative and affricates /ʂ, tʂ, tʂʰ/, they were acquired by both groups at 4;6–4;11. The bilingual children acquired alvelo-palatal fricative /ʐ/ only by age five and later than the Putonghua monolingual children. While 75% of the Putonghua monolingual children completed their phonemic acquisition by 5;0, 75% of the bilingual children do not complete their phoneme acquisition until after five years old (So & Zhou, 2000).

Age of emergence of Putonghua vowel phonemes

A Putonghua vowel phoneme was judged to be acquired if 75% of the children in the same age-group produced the phoneme correctly in at least three words. The age of acquisition of vowel phonemes of bilingual children was compared to that of Putonghua monolingual children shown in Table 16.5. The results indicated that the age of acquisition of vowels of the bilingual and Putonghua monolingual was the same except for four tripthongs /uai, uei, iau, iou/ which were not acquired until 3;5 by the bilingual children.

Comparison of Putonghua phonological rules

The percentages of the bilingual children using different error patterns affecting syllable-initial, syllable-final consonants and vowels were shown in Table 16.6. Vowels errors were also identified. Some of the error patterns used by the bilingual children were similar to those used by the Putonghua monolingual children while other error patterns were not. The common error patterns of stopping, aspiration and backing lasted beyond age five while the error patterns of deaspiration and affrication lasted until age five and fronting till age four and a half. The bilingual children also used error patterns such as nasalization beyond age five, deretroflexion until age five, deaffrication until age four and a half and final consonant deletion until age three and a half. Vowel errors exist even beyond age five.

Table 16.5 Comparison of age of acquisition of Putonghua vowels: Bilingual and Putonghua monolingual children ($n = 40$) (75% criterion)

Age	Bilingual children	Putonghua monolingual children
2;6–2;11	i, y, u, A, ɤ, o, ɚ, ə, ɛ ae, ao, ei oʊ, ia, iɛ, ua, uo, yɛ	i, y, u, A, ɤ, o, ɚ, ə, ɛ ae, ao, ei oʊ, ia, iɛ, ua, uo, yɛ, iao, ioʊ, uae, uei
3;0–3;5	iao, ioʊ, uae, uei	

Table 16.6 Percentage of bilingual children using error patterns affecting Putonghua consonants and vowels

Age	Percentage of children using error patterns						Examples of error
	2;6–2;11	3;0–3;5	3;6–3;11	4;0–4;5	4;6–4;11	5;0+	
No. of subjects	n = 4	n = 9	n = 6	n = 9	n = 7	n = 5	
No errors	–	11	–	–	14	20	
Stopping	25	11	17	–	–	20	s, ɕ, ʂ, tɕ, tɕʰ, tʂ, tʂʰ: [t, tʰ]
Fronting	50	11	34	67	–	–	kʰ, k: [tʰ, t]
Deaspiration	50	11	17	17	28	–	tʰ: [t], kʰ: [k]
Deaffrication	25	11	20	17	–	–	tɕ [ɕ], tʂ: [ʂ]
Final consonant deletion	25	11	–	–	–	–	an: [la]
Aspiration	–	–	17	17	28	20	t: [tʰ], k: [kʰ]
Backing	25	11	–	–	43	20	ts: [tʃ], s: [ʃ]
Deretroflexion	50	33	34	33	14	–	ʂ tʂ, tʂʰ: [s, ts, tsʰ]
Nasalization	50	–	17	55	14	20	l: [n]
Affrication	25	–	–	–	43	–	s:[ts], ɕ:[tʂ], ɕ:[tɕ]
Change vowels	50	33	17	33	28	40	o:[u]

Discussion

The children participating in the study lived in Shenzhen, an immigrant city whose residents often come from different parts of China. Their parents frequently have different mother tongues so that children can be exposed to two languages from birth (most fathers spoke Cantonese while mothers spoke Putonghua). The bilingual children had to acquire two different phonological systems. It is not surprising, then, that the results indicated that the bilingual children showed a general delay in the phonological acquisition in both languages when compared to monolingual children of either language. This may be due to the fact that the bilingual children have less exposure to each language compared with monolingual children of either language (Dodd *et al.*, 1996; Watson, 1991). Bilingual development also seemed to be characterised by linguistic behaviour specific to the languages of the bilingual speaker, such as the use of atypical error patterns in backing (/t/[k]) and in aspiration (/p, t, k/ [p^h, t^h, k^h]).

Putonghua is the official language in China and consequently, it is the dominant language for most bilingual children in China. They used Putonghua at school, with peers and sometimes at home. From the data collected from the questionnaires, 70% of the bilingual families used both languages to communicate with their children. Fifty percent of bilingual children used both languages at home. The questionnaire also found that 70% of the bilingual children used only Putonghua with their peers and all the bilingual children used Putonghua at school. The bilingual children used Putonghua more often than Cantonese and therefore their acquisition of Putonghua was much faster than their acquisition of Cantonese. When children are small, their exposure to their mother tongue is likely to be extensive but as children grow older, the dominance of Putonghua is likely to increase as they interact with a wider language community. Teachers and peers will play an important role in the bilingual child's language development.

Examples of phonological interference

The bilingual children's age of acquisition of the phonemes of each language was slower than that of monolingual children. The following examples suggest that the phonological features of one language may influence bilingual children's realisation of the phonological features of their other language.

(1) Bilingual children acquired the clusters /kw, $k^h w$/ only by the age of 4;0, which is delayed compared to Cantonese monolingual children who acquire clusters at 3;0 (So & Dodd, 1995). There are no clusters in

Putonghua, and consequently bilingual children's acquisition of clusters might suffer interference from Putonghua phonology.

(2) One surprising finding was that the bilingual children acquired Putonghua affricates /ts, ts^h/ and liquid /l/ (at 4;0), earlier than monolingual Putonghua-speaking children who do not acquire these sounds until 4;6. This may be because /ts, ts^h/ and liquid /l/ are also phonemes in Cantonese. When the bilingual children learned Cantonese as a mother tongue, they were exposed to these sounds and the increased exposure may have enhanced their acquisition rate in Putonghua. However, retroflex /ʐ/ was acquired much more slowly by bilingual children than the Putonghua monolingual children. There is no retroflex in Cantonese and the acquisition of this phoneme may be affected by the Cantonese phonological system.

(3) Bilingual children's acquisition of Putonghua triphthongs was slower than that of Putonghua monolingual children. This may be due to the fact that there are no triphthongs in Cantonese. The bilingual children seemed to need more time to learn to separate the vowel systems of the two different languages.

(4) The error pattern of retroflexion is not evident in bilingual children's speech though it is common for Putonghua monolingual children (So & Zhou, 2000). This may be due to the influence of the Cantonese phonological system where there is no retroflex sound. Bilingual children also have a de-retroflexion error pattern and again this may be due to the fact that there is no retroflex sound in Cantonese. When bilingual children attempt to produce a Putonghua retroflex target, they may delete the retroflex feature due to interference from Cantonese.

Error patterns

There was no significant difference between the total number of errors produced by bilingual children and that of the Putonghua monolingual children perhaps because the bilingual children in this study have Putonghua as their dominant language. In contrast, the bilingual children made more errors in Cantonese than did the Cantonese-speaking monolingual children. Therefore, the more dominant language, Putonghua, was less influenced by bilingualism than the less dominant language, Cantonese.

Bilingual children often use some phonological features of the more dominant language when speaking the less dominant one (Abudarham, 1987). Hence, dominance of the languages concerned would affect the degree and nature of interference, and the type of atypical error patterns. The age at which bilingual children are exposed to the second language, parental and environmental influences also contribute towards the bilingual results (Abudarham, 1987). Some examples of atypical error behaviour are discussed below.

(1) Bilingual children made vowel errors in both Cantonese and Putonghua. This is in contrast to monolingual children who usually acquire accurate vowels as early as two and a half years of age. There is no precise place of articulation for a particular vowel, and both languages have complex vowel systems where vowels are highly salient. The bilingual children used Cantonese vowels when speaking Putonghua and Putonghua vowels when speaking Cantonese. This may be a result of interference (Romaine, 1995) in the sense that two complex vowel systems may be hard to differentiate.

(2) *Atypical consonant patterns.* Some errors made by bilingual children are different from monolinguals. For Cantonese, the bilingual children made errors such as initial consonant deletion, frication, aspiration, gliding, backing and final glide deletion. These errors were made by less than 10% of the Cantonese monolinguals in any age groups. For Putonghua, the bilingual children also made errors different from the Putonghua monolinguals. The unusual errors included final consonant deletion, deaffrication and nasalisation. The cause of such errors might be due to negative transfer of the mother tongue.

The results indicated that, compared to monolinguals, the bilingual children exhibited non-developmental, as well as delayed error patterns. It is impossible for all bilingual children to have disordered phonology. Bilingualism gives rise to error patterns that may be atypical for monolingual acquisition, but are typical for bilingual phonological development (Dodd *et al.*, 1996; Holm & Dodd, 1999a). These findings are of particular relevance for speech and language pathologists and teachers of bilingual children in Hong Kong and China. They will contribute to the understanding of the phonological abilities of bilingual children and will provide data for language teaching and intervention programmes for bilingual children. The findings may also support second language teachers' understanding of developmental patterns in Putonghua and Cantonese language learners.

Notes

1. Some phonologists view the labialised velar clusters /k^hw, kw/ as labialised velar stops /k^h, k/.
2. Some phonologists take the new that there are eleven vowels /i, y, ɪ, e, œ, ɵ, a, ɐ, ɔ, ʊ/ and 11 diphthongs /ai, ɐi, au, ɐu, ei, ɵy, ɔi, ui, iu, ou, eu/ in Cantonese.

Appendix

<u>問卷</u>

兒童姓名：＿＿＿＿＿＿＿＿＿＿＿　　出生日期：＿＿＿日＿＿＿月＿＿＿＿年

以下問題有助我們了解 貴子女的語言使用情況。有關內容絕對保密。請在適當的空格內加上「√」號：

1. 父母的母語：
    父：☐ 廣州話 ☐ 普通話 ☐ 其他＿＿＿＿＿＿
    母：☐ 廣州話 ☐ 普通話 ☐ 其他＿＿＿＿＿＿

2. 貴子女在家中較多用的語言：
    ☐ 廣州話 ☐ 普通話 ☐ 廣州話和普通話 ☐ 其他＿＿＿＿＿＿

3. 父母在家中對 貴子女所用的語言：
    父：☐ 廣州話 ☐ 普通話 ☐ 廣州話和普通話 ☐ 其他＿＿＿＿＿＿
    母：☐ 廣州話 ☐ 普通話 ☐ 廣州話和普通話 ☐ 其他＿＿＿＿＿＿

4. 貴子女有否兄弟姊妹：
    ☐ 有 (請到第五題) ☐ 沒有 (請到第六題)

5. 他們會和貴子女說哪一種語言：
    ☐ 廣州話 ☐ 普通話 ☐ 廣州話和普通話 ☐ 其他＿＿＿＿＿＿

6. 在家中，由誰來照顧貴子女：☐ 父 ☐ 母 ☐ 其他＿＿＿＿＿＿
    如是其他的話，此人會用甚麼語言和貴子女溝通？
    ☐ 廣州話 ☐ 普通話 ☐ 廣州話和普通話 ☐ 其他＿＿＿＿＿＿

7. 貴子女在學校所用的語言：
    ☐ 廣州話 ☐ 普通話 ☐ 廣州話和普通話 ☐ 其他＿＿＿＿＿＿

8. 貴子女何時學習廣州話？＿＿＿＿＿＿歲
9. 貴子女何時學習普通話？＿＿＿＿＿＿歲
10. 貴子女有否聽覺問題？☐ 有 ☐ 否
11. 貴子女有否健康問題？☐ 有 ☐ 否

家長簽名 ＿＿＿＿＿＿＿＿＿　　家長姓名 ＿＿＿＿＿＿＿＿＿＿　　日期 ＿＿＿＿＿＿＿＿

Questionnaire English Version

Name of child:_____   Date of birth: _____

The following questions are for understanding the languages your child use in different communication contexts. The information will be useful for the bilingual speech production research project. All data collected will be treated in confidence and restricted to research purpose ONLY.

Please read the items carefully and put a ✓ in the appropriate boxes:

(1) Parents' native language
Father: ☐ Cantonese ☐ Putonghua ☐ Others: _____
Mother: ☐ Cantonese ☐ Putonghua ☐ Others: _____

(2) The language your child use at home is
☐ Cantonese   ☐ Putonghua
☐ Cantonese and Putonghua   ☐ Others: _____

(3) The language parents use with the child at home is
Father: ☐ Cantonese ☐ Putonghua ☐ Others:_____
Mother: ☐ Cantonese ☐ Putonghua ☐ Others:_____

(4) Your child has brothers or sisters
☐ Yes, (please go to item 5)   ☐ No, (please go to item 6)

(5) The language brothers/sisters use with your child:
☐ Cantonese   ☐ Putonghua
☐ Cantonese and Putonghua   ☐ Others: _____

(6) The caregiver at home is: ☐ Father ☐ Mother ☐ Others:_____

If there is another caregiver at home apart from father or mother, the language used by that caregiver with the child is
☐ Cantonese   ☐ Putonghua   ☐ Others:_____

(7) The language your child uses at school is
☐ Cantonese   ☐ Putonghua   ☐ Others:_____

(8) At what age does your child start learning Cantonese? __ years old

(9) At what age does your child start learning Putonghua? __ years old

(10) Has your child got any hearing problems? _____ yes, _____ No

(11) Has your child got any health problems? _____ yes, _____ No

Parent's signature: _____   Parent's Name: _____
Date:_____

Part 4
Coda

Chapter 17
Towards Developmental Universals

ZHU HUA and B. DODD

This volume has examined the phonological development and disorders of monolingual children acquiring eight different languages and of bilingual children acquiring six different language pairs. While there are many things in common among the phonologies studied, they also differ greatly from each other. The commonalities and differences, which make cross-linguistic comparison feasible and interesting, are summarised below (see Table 17.1 for an overview).

Similarities in the Phonologies

Similarities in the phonological system of the following languages: English, German, Putonghua, Cantonese, Maltese, Telugu, Colloquial Egyptian Arabic, Turkish, Spanish, Mirpuri/Punjabi/Urdu, and Welsh:

(1) All the above-mentioned languages share the following consonants: voiceless plosive /p/, nasals /m, n/, voiceless fricative /f, s/.
(2) All the languages except one or two share the following consonants: voiceless plosives /t, k/ and voiceless fricative /h/, (/t/ does not exist in Mirpuri/Punjabi/Urdu, /k/ in Colloquial Egyptian Arabic; /h/ in Putongha).
(3) Nearly all the languages have /r/ in different forms: as an approximant in English and Putonghua, a trill in Maltese, Telugu, Colloquial Egyptian Arabic and Welsh, and a flap in Mirpuri/Punjabi/Urdu.
(4) Almost all the vowel inventories include /i, u, a/.
(5) The velar nasal /ŋ/ tends to occur at syllable-final position, not at syllable-initial position. This is the case for all the languages except Cantonese.
(6) For all the languages studied in this volume, consonants are optional at syllable-final and -initial position with the exception of German and Colloquial Egyptian Arabic. In these two languages, consonants are compulsory at syllable-initial position.

Table 17.1 An overview of phonologies of the languages studied in this volume

Language	British English	German	Putonghua	Cantonese	Maltese	Telugu	CEA	Turkish	Spanish	Punjabi	Welsh
Consonant (in total)	24	23	22	17	22	33	27	20	20	35	25
SI	23	21	21	17	?	?	?	?	?	?	22
SF	21	14	2	8	?	?	?	?	?	?	21
Vowel (in total)	26	16	22	8	18	12	8	8	?	12	19
Simple vowel	12	13	9	8	11	10	8		5	12	11
Diphthong	9	3	9	None	7	2	None	?	A wide variety	?	8
Triphthong	5		4	None	?	?	None	?	?	?	?
Clusters	49	24 at WI, many at WM/WF	None	2	100+ CC A few CCC	Primarily in WM	Only WF	Only WF	Only stop/f+liquid at SI Only stop/sonorant +s in SFWM	Very few	A few
Syllable shapes	C0-3VC0-4	C1-3VC0-3	[C]V[C] + Tone	[C] [G]V [C/G] + Tone	C0-3VC0-2	?	CVC0-2	[C]V [C0-2]	C0-2VC0-2	?	C0-3VC0-2
Lexical tones	none	None	4	6 contrasting, 3 entering	None	None	None	None	None	None	None

Note: CEA: colloquial Egyptian Arabic; C: consonant; V: vowel; G: glide; ?: information unavailable; SI: syllable-initial; SF: syllable-final; WI: word-initial; WM: word-medial; WF: word-final.

Differences in the Phonologies

The phonologies involved differ greatly from each other. They differ in terms of the number of segments they have, the contrastive features between segments, syllable shapes, phonotactics, tones, etc. Specifically the differences are:

(1) The size of consonants inventories: the largest one is that of Urdu – as many as 42; the smallest is Cantonese with its 17 contrastive consonants.

(2) The size of vowel inventories: English has as many as 26 and three types of vowels (i.e. simple vowels, diphthongs and triphthongs), while languages such as Cantonese and Colloquial Egyptian Arabic have only eight vowels and include only simple vowels.

(3) The way consonants contrast with each other: while voicedness is a contrastive feature for English, German, Maltese, Turkish, Spanish and Welsh, aspiration is a contrastive feature for Putonghua and Cantonese. However, in Mirpuri/Punjabi/Urdu, both voicedness and aspiration are contrastive features. Examples of their sound inventory are: /p, p^h, b, b^h, t̪, $t̪^h$, d̪, $d̪^h$, t, t^h, d, d^h, k, k^h, g, g^h/.

(4) Syllable shapes: while the vowel is a compulsory part of the syllable in all the languages, consonant use varies in that:
- it is optional at syllable-final position in all the languages. All the languages can end the syllable with a vowel, and
- it is optional at syllable-initial position in all the languages except German and Colloquial Egyptian Arabic.

(5) Clusters: there are considerable differences among languages in terms of whether and where clusters are permissible and the maximum length. For example, while there is no cluster in Putonghua and only two clusters in Cantonese, English allows a maximum number of three consonants to co-occur at syllable-initial position and four consonants at syllable-final position. In Spanish, coda clusters can only occur within a word, not at word-final position. It is difficult to compare the total number of phonotactically permissible clusters across the languages due to the lack of relevant information (cf. it is reported that Maltese has over 100 consonant clusters, mainly in the form of CC).

(6) Two tonal languages: Putonghua and Cantonese are the only tonal languages among the languages studied. In these two languages, tones carried by each syllable are lexical in the sense that different tones result in different lexical meanings for the same syllable. Therefore, tones are regarded as a compulsory part of the syllable in these tonal languages.

(7) Other language-specific features: for example, mutations in Welsh (phonological changes to word-initial consonants triggered by a range of morphosyntactic contexts); the contrastive feature of vowel length in Telugu and Colloquial Egyptian Arabic where the length of the vowel differentiates lexical meaning; vowel harmony in Turkish where generally all vowels in a word agree in the degree of place of articulation (either all front vowels or all back vowels), and germination in Maltese where a consonant is prolonged to cover two segments' length when two identical consonants are adjacent to each other.

Similarities and Differences in Developmental Patterns Across the Languages

The similarities and differences in the phonologies studied allow comparison between developmental patterns of children speaking different languages or language pairs in both typical and atypical development.

The following patterns are observed across the findings reported in different chapters in this volume. Possible theoretical explanations are also proposed.

1. *The earlier acquisition of vowels in comparison to consonants.* Vowels are acquired earlier than consonants and are resistant to phonological disorder. Among the languages reported, English has the most complicated vowel inventory. It has 26 vowels in three categories: simple vowels, diphthongs and triphthongs. However, the youngest age group of English-speaking children studied (3;0–3;11) had already reached well over 96% on PVC (percent vowel correct, i.e. the percentage of vowels used correctly against the number of opportunities). The early acquisition of vowels can possibly be explained by the concept of phonological saliency and that of sonority. Both concepts believe vowels have higher ranking than consonants and would therefore be expected to be acquired earlier than consonants. In contrast, the study of Cantonese/Putonghua-speaking bilingual children found that bilingual children, unlike their monolingual peers, made vowel errors in both Cantonese and Putonghua, perhaps as the result of interference of the two vowel systems of the two relatively similar phonological systems.

2. *Completion of phonetic acquisition.* Since various youngest age groups were examined in different studies, it is difficult to compare the onset of sound acquisition in monolingual speakers of different languages. However, relatively comparable data are available on the age of completion of phonetic acquisition in languages such as English, German,

Putonghua, Maltese and Turkish (Table 17.2 summarises the available information on these languages). Sound inventory acquisition was complete by 3;0. The earliest completion reported was for Turkish-speaking children (despite the slightly stricter criteria of a sound having to occur twice in word context rather than once). Completion of sound inventories was 3;11 for Maltese-speaking children; by 4;5 for Putonghua-speakers; 4;11 for German-speakers but not until 7;0 for English-speaking children. The late completion of the acquisition of the sound inventory in English is mainly due to the fact that three sounds /ɹ, θ, ð/ only appeared in the sound inventory of 90% of the children aged 6;0–7;0 while the acquisition of the rest of the sounds was completed just after five years of age. It is worth noting that while /ɹ/ is common to all the languages studied in this volume, /θ, ð/ only occur in English. The data provides evidence against Jakobson's claim on the correlation between the order of phonological acquisition and the distribution of the sounds among the world's languages. While these different ages of completion in different languages suggests that phonetic acquisition is subject to language-specific influences, indeed more so than has been assumed in previous studies (an argument against biological model and articulatory complexity accounts of phonological acquisition), the picture is complicated by the findings from a socio-phonetic analysis of speech data from Arabic-English bilingual children reported in Chapter 15. This study suggests that children's phonology, especially the phonetic shape, continues to develop after the age of five.

3. *Phonemic acquisition.* Although it is difficult to make a direct comparison of age of phonetic acquisition of segments across different languages, due to the diversity in the criteria used, it is clear that some sounds tend to occur earliest in all languages (i.e. children usually use these sounds correctly in word contexts). These are nasals /m, n/ and plosives such as /p, b, t, d, k, g/. These sounds are also common to all or most of the languages studied. The acquisition of other sounds common to the languages studied such as /f, s/ seems to be more complicated. In those studies that included children as young as two, /f, s/ are not among the first group of sounds to be acquired phonetically. They often appeared in the inventory of the second youngest age group (e.g. German, Putonghua, Maltese) or even the third youngest age group (Turkish). These discrepancies in the age of acquisition of sounds common to all the languages studied confirmed the failure of Jakobson's 'laws of irreversible solidarity' in accounting for language variations in acquisition of the same sounds.

4. *Aspirated versus unaspirated sounds.* Unaspirated phonemes tend to be acquired earlier than their aspirated pairs, if not at the same time. This is confirmed by Putonghua, Cantonese and Mirpuri/Punjabi/Urdu in which aspiration serves as a lexical feature. Using the framework of

Table 17.2 An overview of phonetic acquisition in English, German, Putonghua, Turkish and Punjabi*

Language	English	German	Putonghua	Maltese	Turkish	Punjabi
Age group criteria	90%	90%	90%	75%	90%	90%
Opportunities criteria	Once	twice	once	once in any 25 phonetic forms	twice	once
1;3–1;6	NA	NA	NA	NA	p, b, t, d, k, c m, n, j	NA
1;6–1;11	NA	m b d t n	t, tʰ, k, m, n, ŋ, x, tɕ, tɕʰ, ɕ	NA	g, ɟ, ʃ, tʃ, dʒ, ʋ, l, ɫ,	
2;0–2;5	NA	p f v l	f, s, tʂ	m, n, p, b, t, d, k, ʔ h w, l, j	s, f, ɾ	
2;6–2;11	NA	x g k h ʁ pf	p, l	f, s, ʃ ɾ	v, z, h	
3;0–3;5	p, b, t, d, k, g m, n, ŋ f, v, s, z, h w, l, j	j ŋ	pʰ, kʰ, tʂʰ	g v tʃ		

Towards Developmental Universals

	tʃ	ɕ	ʂ	z, dʒ	
3;6–3;11					
4;0–4;5	ʒ, dʒ			ts, tsʰ, ɹ	
4;6–4;11		ɕ	ʃ		
5;0–5;5	ʃ				m, n, p, b, t, d, k, f, s, ʃ, t, l
5;6–5;11					n̪, t̪, dʒ, r
6;0–6;5	ɹ				
6;6–6;11					pʰ, t̪ʰ
7;0 above	θ, ð				

Note: Information on other languages studied in this volume is unavailable, either because phonemic acquisition is reported, or because the data were not comparable. The youngest age group in each language is the youngest one studied in each language. It does not represent the onset of sound acquisition.

markedness, this suggests that unaspirated sounds are unmarked compared with aspirated sounds. This is confirmed with the predominance of de-aspiration error patterns found in these languages (see later).

5. *Tonal acquisition.* Both studies on Putonghua and Cantonese monolingual children found that tones were acquired by the age of two, earlier than segments. The same pattern has also been reported in the study on Putonghua/Cantonese-speaking bilingual children – one of the few studies on the phonological development of children acquiring two tonal languages: only 5% of a total of 40 Putonghua/Cantonese-speaking subjects made several tonal errors in Cantonese (So & Leung, this volume, no information is provided on Putonghua in the study). Since monolingual children rarely make vowel errors, errors in the speech of these bilingual children may result from similarities between the phonological systems of Putonghua and Cantonese. However, tones seem to be less affected by the interference or interaction of the two languages. Tones are also resistant to phonological impairment as demonstrated in the studies on Putonghua- and Cantonese-speaking children with speech disorders. All these findings strengthen the claim that tones have the highest saliency value in tonal languages such as Cantonese and Putonghua.

6. *Error patterns.* Tables 17.3 and 17.4 summarise both normal and unusual error patterns found in monolingual and bilingual children. Discrepancies exist in the criteria used in deciding whether an error pattern exists. For example, in English: at least five occurrences for an error was used as a criterion for error pattern use; in German: three occurrences; in Putonghua and Cantonese: two; in colloquial Egyptian Arabic: 25%. Despite these differences, almost all the studies used 10% as a group cut-off point: normal error patterns are those used by 10% or more of the normally developing children in one or several age groups while unusual error patterns are those used by less than 10% of normally developing children in any age group. By putting together error patterns reported for normally developing and phonologically disordered monolingual or bilingual children, Tables 17.3 and 17.4 show both language-specific error patterns and error patterns common to different languages. This provides a rare opportunity to examine the interaction between developmental universals and the role of language-specific features in phonological acquisition.

All the children, regardless of their language background, show a tendency to simplify syllable structure. Cluster reduction is common to all the languages where applicable. Assimilation, weak stress deletion and final consonant deletion have occurred in all the languages except colloquial Egyptian Arabic which focused on the speech development of children aged between 3;0–5;0. These error patterns might have occurred in younger age groups.

There is a tendency to use an unmarked feature to replace a marked feature among children reported in this volume. This is evident in the following error patterns:

- deaspiration in Putonghua and Cantonese monolingual children and Putonghua/Cantonese bilingual children (cf. deaspiration reported as a 'less common' error pattern in bilingual children speaking Mirpuri/Punjabi/Urdu and English bilingual children);
- deaffrication in English, German, Cantonese, Maltese, Turkish monolingual children and Cantonese/English, Putonghua/Cantonese and Mirpuri/Punjabi/Urdu-English bilingual children;
- de-emphasisation in colloquial Egyptian Arabic-speaking monolingual children in which emphatic sounds are replaced with non-emphatic sounds: /bat̪/ [batt];
- de-dentalisation in Punjabi of Punjabi/English bilingual children in which dentalised sounds are produced without a dental feature.

However, the tendency to replace marked sounds with unmarked sounds does not mean that children do not replace unmarked sounds with marked sounds at all. In Putonghua, both deaspiration and aspiration occurred in the children's speech. However, deaspiration is more prevalent and aspiration is suppressed earlier.

Other error patterns such as stopping and fronting are common to most of the languages with the exception of colloquial Egyptian Arabic. This is consistent with the relative early acquisition of stops. However, it is difficult to explain the error pattern of fronting of /k/ in the same way, since /k/ emerges as early as /p, b, t, d/ in children's speech in almost all of the languages. It is observed that while some sounds are stabilised as soon as they have emerged, it takes some time for other sounds to be accurately produced in all words. For example, Putonghua, German and Maltese report data that confirms this observation. While the acquisition of /k/ illustrates that phonological acquisition involves more than developing an ability to articulate a sound in a word context, it is unclear why some sounds need more time than others to become stabilised in the children's production. Gibbon (1990, cited by Ball *et al.*, this volume), by using electropalatographic analysis of the fronted velars and intended alveolars, suggested that the dominance of velar fronting in early speech might be related to slow development in the ability to separate front and back tongue gestures.

Language-specific variation is also evident among languages in many ways. In particular, what counts as a typical or an unusual error pattern is language-specific. This applies to the error patterns of initial consonant deletion, backing, liquid gliding, deaffrication, affrication and aspiration, among others. For example, while initial

Table 17.3 Comparison of error patterns in eight languages

	English	German	Putonghua	Cantonese	Maltese	CEA	Turkish	Spanish
Assimilation	N	N	N	N	N	?	N	N
Reduplication	N	?	?	?	N	?	N	?
Cluster reduction	N	N	NA	N	N	N	N	N
Weak syllable deletion	N	N	NA	NA	N	?	N	N
Final consonant deletion	N	N	N	N	N	?	N	N
Initial consonant deletion	U	?	N	U except h deletion	N	?	N	?
Medial consonant deletion	U	?	NA	NA	?	?	?	?
Voicing	N	N	?	U	N	N	N	NA
Stopping	N	N	N	N	N	U	N	N
Fronting	N	N	N	N	N	?	N	N
Backing	U	N	N	U	?	U	U	?
Liquid gliding	N	?	N	U	N	?	?	N
Deaffrication	N	N	U	N	N	NA	N	?
Affrication	U	?	N	N	?	?	N	?
Deaspiration	NA	NA	N	N	NA	NA	NA	NA
Aspiration	NA	NA	N	U	NA	NA	NA	NA

Towards Developmental Universals 441

	English	German	Putonghua	Cantonese	Maltese	CEA	Turkish	Spanish
Denasalisation	U						U	
Favoured sound	d, h, nasal	d, h	velar			w, j		
	Intrusive consonants	Contact assimilation	Triphthong/ diphthong reduction		Compensatory vowel lengthening	De-emphasisation	Stopping of r∫j; nasalisation of fricatives/ liquids fricative gliding	
		Glottal replacement	Consonant addition	Final glide deletion	Germination			
					r-lateralisation	r-deviation (r → l)	Liquid deviation/ vowel lengthening	
		Interdentality (s → θ)				Sibilant derviation (s → θ)		

Notes:
(1) Source: information on all the languages except Spanish in the table are based on the data reported in this volume. Spanish data is cited from Yavaş (1998). Information on error patterns of Telugu-speaking children and unusual error patterns of Maltese-speaking children is unavailable.
(2) Additional language-specific error patterns are listed in the relevant column.
(3) Abbreviations: N = normal error patterns (error patterns used by 10% or more of the normally developing children in one or several age groups); U/Shaded cells = unusual error patterns (error patterns used by less than 10% of normally developing children in any age group); NA = not applicable. ? = error patterns that are not mentioned in the studies for the following possible reasons: not significant for that language (in most cases); data is not available due to the age range of the youngest cohort in the studies (e.g. error pattern of reduplication).

Table 17.4 Comparison of error patterns in bilingual children

Bilingual language pairs	Cantonese/English		Punjabi/English	Putonghua/Cantonese		Welsh/English	
Language in each pair	Cantonese	English	Punjabi	Putonghua	Cantonese	Welsh	English
Assimilation	?	?	N	?	?	?	?
Reduplication	?	?	N	?	?	?	?
Cluster reduction	N	N	?	NA	N	?	N
Weak syllable deletion	NA	N	N	NA	NA		?
Final consonant deletion	U	U	N	N	N	?	N
Initial consonant deletion	NU	NU	NA	?	NU	?	?
Medial consonant deletion	NA	NA	N	?	?	?	?
Voicing	NU	N	N	?	?	?-	?
Stopping	N	N	N	N	N	N	N
Fronting	N	N	N	N	N	N	N
Backing	NU	NU	N	N	NU	?	?
Liquid gliding	NU	N	N	?	NU	U	N
Deaffrication	N	N	?	NU	N	?	?
Affrication	N	NU	U	N	?	?	?
Deaspiration	N	NA	U	N	N	NA	NA

Towards Developmental Universals

Bilingual language pairs	Cantonese/English		Punjabi/English	Putonghua/Cantonese		Welsh/English	
Aspiration	NU	NA	?	NU	?	NA	NA
Intrusive consonants	?	?	N	?	?	?	?
Denasalisation	?	?	N	?	?	?	?
Frication	?	N	?	?	N	?	?
De-retrolex	?	?	N	N	?	?	?
Nasalisation	?	N	?	N	?	?	?
			De-dentalisation			Trill fricativisation/approximantisation (r → ð)	
			Use of lateral fricative (ʃ → ɬ)			Lateral fricative simplification/decoupling ɬ → x	
						Fricative simplification	

Notes:
(1) Source: information on all the languages in the table are based on the data reported in this volume.
(2) Additional language-specific error patterns are listed in the relevant column.
(3) Abbreviations: N = normal error patterns (error patterns used by 10% or more of the normally developing children in one or several age groups); NU = normal error patterns but considered atypical for monolingual children; U/shaded cells = unusual error patterns (error patterns used by less than 10% of normally developing children in any age group with the exception of Welsh data for which unusual error patterns are based on the two children described in the chapter). NA = not applicable. ? = error patterns that are not mentioned in the studies for the following possible reasons: not significant in that language and hence no mention in the findings (in most cases); data is not available due to the age range of the youngest cohort in the studies (e.g. error pattern of reduplication) or small sample size.

consonant deletion is an unusual error pattern in English and Cantonese (except /h/ deletion), it is a common error pattern for monolingual speakers of the languages such as Putonghua, Maltese and Turkish and also for English/Cantonese bilingual children and Putonghua/Cantonese bilingual children.

There are several explanations for the language-specific nature of typical error patterns. It may reflect the interaction between language developmental universals and the nature of an individual language. Alternatively, specific to bilingual children, it may reflect the interaction between the two phonological systems being acquired. As discussed in Chapter 1, there are phonological errors in the speech of bilingual children that are not typical of monolingual children. The differences might result from the methodologies used in the studies. Since whether an error pattern will be classified as typical or unusual is based on a 10% cut-off point, the classification is subject to potential bias of sampling and the sample size of children studied. The 10% cut-off point is arbitrary, and based on incidence figures for developmental speech disorders in English.

The role of an individual language in language acquisition is also manifested in different acquisition patterns of the same sound or feature. One example is clusters. Various patterns associated with clusters have been reported in the previous literature and in this volume. In terms of order of acquisition, it is found that two-member clusters are acquired earlier than three-member clusters (English: Stoel-Gammon & Dunn, 1985; German: this volume); and syllable-initial clusters are acquired earlier than syllable-final clusters (English: Stoel-Gammon & Dunn, 1985; Maltese: this volume). In terms of error patterns, the common cluster reduction pattern in English is that the member that is deleted is generally the one that is acquired late as a single consonant (Yavaş, 1998), for example, [bu] for /blue/, [tap] for /strap/. Alternatively, in reducing clusters, a child might follow the Sonority Sequencing Principle and delete the segment with the lower sonority index (Yavaş & Goldstein, this volume). While the child tends to produce a single consonantal segment in place of a cluster, Lleo and Prinz (1996) report that the segment is not necessarily identical to one of the target segments. This finding is confirmed in Maltese data reported in this volume. Another language-specific pattern came from Telugu: consonant clusters tend to be realised as geminates and the consonants involved tend to be assimilated into each other during acquisition in Telugu (Nirmala, 1981b, reported in Vasanta, this volume).

Another manifestation of the role of an individual language in language acquisition is the sound /r/. Nearly all the languages studied have /r/ in different forms (as an approximant in English, Putonghua, a trill in Maltese, Telugu, colloquial Egyptian Arabic and Welsh; a flap in

Mirpuri/Punjabi/Urdu). However, each language differs in its replacement patterns:

- English: r → w/ʋ
- Putonghua: r → j
- Maltese: lateralisation of r → l
- Colloquial Egyptian Arabic: r → l
- Turkish: r → j/vowel
- Welsh by Welsh/English bilingual: trill fricativisation/approximantisation r → ð/r (approximant)
- Mirpuri/Punjabi/Urdu: r → l or deleted
- Italian, Hindi, Igbo, Portuguese, Quiche, Spanish: r → l (Bortolini & Leonard, 1991)

The Welsh trill seems to have the most distinctive realisation pattern: the Welsh–English bilingual children used either the approximant-r as in English to replace the trill as the result of interaction between Welsh and English, or to use a voiced fricative in place of the trill. The realisation of /r/ as a fricative might be due to the acoustic similarity between fricatives and the target trill (Ball et al., this volume). Using an acoustic analysis approach, Khattab (this volume) also found that Arabic–English bilingual children seem to have a wider repertoire of /r/ sounds than that of the monolinguals due to the interaction between Arabic, English and other non-native varieties of English that the children are exposed to.

7. Bilingual versus monolingual acquisition. Studies of bilingual children reported in the volume present a complicated picture of bilinguals' phonological acquisition: different and sometimes conflicting findings are reported with regard to the central issue of whether the phonological acquisition of bilingual children is qualitatively and/or quantitatively the same or different from that of monolingual children.

Evidence for the argument that bilingual children's phonological acquisition is quantitatively and qualitatively the same as monolingual children came from Spanish (Yavas & Goldstein, this volume). Measured in terms of speech accuracy, the Spanish/English-speaking bilingual children's accuracy for sound classes was similar to or even exceeded that of monolingual children. They also demonstrated the same strategy in learning phonological rules of cluster reduction as their monolingual counterparts: when reducing two consonant cluster codas, they deleted the segment with the lower sonority index so that the one retained provided the minimum descent in sonority from the nucleus to the coda.

However, counter-evidence came from the Putonghua/Cantonese bilingual study (So & Leung, this volume) and Mirpuri/Punjabi/Urdu and English-speaking bilingual study (Stow & Pert, this volume), though the findings are less conclusive. It was reported that

Putonghua/Cantonese-speaking bilingual children seemed to exhibit a general delay in comparison to monolinguals in the phonological acquisition of both languages. For example, the four tripthongs in Putonghua were not acquired until 3;5 by Putonghua/Cantonese-speaking children while monolingual children would have acquired the vowels by 2;11 – although bilingual children acquired Cantonese vowels more or less at the same time. However, as the authors point out, the picture is not clear-cut, since bilingual children acquired some phonemes earlier than monolingual children. For example, bilingual children acquired Putonghua affricates /ts, ts^h/ and liquids at 4;6, earlier than monolingual Putonghua-speaking children who do not acquire these sounds until 4;6. This may be due to the fact that these sounds are also part of Cantonese inventory the children are acquiring and thus the acquisition of these shared sounds benefits from increased exposure.

A relatively late establishment of Mirpuri/Punjabi/Urdu consonants in bilingual children speaking Mirpuri/Punjabi/Urdu and English was also reported (Stow & Pert, this volume). However, the delay is viewed as a reflection of the relative difficulty of eliciting speech samples rather than an overall delay.

While the different measures used in the above-mentioned studies makes it difficult to compare across studies, a much clearer picture came from the Cantonese/English bilingual study (Holm & Dodd, this volume). Using various measures including phonetic inventory, speech accuracy and error patterns, the study found that in general, the phonetic development of the bilingual children did not differ from monolingual children in that phonemes were acquired in similar sequences and at similar times in both languages and shared phonemes were stimulable in both languages. In terms of speech accuracy, while the bilingual children's speech accuracy was better in Cantonese than English, there was no difference in the Cantonese accuracy between the monolingual and bilingual children and the bilingual children's English accuracy was significantly lower than the monolingual children's. The differences may be due to the fact that all the bilingual children were mainly exposed to Cantonese in their early years.

In terms of error patterns, more evidence for the existence of qualitative and quantitative differences between the phonological acquisition of bilingual children and that of monolingual children were found. Atypical error patterns are reported in two bilingual studies in this volume, which compared the error patterns of the bilingual children's speech with available information on that of monolinguals: Cantonese/English, Putonghua/Cantonese (for bilingual error patterns, see Table 17.4). These two groups of bilingual children both produced error patterns that rarely occur in the speech of monolingual children. Further comparison of the bilingual children's Cantonese in the two studies showed significant similarities. Error patterns, 'atypical' of monolingual development, such as initial consonant deletion, backing, liquid gliding and aspiration were evident in the Cantonese speech production of two groups of bilingual children who differed in the other language they are acquiring. In contrast, there were also differences in the type of error patterns used between the two groups of bilingual children who shared Cantonese as one of their languages, demonstrating the influence of the other language on Cantonese. For example, while final consonant deletion was a common error pattern in the Cantonese speech of Putonghua/Cantonese-speaking bilingual children, it was an atypical error pattern in the Cantonese speech of Cantonese/English-speaking bilingual children. The same pattern also existed in the non-Cantonese language of the bilingual children (i.e. English in Cantonese/English-speaking children and Putonghua in Putonghua/Cantonese-speaking children). It is interesting to note that no atypical patterns are reported in the speech of either language of Welsh/English-speaking bilinguals. This may be partly due to the lack of normative data on Welsh-speaking monolinguals.

8. *Disordered phonology versus normal phonology.* The studies of children with speech disorders reported in the volume show that disordered phonology, irrespective of language and irrespective of the monolingual and bilingual context, are characterised by persistent delayed error patterns, atypical error patterns, variability, restricted phonetic or phonemic inventory, and systematic sound or syllable preference. The data from Telugu-speaking children with pre-lingual hearing loss (Vasanta, this volume) suggested that their phonology may also demonstrate phonotactic limitations.

In addition, four subgroups of children with speech disorders (articulation disorder, phonological delay, consistent phonological disorder, and inconsistent phonological disorder) are reported in English, German, Putonghua, Cantonese and Turkish (for a definition of these subgroups, see Chapter 3). Children with symptoms of more than one type of speech disorder have been reported in languages such as German, Cantonese and Welsh. Among these children, articulation impairment co-occurs with other types of speech disorder. For example, the study on Welsh/English-speaking bilingual children reported a case study of a child with speech characterised by both an articulation disorder and inconsistent speech disorder.

Despite their language backgrounds, phonologically disordered children resemble the normally developing children speaking the same language in that they show similar sensitivity to the target phonological system. Their phonology more often than not operates within the constraints of the target phonology. For example, 'illegal' phonemes were very rarely used to replace the target phonology; the syllable shapes in their production tends to conform to the phonotactic rules of the target languages; vowels and tones which tend to be acquired early by normally developing children were resistant to phonological impairment.

9. *Issues specific to bilingual children with speech disorder.* A number of issues specific to bilingual children with speech disorder were raised in Chapter 1.

What criteria can be used in diagnosing bilingual children with speech disorder? The answer to this question is that they should be compared with their normally developing bilingual peers rather than monolingual peers. However, the lack of normative data on bilingual children is repeatedly reported in the bilingual literature. When bilingual normative data is not available, great caution needs to be taken in comparing bilingual children with monolingual children. Error patterns, speech accuracy and phoneme inventories, which are often employed to compare monolingual children with speech disorder with their normally developing peers, are less reliable when it comes to comparing bilingual children with 'suspected' speech disorder and their monolingual peers for the reason previously discussed on the characteristics of normally developing bilingual children. Yavas and Goldstein (this volume) also pointed out that when a bilingual child reveals developmental patterns that are different from monolinguals, it is crucial to determine whether these nonconforming patterns are due to the influence of the child's other languages, or if they are indications of a disorder.

Do bilingual children have the same type of speech disorder in both languages? Evidence from case studies of a Cantonese/English-speaking bilingual child and two Welsh/English-speaking bilingual children seems to suggest that a single deficit underlines disorder in the two phonological systems of bilingual children and, therefore, bilingual children tend to demonstrate similar types of surface errors in both languages (though not identical errors).

Will the therapy on one language affect the other language? The treatment study of a Cantonese/English-speaking bilingual child seems to suggest that effects of articulation therapy in one language will be generalised to the other language. However, in the same case study, phonological therapy on one language, that targeted phonological errors, failed to affect the other phonological system. In contrast, examples of intra-language generalisation are found in a Welsh/English bilingual child's post-therapy speech (Ball *et al.*, this volume). These contradictory findings suggest that more clinical studies are needed to test intra-language generalisation of phonological therapy.

Conclusion

This volume attempted to set up a paradigm for identifying developmental universals and language-specific features in phonological acquisition. By systematically comparing the data from normally and atypically developing multilingual children including monolingual and bilingual children, it derived a set of similarities in the phonological acquisition of children with various language backgrounds that will, in turn, become candidates for developmental universals. It is primarily for this purpose of cross-linguistic comparison and generalisation and secondly for clinical rigorousness that there is an urgent need for using comparable criteria in multilingual studies.

However, in some areas such as bilingual phonological acquisition where findings are tentative and in some cases conflicting, the work has only begun and it is hoped that the volume will inspire more studies in that direction. The book also examines empirical clinical issues and includes clinical cases where the data are available. These cases studies, though limited in scope, are much needed for clinicians who are working with children speaking languages other than English. A list of websites for speech and language therapists' professional organisations in each country is provided in the Appendix.

One finding has clearly emerged. Different languages and different language pairs seem to give rise to different findings. That is, data from the study of one language does not necessarily hold for other languages; data from the study of one language pair spoken by a bilingual child does not necessarily predict findings for other language pairs, even when one language of the pair is the same. The research effort needed to identify the boundaries of the effect of language specificity on phonological acquisition is enormous and of great theoretical and clinical importance.

References

Abdalla, A.G. (1960) An instrumental study of the intonation of Egyptian Colloquial Arabic. PhD thesis, University of Michigan.

Abudarham, S. (1987) Fact and friction. In S. Abudarham (ed.) *Bilingualism and the Bilingual: An Interdisciplinary Approach to Pedagogical and Remedial Issues* (pp.15–34). Birshire: NFER-NELSON Publishing Co. Ltd.

Acarlar, F. (1995) Normal ve fonolojik bozukluğu olan çocukların karşılaştırılması (Comparative study on normally developing and phonologically disordered children). Hacettepe University Doctoral Dissertation, Ankara, Turkey.

Acarlar, F. and Ege, P. (1996) Türkçe kazanımda kullanılan fonolojik süreçlerin incelenmesi (Phonological processes in the acquisition of Turkish). *Tηrk Psikoloji Dergisi* 38, 35–43.

Acevedo, M. (1993) Development of Spanish consonants in preschool children. *Journal of Childhood Communication Disorders* 15, 9–15.

Al-Ani, S.H. and El-Dalee, M.S. (1984) Tafkhim in Arabic: The acoustic and psychological parameters. In M.P.R. Van den Broecke and A. Cohen (eds) *Proceedings of the Tenth International Congress of Phonetic Sciences.* Dordrecht: Holland: Cinnaminson: USA: Foris Publications.

Allen, G. (1985) How the young French child avoids the pre-voicing problem for word-initial voiced stops. *Journal of Child Language* 12, 37–46.

Allen, G. and Hawkins, S. (1980) Phonological rhythm: Definition and development. In G. Yeni-Komshian, J. Kavanagh and C. Ferguson (eds) *Child Phonology, Volume 1* (pp. 227–56). New York: Academic Press.

Allman, T.M. (2002) Patterns of spelling in young deaf and hard of hearing students. *American Annals of the Deaf* 147(1), 46–64.

Al-Shareef, J. (2002) Language change and variation in Palestine: A case study of Jabalia refugee camp. Unpublished PhD dissertation, University of Leeds.

Amayreh, M.M. and Dyson, A.T. (1998) The acquisition of Arabic consonants. *Journal of Speech and Language Hearing Research* 41, 642–53.

Amayreh, M.M. and Dyson, A.T. (2000) Phonological errors and sound changes in Arabic-speaking children. *Clinical Linguistics and Phonetics* 14, 79–109.

American Speech Language-Hearing Association (ASHA) (1985) Clinical management of communicatively handicapped minority language populations. *ASHA* 27, 29–32.

Ammar, W. (1992) Articulation disorders in Arabic. Unpublished PhD thesis, University of Alexandria.

Ammar, W. (1999) The acquisition of consonant clusters in Egyptian children from two to four years. *Language Sciences* 2(3), 10–37.

Ammar, W. (2002) Acquisition of syllabic structure in Egyptian Colloquial Arabic. In F. Windsor, M. Louise Kelly and N. Hewlett (eds) *Investigations in Clinical Phonetics and Linguistics.* Mahwah, New Jersey, London: Lawrence Erlbaum Associates.

Ammar, W. and Rifaat, K. (1998) The phonetic inventory of consonants of normal three to four-year-old normal Egyptian children. *Langues et Linguistique. Revue Internationale de Linguistique* 3, 61–81.

References

Anani, M. (1985) Differences in the distribution between Arabic /l/, /r/, and English /l/,/r/. *Papers and Studies in Contrastive Linguistics* 20, 129–33.

Anderson, J.L. (1983) The markedness differential hypothesis and syllable structure difficulty. In G.S. Nathan (ed.) *Articulation and Phonological Disorders* (pp. 172–232). Boston: Allyn and Bacon.

Anderson, R. and Smith, B. (1987) Phonological development of two-year-old monolingual Puerto Rican Spanish-speaking children. *Journal of Child Language* 14, 57–78.

Anthony, A., Bogle, D., Ingram, T. and McIsacc, M. (1971) *Edinburgh Articulation Test*. Edinburgh: Churchill Livingstone.

Aquilina, J. (1959) *The Structure of Maltese*. Malta: University of Malta.

Aquilina, J. (1987) *Maltese-English Dictionary* (Vol. 1). Malta: Midsea Books Ltd.

Awbery, G. (1984) Phonotactic constraints in Welsh. In M.J. Ball and G.E. Jones (eds) *Welsh Phonology: Selected Readings* (pp. 65–104). Cardiff: University of Wales Press.

Azzopardi, M. (1981) The phonetics of Maltese: Some areas relevant to the deaf. Unpublished PhD thesis, University of Edinburgh.

Azzopardi, S. (1997) Phonological development of consonants in 4-year-old Maltese children. Unpublished dissertation, University of Malta.

Badar, R. (2002) Factors affecting the consistency of word production: Age, gender and word characteristics. Unpublished MSc dissertation, University of Newcastle upon Tyne, UK.

Baker, C. (1988) Normative testing and bilingual populations. *Journal of Multilingual and Multicultural Development* 9, 399–409.

Baker, C. and Prys Jones, S. (1998) *Encyclopedia of Bilingualism and Bilingual Education*. Clevedon: Multilingual Matters.

Ball, M.J. (1988) LARSP to LLARSP. Designing a Welsh grammatical profile. *Clinical Linguistics and Phonetics* 2, 55–73.

Ball, M.J. (1989) Transcribing the suprasegmentals of Welsh. *Journal of the International Phonetic Association* 19, 89–96.

Ball, M.J. (1994) Using dependency phonology in the analysis of disordered speech. *Australian Journal of Human Communication Disorders* 22, 22–30.

Ball, M.J. (in press) Welsh. In D. Britain (ed.) *Language in the British Isles* (2nd edn). Cambridge: Cambridge University Press.

Ball, M.J. and Kent, R. (1997) *The New Phonologies*. San Diego: Singular Publishers.

Ball, M.J. and Müller, N. (1992) *Mutation in Welsh*. London: Routledge.

Ball, M.J., Müller, N. and Munro, S. (2001a) Patterns in the acquisition of the Welsh lateral fricative. *Clinical Linguistics and Phonetics* 15, 3–7.

Ball, M.J., Müller, N. and Munro, S. (2001b) The acquisition of the lateral fricative in Welsh-English bilinguals. *Multilingua* 20, 269–84.

Ball, M.J., Müller, N. and Munro, S. (2001c) The acquisition of the rhotic consonants by Welsh-English bilingual children. *International Journal of Bilingualism* 5, 71–86.

Ball, M.J. and Munro, S.M. (1981) Language assessment procedures for linguistic minorities: An example. *Journal of Multilingual and Multicultural Development* 2, 231–41.

Ball, M.J. and Williams, B. (2001) *Welsh Phonetics*. Lewiston, NY: Edwin Mellen Press.

Bankson, N. and Bernthal, J. (1998) Analysis and interpretation of assessment data. In J. Bernthal and N. Bankson (eds) *Articulation and Phonological Disorders* (pp. 270–98). Boston: Butterworth-Heinemann.

Barbour, S. and Stevenson, P. (1990) *Variation in German*. Cambridge: Cambridge University Press.

Barlow, J. (2001) Error patterns and transfer in Spanish-English bilingual phonological production. Paper presented at the 26th Annual Boston University Conference on Language Development, Boston, MA.

Bates, E., Marchman, V., Thal, D., Fenson, L., Dale, P., Reznick, S., Reilly, J. and Hartung, J. (1994) Developmental and stylistic variation in the composition of early vocabulary. In K. Perera, G. Collis and B. Richards (eds) *Growing Points in Child Language* (pp. 85–124). Cambridge: Cambridge University Press.

Battacchi, M.W., Facchini, G.M., Manfredi, M.M. and Rubatta, C.O. (1964) Presenatzione di un reattivo per l'esame dell'articolazione fonetica nei fanciulli in eta prescolare di lingua italiana. *Bollettino della Societa Italiana di Fonetica, Foniatria e Audiologia* 13, 441–86.

Bauman-Waengler, J. (1994) Normal phonological development. In R.J. Lowe (ed.) *Phonology: Assessment and Intervention Applications in Speech Pathology*. Baltimore: Maryland.

Beckman, M.E. and Edwards, J. (2000) The ontogeny of phonological categories and the primacy of lexical learning in linguistic development. *Child Development* 71(1), 240–49.

Bellin, W. (1984) Welsh phonology in acquisition. In M. Ball and G. Jones (eds) *Welsh Phonology: Selected Readings* (pp. 156–75). Cardiff: University of Wales Press.

Bellin, W. (1988) The development of pronunciation. In M.J. Ball (ed.) *The Use of Welsh* (pp. 213–28). Clevedon: Multilingual Matters.

Bhardwaj, M.R. (1995) *Colloquial Panjabi*. London: Routledge.

Bhaskara Rao, P. (1982) A reexamination of consonantal sandhi in modern colloquial Telugu. *Bulletin of the Deccan College Research Institute* 41, 16–26.

Bhatia, T.K. (1993) *Punjabi: A Cognitive-Descriptive Grammar*. London: Routledge.

Bhatia, T.K. and Koul, A. (2000) *Colloquial Urdu*. London: Routledge.

Bialystok, E. (ed.) (2001) *Bilingualism in Development: Language, Literacy, and Cognition*. Cambridge: Cambridge University Press.

Bird, S. and Blackburn, B. (1990) A logical approach to Arabic phonology. *Proceedings of the Fifth Conference of the European Chapter of the Association for Computational Linguistics*.

Bishop, D. (1997) *Uncommon Understanding: Development and Disorders of Language Comprehension in Children*. Hove: Psychology Press.

Bleile, K.M. (1995) *Manual of Articulation and Phonological Disorders: Infancy Through Adulthood*. San Diego, California: Singular Publishing Group, Inc.

Bloomfield, L. (1933) *Language*. New York: Holt, Reinhart and Winston.

Bond, Z.S., Eddey, J.E. and Bermejo, J.J. (1980) VOT del espanol to English: Comparison of a language-disordered and normal child. *Journal of Phonetics* 8, 287–90.

Boothroyd, A. (1984) Auditory perception of speech contrasts by subjects with sensorineural hearing loss. *Journal of Speech and Hearing Research* 27, 134–44.

Borg, A.J. (1973) The segmental phonemes of Maltese. *Linguistics* 109, 5–11.

Borg, A.J. (1975) Maltese morphophonemics. *Journal of Maltese Studies* IV, 11–28.

Borg, A.J. (1980) Language and socialisation in developing Malta. *Work in Progress* 13, 60–71; Department of Linguistics, University of Edinburgh.

Borg, A.J. (1988) *Ilsienna*. Malta: Has-Sajjied.

Borg, A.J. and Azzopardi-Alexander, M. (1997) *Maltese*. London: Routledge.

Bortolini, U. and Leonard, L. (1991) The speech of phonologically disordered children acquiring Italian. *Clinical Linguistics and Phonetics* 5, 1–12.

Boysson-Bardies, B. and Vihman, M.M. (1991) Adaptation to language: Evidence from babbling and first words in four languages. *Language* 67(2), 297–319.

Bradford, A. (1990) The motor planning skills of subgroups of speech disordered children. Unpublished Honours thesis, University of Queensland, Brisbane.

Bradford, A. and Dodd, B. (1994) The motor planning abilities of phonologically disordered children. *European Journal of Disorders of Communication* 23, 349–69.

Bradford, A. and Dodd, B. (1996) Do all speech-disordered children have motor deficits? *Clinical Linguistic and Phonetics* 10, 77–101.

Braun, A. (2002) Behandlung phonologischer Störungen im Kindesalter: Ein Vergleich der Effektivität von artikulatorischer und phonologischer Therapie. Unpublished MSc dissertation, RWTH, Aachen University.

Broomfield, J. (2003) Developmental speech and language disability: Epidemiology and clinical effectiveness. Unpublished PhD thesis, University of Newcastle upon Tyne.

Broomfield, J. and Dodd, B. (2001) Mainstream paediatric speech and language therapy service population: Epidemiology. *International Journal of Language and Communication Disorders* 36 (Supplement), 447–52.

Broomfield, J. and Dodd, B. (2004) Children with speech and language disability: Caseload characteristics. *International Journal of Language and Communication Disorders* 39(3), 303–24.

Broselow, E.I. (1976) The phonology of Egyptian Arabic. PhD thesis, University of Massachusetts.

Burling, R. (1959/1978) Language development of a Garo and English Child. *Word*, 15, 45–68. Reprinted in E. Hatch (ed.) (1978) *Second Language Acquisition* (pp. 54–75). Rowley: Newbury House.

Burt, L., Holm, A. and Dodd, B. (1999) Phonological awareness skills of 4-year-old British children: An assessment and developmental data. *International Journal of Language and Communication Disorders* 34, 311–35.

Butcher, A. (1989) The use and abuse of phonological assessment. *Child Language Teaching and Testing* 5(3), 262–77.

Butler, C. (1985) *Statistics in Linguistics*. Oxford: Blackwell.

Campbell, G.L. (1995) *Concise Compendium of the World's Languages*. London: Routledge.

Caramazza, A., Yeni-Komshian, G.H., Zurif, E.B. and Carbone, E. (1973) The acquisition of a new phonological contrast: The case of stop consonants in French-English bilinguals. *Journal of the Acquisitional Society of America* 54(2), 421–28.

Carrow, E. (1974) *Austin Spanish Articulation Test*. Austin, TX: Learning Concepts.

Carrow-Woolfolk, E. (1985) *Test for Auditory Comprehension of Language – Revised*. Texas: DLM Teaching Resources.

Catford, J.C. (1988) Functional load and diachronic phonology. In Y. Tobin (ed.) *The Prague School and its Legacy*. Amsterdam: John Benjamins.

Chambers, J. (2003) *Sociolinguistic Theory* (2nd edn). Oxford: Blackwell.

Chao, Y.R. (1947) *Cantonese Primer*. Cambridge: Harvard University Press.

Chao, Y.R. (1951/1973) The Cantian Idiolect: An analysis of the Chinese spoken by a twenty-eight-month-old child. In C.A. Ferguson and D.I. Slobin (eds) *Studies of Child Language Development*. New York: Holt, Rinehart and Winston, Inc.

Cheng, L.L.-R. (2001) Educating speech-language pathologists to work in multicultural populations – An Asian-Pacific perspective. *Speech and Hearing Review* 2, 192–213.

Cheung, K.H. (1986) The phonology of present day Cantonese. Unpublished doctoral thesis, University of London.

Cheung, P. and Abberton, D. (2000) Patterns of phonological disability in Cantonese-speaking children. *International Journal of Language and Communication Disorders* 35, 451–74.

Chiat, S. (1989) The relation between prosodic structure, syllabification and segmental realisation: Evidence from a child with fricative stopping. *Clinical Linguistics and Phonetics* 3(3), 223–42.

Christman, S.S. (1992) Uncovering phonological regularity in neologisms: Contributions of sonority theory. *Clinical Linguistics and Phonetics* 6(3), 219–47.

Clements, G.N. (1990) The role of sonority cycle in core syllabification. In J. Kingston and M.E. Beckman (eds) *Papers in Laboratory Phonology* (pp. 283–333). Cambridge, UK: Cambridge University Press.

Clements, G.N. and Keyser, S.J. (1983) *Phonology: A Generative Theory of the Syllable*. Linguistics Inquiry Monographs 9, Cambridge, MA: The M.I.T. Press.

Clumeck, H. (1977) Studies in the acquisition of Mandarin phonology. Unpublished PhD thesis, University of California, Berkeley.

Clumeck, H. (1980) The acquisition of tone. In G. Yeni-Komshian, J. Kavanagh and C. Ferguson (eds) *Child Phonology 1*, New York: Academic Press.

Cook, V. (ed.) (2003) *Effects of the Second Language on the First*. Clevedon: Multilingual Matters.

Coulmas, F. (1999) *The Blackwell Enclyclopedia of Writing Systems*. Oxford, UK: Blackwell.

Crary, M. (1983) Phonological process analysis from spontaneous speech: The influence of sample size. *Journal of Communication Disorders* 16, 133–41.

Creaghead, N., Newman, P.W. and Secord, W.A. (1989) *Assessment and Remediation of Articulatory and Phonological Disorders* (2nd edn). Columbus: Merrill Pub. Co.

Cruttenden, A. (2001) *Gimson's Pronunciation of English* (6th edn). London: Arnold.

Crystal, D. (1985) Things to remember when transcribing speech. *Child Language Teaching and Therapy* 1, 235–39.

Crystal, D. (1995) *The Cambridge Encyclopaedia of the English Language*. Cambridge: Cambridge University Press.

Crystal, D. (1997) *The Cambridge Encyclopedia of Language* (2nd edn). Cambridge: Cambridge University Press.

Crystal, D., Fletcher, P. and Garman, M. (1989) *Grammatical Analysis of Language Disability* (2nd edn). London: Whurr.

Cutler, A., McQueen, J.M. and Norris, D. (2001) The roll of the silly ball. In E. Dupoux (ed.) *Language, Brain and Cognitive Development* (pp. 181–94). Cambridge, MA: The M.I.T. Press.

Cutler, A., Otake, T. and Murthy, L. (2003) Rhythmic effects in non-native listening. Paper presented at the 18th International Congress of Phonetic Sciences held in Barcelona, Spain.

De Houwer, A. (1995) Bilingual language acquisition. In P. Fletcher and B. MacWhinney (eds) *Handbook of Child Language*. Oxford: Blackwell.

De la Fuente, M.T. (1985) The order of acquisition of Spanish consonant phonemes by monolingual Spanish speaking children between the ages of 2.0 and 6.5. Unpublished doctoral dissertation, Georgetown University, Washington, DC.

DeFrancis, J. (1984) *The Chinese Language: Fact and Fantasy*. Honolulu: University of Hawaii Press.

Department for Education and Employment (1999) *Sure Start Planning Pack: Sure Start for All: Guidance on Involving Minority Ethnic Children and Families*. Nottingham: DfEE Publications.

Derwing, B.L. and Yoon, Y.B. (1999) The effect of orthographic knowledge on syllable segmentation: A cross-linguistic study. Paper presented at the 14th International Congress of Phonetic Sciences held in San Francisco, California.

Deuchar, M. and Clark, A. (1995) Early billigual acquisition of the voicing contrast in English and Spanish. *Bangor Research Papers in Linguistics* 6, 24–37.

Dinnsen, D. (1992) Variation in developing and fully developed phonetic inventories. In C.A. Ferguson, L. Menn and C. Stoel-Gammon (eds) *Phonological Development Models, Research and Implications*. Maryland: York Press.

Dinnsen, D. (1996) Context-sensitive underspecification and the acquisition of phonemic contrasts. *Journal of Child Language* 23, 57–79.

Dinnsen, D. and Chin, S. (1994) Independent and relational accounts of phonological disorders. In M. Yavaş (ed.) *First and Second Language Phonology* (pp. 135–48). San Diego, CA: Singular Publishing Group.

Dinnsen, D., Chin, S., Elbert, M. and Powell, T. (1990) Some constraints on functionally disordered phonologies: Phonetic inventories and phonotactics. *Journal of Speech and Hearing Research* 33, 28–37.

Dinnsen, D., Elbert, M. and Weusner, G. (1979) On the characterisation of functional misarticulations. Paper presented to the Annual Convention of the ASHLA. Atlanta.

Dobrich, W. and Scarborough, H. (1992) Phonological characteristics of words young children try to say. *Journal of Child Language* 19, 597–616.

Docherty, G.J. (1992) *The Timing of Voicing in British English Obstruents*. Berlin & New York: Foris Publications.

Docherty, G.J. and Foulkes, P. (2000) Speaker, speech and knowledge of sounds. In N. Burton-Roberts, P. Carr and G.J. Docherty (eds) *Phonological Knowledge. Conceptual and Empirical Issues* (pp. 105–29). Oxford: Oxford University Press.

Docherty, G.J. and Foulkes, P. (2004) Glottal variants of (t) in the Tyneside variety of English: An acoustic profiling study. In J.M. Beck and W. Hardcastle (eds) *Figure of Speech – a Festschrift for John Laver*. London: Lawrence Erlbaum.

Docherty, G.J., Foulkes, P., Tillotson, J. and Watt, D.J.L. (2005) On the scope of phonological learning: Issues arising from socially structured variation. In C.T. Best, L. Goldstein and D.H. Whalen (eds) *Laboratory Phonology 8*. Berlin: Mouton de Gruyter.

Dodd, B. (1993) Speech disordered children. In G. Blanken, H. Dittmann, H. Grimm, J. Marshall and C.W. Wallesch (eds) *Linguistic Disorders and Pathologies* (pp. 825–34). Berlin, Germany: De Gruyter.

Dodd, B. (1995) *Differential Diagnosis and Treatment of Children with Speech Disorder*. London: Whurr.

Dodd, B. and Bradford, A. (2000) A comparison of three therapy methods for children with different types of developmental speech disorders. *International Journal of Language and Communication Disorders* 35, 189–209.

Dodd, B., Holm, A. and Li, W. (1997) Speech disorder in pre-school children exposed to Cantonese and English. *Clinical Linguistics and Phonetic* 11, 229–43.

Dodd, D. Holm, A., Zhu Hua and Sharon Crosbie (2003) Phonological development: Normative data from English-speaking children. *Clinical Linguistics and Phonetics* 17, 617–43.

Dodd, B., Leahy, J. and Hambly, G. (1989) Phonological disorders in children: Underlying cognitive deficits. *British Journal of Developmental Psychology* 7, 55–71.

Dodd, B. and Iacono, T. (1989) Phonological disorders in children: Changes in phonological process use during treatment. *British Journal of Disorders of Communication* 24, 333–51.

Dodd, B. and McCormack, P. (1995) A model of speech processing for differential diagnosis of phonological disorders. In B. Dodd (ed.) *Differential Diagnosis and Treatment of Children with Speech Disorder* (pp. 65–90). London: Whurr.

Dodd, B., So, L. and Li, W. (1996) Symptoms of disorder without impairment: The written and spoken errors of bilinguals. In B. Dodd, R. Campblell and L. Worrall (eds) *Evaluating Theories of Language* (pp. 119–39). London: Whurr.

Dodd, B., Zhu Hua, Crosbie, S., Holm, A. and Ozanne, A. (2002) *Diagnostic Evaluation of Articulation and Phonology*. London: The Psychological Corporation.

Donegan, P.J. and Stampe, D. (1979) The study of natural phonology. In D.A. Dinnsen (ed.) *Current Approaches in Phonological Theory*. Bloomington, IN: Indiana University Press.

Duckworth, M., Allen, G., Hardcastle, W. and Ball, M. (1990) Extensions to the International Phonetic Alphabet for the transcription of atypical speech. *Clinical Linguistics and Phonetics* 4(4), 273–86.

Durell, M. (1992) *Using German*. Cambridge: Cambridge University Press.

Dyson, A.T. and Amayreh, M.M. (2000) Phonological errors and sound changes in Arabic-speaking children. *Clinical Linguistics and Phonetics* 14(2), 79–109.

Eckman, F.R. (1977) Markedness and the contrastive analysis hypothesis. *Language Learning* 27, 315–30.

Edwards, J. (1979) Social class difference and the identification of sex in children's speech. *Journal of Child Language* 1, 205–209.

Edwards, M. (1973) The acquisition of liquids. *Ohio State University Working Papers in Linguistics* 15, 1–54.

Edwards, M. (1974) Perception and production in child phonology: The testing of four hypotheses. *Journal of Child Language* 1, 205–19.

Edwards, M. (1992) Phonological assessment and treatment in support of phonological processes. *Language, Speech and Hearing Services in Schools* 23, 233–40.

Elbert, M. (1992) Clinical forum: Phonological assessment and treatment consideration of error types. A response to Fey. *Language, Speech and Hearing Services in Schools* 23, 241–46.

Ellis, R. (1994) *The Study of Second Language Acquisition*. Oxford: Oxford University Press.

Elman, J., Diehl, R. and Buchwald, S. (1977) Perceptual switching in bilinguals. *Journal of the Acoustical Society of America* 62, 971–74.

Elsen, H. (1991) *Erstspracherwerb – Der Erwerb des deutschen Lautsystems*. Wiesbaden: Deutscher Universitäts Verlag.

Enderby, P. and John, A. (1997) *Therapy Outcome Measures for Speech and Language Therapists*. San Diego: Singular Publishing.

Enderby, P. and Philipp, R. (1986) Speech and language handicap: Towards knowing the size of the problem. *British Journal of Disorders of Communication* 21, 151–65.

Ethnologue (2003) On WWW at http://www.ethnologue.com. Accessed 23.9.03.

Fantini, A.F. (1985) *The Language Acquisition of a Bilingual Child*. Clevedon: Multilingual Matters.

Fee, E.J. (1995) Segments and syllables in early language acquisition. In J. Archibald (ed.) *Phonological Acquisition and Phonological Theory*. Hillsdale: LEA.

Ferguson, C.A. (1956) The emphatic *l* in Arabic. *Language* 23(3), 446–552.

Fey, M.E. (1992) Clinical Forum: Phonological assessment and treatment. Articulation and phonology: Inextricable constructs in speech pathology. *Language, Speech, Hearing Services in Schools* 23(3), 225–32.

Flege, J.E. (1995) Second language speech learning: theory, findings, and problems, In W. Strange (ed.) *Speech Perception and Linguistic Experience: Theoretical and Methodological Issues* (pp. 233–72). Baltimore: York Press.

Flege, J.E. and Port, R. (1981) Cross-language phonetic interference: Arabic to English. *Language & Speech* 24(2), 125–45.

Fongaro-Leverin, S. (1992) Der Erwerb des Lautsystems und die Phonologischen Prozesse sich normal entwickelnder Kinder: Ein Interlinguistischer Vergleich Deutsch/Portugiesisch. Unpublished PhD thesis, Ludwig-Maximilian-Universität.

Foulkes, P., Docherty, G.J. and Watt, D. (2005) Phonological variation in child directed speech. *Language* 81, 177–206.

Foulkes, P., Docherty, G.J. and Watt, D. (1999) Tracking the emergence of sociophonetic variation: Realisations of (t) by Newcastle children. *Leeds Working Papers in Linguistics and Phonetics* 7, 1–25; University of Leeds.

Fox, A.V. (2000) The acquisition of phonology and the classification of speech disorders in German-speaking children. Unpublished PhD thesis, Newcastle upon Tyne.

Fox, A.V. (2002) *PLAKSS – Psycholinguistische Analyse kindlicher Sprechstörungen.* Frankfurt: SWETS – Test Services.

Fox, A.V. (2003) *Kindliche Aussprachestörungen – Phonologische Entwicklung, Differentialdiagnostik und Therapie.* Idstein: Schultz Kirchner Verlag.

Fox, A.V. and Dodd, B.J. (1999) Der Erwerb des phonologischen Systems in der deutschen Sprache. *Sprache – Stimme – Gehör* 23, 183–91.

Fox, A.V. and Dodd, B.J. (2001) Phonological disorders in German-speaking children. *American Journal of Speech and Language Pathology* 10, 291–307.

Fox, A.V., Dodd, B. and Howard, D. (2002) Risk factors for speech disorders in children. *International Journal of Language and Communication Disorders* 37, 117–31.

Frendo, G. (2002) The phonology of three-year old Maltese speaking twins. Unpublished dissertation, University of Malta.

Gaber, A. (1986) *Sounds of Arabic.* Egypt: Giza, Omraniya: New Offset Printing Shop.

Gan, R., Ezrati, R. and Tobin, Y. (1996) Phonological processes in Hebrew-English bilingual children (3:0–4:6). *Journal of The Israeli Speech and Language Association* 19, 247–54.

Genesee, F. (1989) Early bilingual development, one language or two? *Journal of Child Language* 16, 161–79.

Genesee, F. (1993) Bilingual language development in pre-school children. In D. Bishop and K. Modford (eds) *Language Development in Exceptional Circumstances* (pp. 62–79). Hove: Laurence Erlbaum.

Genesee, F., Nicoladis, E. and Paradis, J. (1995) Language differentiation in early bilingual development. *Journal of Child Language* 22, 611–31.

Gibbon, F. (1990) Lingual activity in two speech disordered children's attempts to produce velar and alveolar stop consonants: Evidence from electropalatographic (EPG) data. *British Journal of Disorders of Communication* 25, 329–40.

Gierut, J. (1990) Differential learning of phonological oppositions. *Journal of Speech and Hearing Research* 33, 540–49.

Gierut, J. (1999) Syllable onsets, clusters and adjuncts in acquisition. *Journal of Speech Language Hearing Research* 42, 708–26.

Gierut, J., Simmermann, C. and Neumann, H. (1994) Phonemic structures of delayed phonological systems. *Journal of Child Language* 32, 291–316.

Gilbert, J.H.V. (1977) A voice onset time analysis of apical stop production in three-year-olds. *Journal of Child Language* 4, 103–10.

Gildersleeve-Neumann, C. and Davis, B. (1998) Learning English in a bilingual preschool environment: Change over time. Paper presented at the convention of the American Speech-Language-Hearing Association, San Antonio, TX.

Gildersleeve, C., Davies, B. and Stubbe, E. (1996) When monolingual rules don't apply: Speech development in bilingual environment. Paper presented at the annual convention of the American Speech-Language-Hearing Association, Seattle, WA.

Goldman, R. and Fristoe, M. (1987) *Goldman-Fristoe Test of Articulation.* Circle Pines: American Guidance Service.

Goldstein, B. (1996) The role of stimulability in the assessment and treatment of Spanish-speaking children. *Journal of Communication Disorders* 29, 299–314.

Goldstein, B. (1999) Phonological assessment of Latino children. Unpublished assessment tool.

Goldstein, B. (2001) Assessing phonological skills in Hispanic/Latino children. *Seminars in Speech and Language* 22, 39–49.

Goldstein, B. and Iglesias, A. (1996) Phonological patterns in Puerto Rican Spanish-speaking children with phonological disorders. *Journal of Communication Disorder* 29, 367–87.

Goldstein, B. and Washington, P. (2001) An initial investigation of phonological patterns in 4-year-old typically developing Spanish-English bilingual children. *Language, Speech and Hearing Services in the Schools* 32, 153–64.

Goltz, R. and Walker, A. (1961) North Saxon. In R.E. Keller (ed.) *German Dialects.* Manchester: Manchester University Press.

Gonzalez, A. (1981) A descriptive study of phonological development in normal speaking Puerto Rican preschoolers. Unpublished doctoral dissertation, Pennsylvania State University, State College, PA.

Gonzalez, G. (1983) The acquisition of Spanish sounds in the speech of two-year-old Chicano children. In R. Padilla (ed.) *Theory Technology and Public Policy on Bilingual Education* (pp. 73–87). Rosslyn, VA: National Clearinghouse for Bilingual Education.

Gonzalez, M.M. (1978) *Cómo Detectar Al Niño Con Problemas Del Habla (Identifying Speech Disorders in Children).* México: Editorial Trillas.

Goswami, U. (1999a) The relationship between phonological awareness and orthographic representations in different orthographies. In M. Harris and G. Hatano (eds) *Learning to Read and Write: A Cross-linguistic Perspective.* Cambridge, UK: Cambridge University Press.

Goswami, U. (1999b) Integrating orthographic and phonological knowledge as reading develops: Onsets, rimes and analogies in children's reading. In R.M. Klein and P.A. McMullen (eds) *Converging Methods for Understanding Reading and Dyslexia.* Cambridge, MA: The M.I.T. Press.

Goswami, U., Gombert, J.E. and De Barrera, L.F. (1998) Children's orthographic representations and linguistic transparency: Nonsense word reading in English, French and Spanish. *Applied Psycholinguistics* 19, 19–52.

Grech, H. (1998) Phonological development of normal Maltese speaking children. Unpublished PhD thesis, University of Manchester.

Grech, H. and Hesketh, A. (1996) Conventions applicable in transcription and analysis of speech of children exposed to a bilingual environment. *Journal of The Israeli Speech and Language Association* 19, 255–68.

Greenberg, J.H. (1978) *Universals of Human Languages. Phonology* (Vol. 2). Stanford, CA: Stanford University Press.

Grohnfeldt, M. (1980) Erhebung zum altersspezifischen Lautbestand bei drei- bis sechsjährigen Kindern. *Die Sprachheilarbeit* 5, 169–77.

Grosjean, F. (1992) Another view of bilingualism. In R.J. Harris (ed.) *Cognitive Processing in Bilinguals* (pp. 51–62). North Holland: Elsevier.

Grosjean, F. (1995) A psycholinguistic approach to codeswitching: The recognition of guest words by bilinguals. In L. Milroy and P. Muysken (eds) *One Speaker, Two Languages: Cross-disciplinary Perspectives on Codeswitching* (pp. 259–75). Cambridge: Cambridge University Press.

Grosjean, F. (1998) Studying bilinguals: Methodological and conceptual issues. *Bilingualism: Language and Cognition* 2, 131–49.

Grosjean, F. (2001) The bilingual's language modes. In J.L. Nicol (ed.) *One Mind, Two Languages* (pp. 1–22). Oxford: Blackwell.

Grundy, K. (1989) *Linguistics in Clinical Practice*. London: Taylor & Francis.

Grunwell, P. (1977) The analysis of phonological disability in children. Unpublished PhD thesis, University of Reading.

Grunwell, P. (1981a) The development of phonology. *First Language* 3, 161–91.

Grunwell, P. (1981b) *The Nature of Phonological Difficulty in Children*. London: Academic Press.

Grunwell, P. (1982) *Clinical Phonology*. London: Croom Helm.

Grunwell, P. (1985) *Phonological Assessment of Child Speech*. Windsor: NFER-Nelson.

Grunwell, P. (1987) *Clinical Phonology* (2nd edn). London: Croom Helm.

Grunwell, P. (1992) Processes of phonological change in developmental speech disorders. *Clinical Phonetics and Linguistics* 6, 101–102.

Grunwell, P. (1997) Natural Phonology. In M.J. Ball and R.D. Kent (eds) *The New Phonologies* (pp. 35–75). San Diego: Singular.

Guitart, J. (1978) A proposito del Espanhol de Cuba y Puerto Rico: Hacia un modelo no sociolinguistico de lo sociodialectal (Regarding the Spanish of Cuba and Puerto Rico: Towards a non-sociolinguistic model of the social dialectic). In H. Lopez Morales (ed.) *Corrientes actuales en la dialectologia de Caribe Hispanico* (pp. 77–92). Rio Piedras: Editorial Universiataria, Universidad de Puerto Rico.

Hacker, D. and Weiss, K.H. (1986) *Zur phonemischen Struktur funktioneller Dyslalien*. Oldenburg: Arbeiter Wohlfahrt Verlag.

Hamers, J.F. and Blanc, M.H.A. (2000) *Bilinguality and Bilingualism* (2nd edn). Cambridge: Cambridge University Press.

Hammond, R. (1976) Phonemic restructuring of voiced obstruents in Miami-Cuban Spanish. In F. Aid, M. Resnick and B. Saciuk (eds) *1975 Colloquium on Hispanic Linguistics* (pp. 42–51). Washington, DC: Georgetown University Press.

Harrell, R.S. (1957) *The Phonology of Colloquial Egyptian Arabic*. New York: American Council of Learned Societies.

Harrison, G. and Thomas, C. (1975) *The Acquisition of Bilingual Speech by Infants*. London: Final Report on SSRC Grant HR2104/1.

Hashimoto, A. (1972) *Studies in the Yue Dialect*. Cambridge: The University Press.

Hatton, L. (1988) The development of the nasal mutation in the speech of schoolchildren. In M.J. Ball (ed.) *The Use of Welsh* (pp. 239–57). Clevedon: Multilingual Matters.

Heselwood, B. (1998) An unusual kind of sonority and its implications for phonetic theory. *Leeds Working Papers in Linguistics and Phonetics* 6, 66–80.

Heselwood, B. and McChrystal, L. (2000) Gender, accent features and voicing in Punjabi-English bilingual children. *Leeds Working Papers in Linguistics and Phonetics* 8, 45–70.

Hodson, B. (1986) *The Assessment of Phonological Processes – Revised* (2nd edn). Danville, IL: The Interstate Printers & Publishers.

Hodson, B. and Paden, E. (1978) Phonological feature competencies of normal four-year olds. *Acta Symbolica* 9, 37–49.

Hodson, B. and Paden, E. (1981) Phonological processes which characterize unintelligible and intelligible speech in early childhood. *Journal of Speech and Hearing Disorders* 46, 369–73.

Hoffmann, C. (1991) *An Introduction to Bilingualism*. New York: Longman.

Hogg, R. and McCully, C. (1987) *Metrical Phonology: A Coursebook*. New York: Cambridge University Press.

Holm, A. (1998) Speech development and disorder in bilingual children. Unpublished PhD dissertation, University of Newcastle upon Tyne.

Holm, A. and Dodd, B. (1999a) A longitudinal study of the phonological development of two Cantonese-English bilingual children. *Applied Psycholinguistics* 20, 349–76.

Holm, A. and Dodd, B. (1999b) Differential diagnosis of phonological disorder in two bilingual children acquiring Italian and English. *Clinical Linguistics and Phonetics* 13, 113–29.

Holm, A., Dodd, B., Stow, C. and Pert, S. (1999) Identification and differential diagnosis of phonological disorder in bilingual children. *Language Testing* 16(3), 271–92.

Holm, A., Ozanne, A. and Dodd, B. (1997) Efficacy of intervention for a bilingual child making articulation and phonological errors. *International Journal of Bilingualism* 1, 55–69.

Hsu, J. (1987) A study of the various stages of development and acquisition of Mandarin Chinese by children in Taiwan milieu. MA dissertation, College of Foreign languages, Fu Jen Catholic University.

Hughes, A. and Trudgill, P.J. (1996) *English Accents and Dialects. An Introduction to Social and Regional Varieties of British English* (3rd edn). London: Arnold.

Hull, G. (1993) *The Maltese Language Question: A Case Study of Cultural Imperialism*. Valletta: Said International.

Ingram, D. (1976) *Phonological Disability in Children*. London: Edward Arnold.

Ingram, D. (1979) Cross-linguistic evidence on the extent and limit of individual variation in phonological development. *Proceedings of the 9th International Congress of Phonetic Sciences* 2, 150–54.

Ingram, D. (1981) *Procedures for the Phonological Analysis of Children's Language*. Baltimore: University Park Press.

Ingram, D. (1981/1982) The emerging phonological system of an Italian-English bilingual child. *Journal of Italian Linguistics* 2, 95–113.

Ingram, D. (1986a) Explanation and phonological remediation. *Child Language Teaching and Therapy* 2, 1–19.

Ingram, D. (1986b) Phonological development: Production. In P. Fletcher and M. Garman (eds) *Language Acquisition* (2nd edn) (pp. 223–239). Cambridge: Cambridge University Press.

Ingram, D. (1989a) *First Language Acquisition: Method Description and Explanation*. Cambridge: Cambridge University Press.

Ingram, D. (1989b) *Phonological Disability in Children* (2nd edn). London: Whurr.

Ingram, D., Christensen, L., Veach, S. and Webster, B. (1980) The acquisition of word-initial fricatives and affricates in English between 2 and 6 years. In G. Yeni-Komshian, J. Kavanagh and C. Ferguson (eds) *Child Phonology* (pp. 169–92). New York: Academic Press.

Irwin, J. and Wong, S. (eds) (1983) *Phonological Development in Children 18–72 Months*. Carbondale: Southern Illinois University Press.

Itoh, H. and Hatch, E. (1978) Second language acquisition: A case study. In E. Hatch (ed.) *Second Language Acquisition: A Book of Readings* (pp. 76–88). Rowley: Newbury House.

Jakobson, R. (1941/1968) *Child Language, Aphasia and Phonological Universals* (A. Keiler, 1968 trans.). The Hague: Mouton.

Jakobson, R. (1969) *Kindersprache, Aphasie und Allgemeine Lautgesetze*. Frankfurt: Edition Suhrkamp.

James, D. (2001) An item analysis of Australian English words for an articulation and phonology test for children aged 2 to 7 years. *Clinical Linguistics and Phonetics* 15, 457–85.

Jeng, Heng-hsiung (1979) The acquisition of Chinese phonology in relation to Jakobson's laws of irreversible Solidarity. *Proceedings of the 9th International Congress of Phonetic Sciences*. University of Copenhagen.

Jimenez, B.C. (1987) Acquisition of Spanish consonants in children aged 3–5 years, 7 months. *Language Speech and Hearing Services in the Schools* 18(4), 357–63.

Joanisse, M.F. (1999) Exploring syllable structure in connectionist networks. Paper presented at the 14th International Congress of Phonetic Sciences held in San Francisco, California.

Johnson, C.E. and Lancaster, P. (1998) The development of more than one phonology: A case study of a Norwegian-English bilingual child. *The International Journal of Bilingualism* 2(3), 265–300.

Kahn, M. (1975) Arabic emphatics: The evidence for cultural determinants of phonetic sex-typing. *Phonetica* 31(1), 38–50.

Kamhi, A. (1992) The need for a broad-based model of phonological disorders. *Language, Speech and Hearing Services in Schools* 23, 261–68.

Karniol, R. (1990) Second language acquisition via immersion in daycare. *Journal of Child Language* 17, 147–70.

Katamba, F. (1989) *Introduction to Generative Phonology*. London: Longman.

Kay, M. (1987) Non-concatenative finite-state morphology. *Proceedings of the Third Meeting of the European Chapter of the Association for Computational Linguistics*, Morristown, NJ, USA: Association for Computational Linguistics.

Kent, R. (1983) The segmental organization of speech. In P. Macneilage (ed.) *The Production of Speech* (pp. 57–89). New York: Springer-Verlag.

Kent, R. (1992) The biology of phonological development. In C.A. Ferguson, L. Menn and C. Stoel-Gammon (eds) *Phonological Development: Models, Research, Implications* (pp. 65–90). Timonium, MD: York Press.

Kewley-Port, D. and Preston, M.S. (1974) Early apical stop production: A voice onset time analysis. *Journal of Phonetics* 2, 195–210.

Khan, F. (1984) Phonological development of Urdu speaking children. *International Review of Applied Linguistics in Language and Teaching* 22(4), 277–86.

Khan, F. (1991) The Urdu speech community. In S. Alladina and V. Edwards (eds) *Multilingualism in the British Isles, 2, Africa, the Middle East and Asia*. London: Longman.

Khattab, G. (1998) Sociolinguistic study of English-Arabic bilinguals. Unpublished MA dissertation, University of Leeds.

Khattab, G. (2002a) Sociolinguistic competence and the bilingual's adoption of phonetic variants: Auditory and instrumental data from English-Arabic bilinguals. Unpublished PhD thesis, University of Leeds.

Khattab, G. (2002b) VOT production in English and Arabic bilingual and monolingual children. In D.B. Parkinson and E. Benmamoun (eds) *Perspectives on Arabic Linguistics XIII-XIV* (pp. 1–38). Amsterdam: John Benjamins.

Khattab, G. (2002c) /r/ production in English and Arabic bilingual and monolingual speakers. *Leeds Working Papers in Linguistics and Phonetics* 9, 95–122.

Kirkpatrick, E. and Ward, J. (1984) Prevalence of articulation errors in N.S.W. primary school. *Australian Journal of Human Communication Disorders* 12, 55–62.

Kohler, K. (1995) *Einführung in die Phonetik* (2nd edn). Berlin: Erich Schmidt Verlag.

Konefal, J.A. and Fokes, J. (1981) Voice onset time: The development of Spanish-English distinction in normal and language disordered children. *Journal of Phonetics* 9, 437–44.

Konrot, A. (1986) İşitme engelli çocuklarda konuşmanın bürünsel özellikleri nasıl geliştirilebilir? (How the prosodic features can be developed in hearing impaired children). *Anadolu Üni. Eğitim Fakültesi Dergisi* 1(1), 119–29.

Kopkallı-Yavuz, H. and Topbaş, S. (1998) Phonological processes of Turkish phonologically disordered children: language specific or universal? In W. Ziegler and K. Deger (eds) *Clinical Phonetics and Linguistics* (pp. 88–97). London: Whurr Publishers.

Kopkallı-Yavuz, H. and Topbaş, S. (2000) Children's preferences in early phonological acquisition: How does it reflect sensitivity to the ambient language? In A. Göksel and C. Kerslake (eds) *Studies on Turkish and Turkic Languages*. Turcologica. Harrassowitz Verlag: Wiesbaden Oxford University.

Kostic, Dj., Mitter, A. and Krishnamurti, Bh. (1977) *A Short Outline of Telugu Phonetics*. Calcutta: Indian Statistical Institute.

Krishnamurti, Bh. and Gwynn, J.P.L. (1985) *A Grammar of Modern Telugu*. New Delhi: Oxford University Press.

Kubozono, H. (1996) Speech segmentation and phonological structure. In T. Otake (ed.) *Phonological Structure and Language Processing: Cross-linguistic Studies*. New York: Mouton DeGruyter.

Ladefoged, P. and Maddieson, I. (1996) *The Sounds of the World's Languages*. Oxford: Blackwell.

Langdon, H. and Cheng, L.R.L. (2002) *Collaborating with Interpreters and Translators*. Eau Claire, WI: Thinking Publications.

Law, J. (1992) *The Early Identification of Language Impairment in Children*. London: Chapman & Hall.

Law, J., Boyle, J., Harris, F., Harkness, A. and Nye, C. (1998) Child health surveillance: Screening for speech and language delay. *Health Technology Assessment* 2(9), 1–184.

Law, J., Boyle, J., Harris, F., Harkness, A. and Nye, C. (2000) Prevalence and natural history of primary speech and language delay: Findings from a systematic review of the literature. *International Journal of Language and Communication Disorders* 35, 165–88.

Lehn, W. (1963) Emphasis in Cairo Arabic. *Language* 39, 29–39.

Leitão, S., Hogben, J. and Fletcher, J. (1997) Phonological skills in speech and language impaired children. *European Journal of Disorders of Communication* 32, 73–93.

Leonard, L. (1985) Unusual and subtle phonological behaviour in the speech of phonologically disordered children. *Journal of Speech and Hearing Disorders* 50, 4–13.

Leonard, L., Schwartz, R., Allen, G., Swanson, L. and Loeb, D. (1989) Unusual phonological behaviour and the avoidance of homonymy in children. *Journal of Speech and Hearing Research* 32, 583–90.

Leopold, W. (1939–1949) *Speech Development of a Bilingual Child: A Linguist's Record* (94 volumes). Evanston: Northwestern University Press.
Leopold, W.F. (1970) *Speech Development of a Bilingual Child: A Linguist's Record* (Vol. 2). New York: AMS Press.
Li, R. (1989) Classification of Chinese dialects. *Dialect* 4, 241–59.
Li, C.N. and Thompson, S.A. (1977) The acquisition of tone in Mandarin-speaking children. *Journal of Child Language* 4, 185–99.
Li, Paul J.-K. (1977) Child language acquisition of Mandarin phonology. In R. Cheng, Y.C. Li and Ting-chi Tang (eds) *Proceedings of the Symposium on Chinese Linguistics: 1977 Linguistic Institute of the Linguistic Society of America*. Taipei: Student Books.
Light, T. (1977) Clairetalk: A Cantonese-speaking child's confrontation with bilingualism. *Journal of Chinese Linguistics* 5, 261–74.
Lindblom, B. (1998) Systemic constraints and adaptive change in the formation of sound structure. In J.R. Hurford, M. Studdert-Kennedy and C. Knight (eds) *Approaches to the Evolution of Language: Social and Cognitve Bases*. Cambridge: Cambridge University Press.
Lisker, L. and Krishnamurti, Bh. (1991) Lexical stress in a stressless language: Judgments by Telugu and English speaking linguists. *Proceedings of the 12th International Congress on Phonetic Sciences* (Vol. 2/5) (pp. 90–93). Aix-En Provence, France.
Lleo, C. and Prinz, N. (1996) Consonantal clusters in child phonology and the directionality of syllable structure assignment. *Journal of Child Language* 23, 31–56.
Local, J. (1983) How many vowels in a vowel? *Journal of Child Language* 10, 449–53.
Locke, A., Ginsborg, J. and Peers, I. (2002) Development and disadvantage: Implications for the early yeas and beyond. *International Journal of Language and Communication Disorders* 37(1), 3–15.
Locke, J. (1980) The prediction of child speech errors: Implications for a theory of acquisition. In G.H. Yeni-komshian, J.F. Kavanagh and C.A. Ferguson (eds) *Child Phonology, 1: Production*. New York: Academic Press.
Locke, J. (1983a) Clinical phonology: The explanation and treatment of speech sound disorders. *Journal of Speech and Hearing Disorders* 48, 339–41.
Locke, J. (1983b) *Phonological Acquisition and Change*. New York: Academic Press.
Lopez Morales, H. (1971) *Estudio sobre el Espanhol de Cuba (Studies on the Spanish of Cuba)*. New York: Las Americas.
Lyovin, A.V. (1997) *An Introduction to the Languages of the World*. Oxford: Oxford University Press.
Macken, M. and Barton, D. (1980a) The acquisition of the voicing contrast in English: A study of voice onset time in word-initial stop consonants. *Journal of Child Language* 7, 41–74.
Macken, M. and Barton, D. (1980b) The acquisition of the voicing contrast in Spanish: A phonetic and phonological study of word-initial stop consonants. *Journal of Child Language* 7, 433–58.
Macken, M. and Ferguson, C. (1983) Cognitive aspects of phonological development: Model, evidence and issues. In K. Nelson (ed.) *Children's Language* (pp. 255–82). Hillsdale: Erlbaum.
Maez, L. (1981) Spanish as a first language. Unpublished doctoral dissertation, University of California, Santa Barbara.
Magnusson, E. (1991) Metalinguistic awareness in phonologically disordered children. In M. Yavas (ed.) *Phonological Disorder in Children*. London: Routledge.
Malta Central Office of Statistics (1995) Education and economic activity. *Census*, Volume 4.

Mann, D.P., Kayser, H., Watson, J. and Hodson, B. (1992) Phonological systems of Spanish-speaking Texas preschoolers. Paper presented at the annual convention of the American Speech-Language-Hearing Association, San Antonio, TX.

Mason, M., Smith, M. and Hinshaw, M. (1976) *Medida Española de articulación (Measurement of Spanish Articulation)*. San Ysidro, CA: San Ysidro School District.

Mattes, L. (1995) *Spanish Articulation Measures* (2nd edn). Oceanside, CA: Academic Communication Associates.

Matthews, D. and Dalvi, M.K. (1999) *Teach Yourself Urdu*. London: Hodder and Stoughton.

McCarthy, J. (1981) A prosodic theory of non-concatenative morphology. *Linguistic Inquiry* 12, 373–413.

McCormick, B. (1992) *Paediatric Audiology: 0-5 years* (2nd edn). London: Taylor & Francis.

McMahon, S. and Dodd, B. (1995) Multiple-birth children's communication. In B. Dodd (ed.) *Differential Diagnosis and Treatment of Children with Speech Disorder* (pp. 211–29). London: Whurr.

McNutt, J.C. (1994) Generalization of /s/ from English to French as a result of phonological remediation. *Journal of Speech Language Pathology and Audiology* 18, 109–14.

McReynolds, L.V. and Elbert, M. (1981) Criteria for phonological process analysis. *Journal of Speech and Hearing Disorders* 46, 197–204.

Meinhold, G. and Stock, E. (1980) *Phonologie der Deutschen Gegenwartssprache*. Leipzig: VEB Bibliographisches Institut.

Menn, L. (1976) Evidence for an interactionist – discovery theory of child phonology. *Papers Rep. Child Language Development* 12, 169–77.

Menyuk, P. (1968) The role of distinctive feature in children's acquisition of phonology. *Journal of Speech and Hearing Research* 11, 138–46.

Mitchell, T. F. (1990/1993) *Pronouncing Arabic*. Oxford: Clarendon Press.

Möhring, H. (1938) Lautbildungsschwierigkeit im Deutschen. *Zeitschrift für Kinderforschung* 47, 185–235.

Morsi, R. (2001) Developmental articulation test for phonologically disordered Egyptian children. Unpublished MA thesis, University of Alexandria.

Morsi, R. (2003) A tentative articulation test for phonologically disordered Egyptian children. Paper presented at Child Language Seminar, July 9–11, Newcastle-upon-Tyne, UK.

Mowrer, D. and Burger, S. (1991) A comparative analysis of the phonological acquisition of consonants in the speech of two and a half and six year old Xhosa- and English-speaking children. *Clinical Linguistics and Phonetics* 5, 139–64.

Munro, S. (1985) An empirical study of specific communication disorders in bilingual children. Unpublished PhD thesis, University of Wales.

Munro, S., Ball, M.J., Müller, N., Duckworth, M. and Lyddy, F. (2005) Phonological acquisition in Welsh-English bilingual children. *Journal of Multilingual Communication Disorders* 3, 24–49.

Nagamma Reddy, K. (1987) Constraints on consonant sequences across some Indian languages. *Osmania Papers in Linguistics* 13, 39–61.

Nasr, R.T. (1966) *Colloquial Arabic: An Oral Approach*. Beirut: Librarie du Liban.

National Statistics Online (2003a) On WWW at http://www.statistics.gov.uk. Accessed 24.9.03.

National Statistics Online (2003b) On WWW at http://tables.neighbourhood.statistics.gov.uk/tables/eng/TableViewer/wdsview/print.asp. Accessed 12.3.03.

Navarro, A., Pearson, B., Cobo-Lewis, A. and Oller, D. (1995) Early phonological development in young bilinguals: Comparison to monolinguals. Paper presented to the American Speech, Language and Hearing Association Conference.
Nettelblad, U. (1983) *Developmental Studies of Dysphonology in Children*. Lund: CWK Gleerup.
Nirmala, C. (1981a) First language (Telugu) development in children. Unpublished Doctoral dissertation submitted to Osmania University, Hyderabad.
Nirmala, C. (1981b) Medial consonant cluster acquisition by Telugu children. *Journal of Child Language* 8, 63–73.
Ohala, D. (1999) The influence of sonority on children's cluster reduction. *Journal of Communication Disorders* 32(6), 397–422.
Ohala, D. (1995) Sonority driven cluster reduction. In E.V. Clark (ed.) *Proceedings of the 27th Annual Child Language Research Forum*, Stanford, CA: Stanford Linguistics Association.
Ohala, J. (1997) The relation between phonetics and phonology. In W.J. Hardcastle and J. Laver (eds) *The Handbook of Phonetic Sciences* (pp. 674–94). Oxford: Blackwell.
Oller, K. and Delgado, R. (2000) *Logical International Phonetics Program* (v. 2.02). Miami, FL: Intelligent Hearing Systems.
Olmsted, D. (1971) *Out of the Mouth of Babes*. The Hague: Mouton.
Olson, A.C. and Nickerson, J.F. (2001) Syllabic organization and deafness: Orthographic structure or letter frequency in reading? *The Quarterly Journal of Experimental Psychology* 54A(2), 421–38.
Omar, M.K. (1973) *The Acquisition of Egyptian Arabic as a Native Language*. Paris: Mouton.
Otake, T., Hatano, G. and Cutler, A. (1993) Mora or syllable? Speech segmentation in Japanese. *Journal of Memory and Language* 32, 258–78.
Pakistan Government (2003) On WWW at http://www.statpak.gov.pk/depts/pco/index.html. Accessed 23.9.03.
Pandolfi, A.M. and Herrera, M.O. (1990) Producción fonológica diastratica de niños menores de tres años (Phonological production in children less than three-years old). *Revista Teorica y Aplicada* 28, 101–22.
Patkowski, M. (1994) The critical age hypothesis in inter-language phonology. In M. Yavas (ed.) *First and Second Language Phonology* (pp. 205–22). San Diego, CA: Singular Publishing Group.
Pert, S. and Letts, C. (2003) Developing an expressive language assessment for children in Rochdale with a Pakistani heritage background. *Child Language Teaching and Therapy* 19(3), 267–290.
Peters, A. (1983) *The Units of Language Acquisition*. Cambridge: Cambridge University Press.
Petheram, B. and Enderby, P. (2001) Demographic and epidemiological analysis of patients refereed to speech and language therapy at eleven centres 1987–95. *International Journal of Language and Communication Disorders* 36, 515–25.
Pierrehumbert, J. (1980) The phonetics and phonology of English intonation. PhD thesis, MIT.
Pilch, H. (1975) Advanced Welsh phonemics. *Zeitschrift für Celtische Philologie* 34, 60–102.
Pinker, S. and Jackendoff, R. (2005) The faculty of language: What's special about it? *Cognition* 95(2), 201–36.
Pisoni, D.B. and Lively, S.E. (1995) Variability and invariance in speech perception: A new look at some old problems in perceptual learning. In W. Strange (ed.)

Speech Perception and Linguistic Experience: Theoretical and Methodological Issues (pp. 433–62). Baltimore: York Press.

Pisoni, D.B. (1997) Some thoughts on normalization in speech perception. In K. Johnson and J.W. Mullennix (eds) *Talker Variability in Speech Processing* (pp. 9–32). San Diego: Academic Press.

Poole, I. (1934) Genetic development of articulation of consonants sounds in speech. *Elementary English Review* 11, 159–61.

Prabhavathi Devi, M. (1990) Vowel length in Telugu – an instrumental study. In T. Balasubramaniam and V. Prakasam (eds) *Sound Patterns for the Phonetician: Studies in Phonetics and Phonology Honour of J.C. Catford*. Madras: T.R. Publications.

Prakasam, V. (1978) Parametric phonetics and functional phonology. Paper presented at a seminar organised by Annamalai University, Annamalai Nagar, Tamil Nadu.

Prather, E., Hedrick, D. and Kern, C. (1975) Articulation development in children aged two to four years. *Journal of Speech and Hearing Disorders* 40, 179–91.

Preisser, D., Hodson, B. and Paden, E. (1988) Developmental phonology: 18–29 months. *Journal of Speech and Hearing Disorders* 53, 125–30.

Preston, M.S., Yeni-Komshian, G. and Stark, R. (1967) Voicing in initial stop consonants produced by children in the pre-linguistic period from different language communities. *Annual Report*, 2, 305–23. Neurocommunications Laboratory, Baltimore, MD: Johns Hopkins University School of Medicine.

Pye, C., Ingram, D. and List, H. (1987) A comparison of initial consonant acquisition in English and Quiche. In K.E. Nelson and A. van Kleeck (eds) *Children's Language* (Vol. 6) (pp. 75–90). Hillsdale, NJ: Lawrence Erlbaum.

Rahman, T. (1998) *Language and Politics in Pakistan*. Karachi: Oxford University Press.

Ramarao, C. (1969) A grammatical sketch of Telugu. Unpublished manuscript submitted to the Census Bureau of India, Calcutta.

Reynell, J.K. (1987) *Reynell Developmental Language Scales Cantonese (Hong Kong) Version*. Windsor, UK: NFER-Nelson.

Reynolds, M. (1986) A qualitative analysis of phonological processes. *Australian Journal of Human Communication Disorders* 14(2), 47–54.

Rhys, M. (1984) Intonation and the discourse. In M. Ball and G. Jones (eds) *Welsh Phonology: Selected Readings* (pp. 125–55). Cardiff: University of Wales Press.

Rifaat, K. (1987) The acoustic correlates of stress in colloquial Egyptian Arabic. MA thesis, University of Alexandria.

Rifaat, K. (1991) The intonation of Arabic: An experimental Study. PhD thesis, University of Alexandria.

Rifaat, K. (1994) The pitch accents of Egyptian Arab children. *Proceedings of the Colloquium on Arabic Linguistics*, University of Bucharest, Center for Arab Studies, Bucharest.

Rifaat, K. (2003) The structure of Arabic intonation. Paper presented at the *17th Arabic Linguistics Symposium*, May 8–9, Alexandria, Egypt.

Roberts, J. (1997) Acquisition of variable rules: A study of (-t, d) deletion in preschool children. *Journal of Child Language* 24, 351–72.

Roberts, J. and Labov, W. (1995) Learning to talk Philadelphian: Acquisition of short a by preschool children. *Language Variation and Change* 7, 101–12.

Roberts, J., Burchinal, M. and Footo, M. (1990) Phonological process decline from 2 to 8 years. *Journal of Communication Disorders* 23, 205–17.

Robertson, K.L. (1998) Phonological awareness and reading acquisition of children from differing socio-economic backgrounds. *Dissertation Abstracts International Section A: Humanities and Social Sciences* 58(8-A), 3066.

Rocca, P.D. and Marcelino, M. (1999) Some characteristics of VOT in plosives produced by speakers of English and Portuguese. *Proceedings of the 14th International Congress of the Phonetic Sciences* (pp. 1425–28). University of California, Berkeley.

Rochdale Borough Profile (2003) On WWW at http://www.rochdale.gov.uk. Accessed 21.9.03.

Romaine, S. (1995) *Bilingulism* (2nd edn). Oxford: Blackwell Publishers Inc.

Romani, C. and Calabrese, A. (1998) Syllabic constraints in the phonological errors of an aphasic patient. *Brain and Language* 64, 83–121.

Romonath, R. (1991) *Phonologische Prozesse an sprachauffälligen Kindern, eine vergleichende Untersuchung an sprachauffälligen und nichtsprachauffälligen Vorschulkindern*. Berlin: Edition Marhold.

Roseberry-McKibbin, C. (1994) Assessment and intervention for children with limited English proficiency and language disorders. *American Journal of Speech-Language Pathology* 3, 77–88.

Rutherford, W. (1983) Language typology and language transfer. In S. Gass and L. Selinker (eds) *Language Transfer in Language Learning*. Rowley, MA: Newbury House.

Saifullah Khan, V. (1977) The Pakistanis: Mirpuri villagers at home and in Bradford. In J.L. Watson (ed.) *Between Two Cultures*. Oxford: Blackwell.

Saifullah Khan, V. (1979) Migration and social stress: Mirpuris in Bradford. In V. Saifullah Khan (ed.) *Minority Families in Britain*. London: Social Science Research Council.

Sailaja, P. (1997) *The Role of Literacy in Syllable Awareness among Telugu Speakers*. Paper presented at the 18th South Asian language analysis round table conference held at the Jawharlal Nehru University, New Delhi.

Sailaja, P. (1998) Orthography and phonological awareness: Phoneme and syllable manipulation abilities of Telugu-English biliterate adults. Paper presented at the 19th South Asian Language Analysis round table conference held at the University of York, York, UK.

Sailaja, P. (1999) *Syllable Structure of Telugu*. Paper presented at the 14th International Congress of Phonetic Sciences held in San Francisco, California, USA.

Sailaja, P. (2000) Writing systems and phonological awareness. Paper presented at a conference organised by the National University of Singapore.

Salama, H. (2003) The phonemic inventory of normal Egyptian children from the age of three to four years in connected speech. Unpublished postgraduate research, University of Alexandria.

Salem, H. (2000) Study of the acquisition of the syllable structure in sentence perspective in the speech of normal Egyptian children. Unpublished PhD thesis, University of Alexandria.

Sancier, M.L. and Fowler, C.A. (1997) Gestural drift in a bilingual speaker of Brazilian Portuguese and English. *Journal of Phonetics* 25, 421–36.

Sander, E. (1972) When are speech sounds learned? *Journal of Speech and Hearing Disorders* 37, 55–63.

Sastry, J.V. (1972) *Telugu Phonetic Reader*. Mysore: Central Institute of Indian Languages.

Sastry, J.V. (1994) *A Study of Telugu Regional and Social Dialects: A Prosodic Analysis*. Mysore: Central Institute of Indian Languages.

Schnitzer, M.L. and Krasinski, E. (1994) The development of segmental phonological production in the bilingual child. *Journal of Child Language* 21, 585–622.

Schnitzer, M.L. and Krasinski, E. (1996) The development of segmental phonological production in a bilingual child: A contrasting second case. *Journal of Child Language* 23, 547–71.

Sciriha, L. (1999) *A Sociolinguistic Survey of the Maltese Islands 111*. Cyclostyled, Department of English, University of Malta.

Sciriha, L. and Vassallo, M. (2001) *Malta – A Linguistic Landscape*. Malta: Socrates Office.

Scobbie, J.M. (2005) Flexibility in the face of incompatible English VOT systems. In Best, C.T., Goldstein, L. and Whalen, D.H. (eds) *Laboratory Phonology 8*. Berlin: Mouton de Gruyter.

Scovel, T. (1988) *A Time to Speak: A Psycholinguistic Inquiry into Critical Period for Human Speech*. New York: Harper and Row.

Selkirk, E.O. (1982) The syllable. In H. Van der Hulst and N. Smoth (eds) *The Structure of Phonological Representations* (Part II). Dordrecht, Holland: Foris.

Sell, D., Harding A. and Grunwell, P. (1994) GOS.SP.ASS: A screening assessment of cleft palate speech. *European Journal of Disorders of Communication* 29, 1–15.

Shaheen, K. (1979) The acoustic analysis of Arabic speech. Unpublished PhD thesis, University of Wales, Cardiff.

Shiu, Huei-shiou (1990) The phonological acquisition by Mandarin-speaking children: A longitudinal case study on children from 9 months through three years old. Unpublished MA thesis, Taiwan Normal University.

Shriberg, L. (1984) Five types of developmental phonological disorders. *Clinics in Communication Disorders* 4, 38–53.

Shriberg, L. (1997) Developmental phonological disorders: One or many? In B. Hodson and M.L. Edwards (eds) *Perspectives in Applied Phonology* (pp. 105–31). Gaithersburg, MD: Aspen Publishers Inc.

Shriberg, L. and Kwiatkowski, J. (1980) *Natural Process Analysis*. New York: John Wiley.

Shriberg, L. and Kwiatkowski, J. (1982) Phonological disorders 1: A diagnostic classification system. *Journal of Speech and Hearing Disorders* 47(3), 226–43.

Shriberg, L., Kwiatkowski, J. and Hoffman, K. (1984) A procedure for phonetic transcription by consensus. *Journal of Speech and Hearing Research* 27, 456–65.

Siegel, G.M., Winitz, H. and Conkey, H. (1963) The influence of testing instruments on articulatory responses of children. *Journal of Speech and Hearing Disorders* 28, 67–76.

Siencyn, S. (1985) Astudiaeth o'r Gymraeg fel Ail Iaith yng Nghylchoedd Meithrin Mudiad Ysgolion Meithrin. Unpublished MEd thesis, University of Wales.

Simon, C. (1976) A developmental study of acoustic pattern production and perception in voiced-voiceless oppositions. Unpublished PhD thesis, University of London.

Sloat, C., Taylor, S. and Hoard, J. (1978) *Introduction to Phonology*. Englewood Cliffs: Prentice Hall Inc.

Smit, A., Hand, L., Freilinger, J., Bernthal, J. and Bird, A. (1990) The Iowa articulation norms project and its Nebraska replication. *Journal of Speech and Hearing Disorders* 55, 779–98.

Smith, B.L. and Kenny, M.K. (1999) A longitudinal study of the development of temporal properties of speech production: Data from four children. *Phonetica*, 56, 73–102.

Smith, N. (1973) *The Acquisition of Phonology: A Case Study*. Cambridge: Cambridge University Press.

Snow, D. (1997) Children's acquisition of speech timing in English: A comparative study of voice onset time and final syllable vowel lengthening. *Journal of Child Language* 24(1), 35–56.

So, L.K.H. (1991) *Cantonese Segmental Phonology Test* (Pilot Version). Department of Speech and Hearing Sciences: University of Hong Kong.

So, L.K.H. (1992) *Cantonese Segmental Phonology Test* (Research Version). Department of Speech and Hearing Sciences: University of Hong Kong.

So, L.K.H. (1993) *Cantonese Segmental Phonology Test*. Hong Kong: Bradford Publishing Company.

So, L.K.H. and Dodd, B. (1994) Phonologically-disordered Cantonese-speaking children. *Clinical Linguistics and Phonetics* 8(3), 235–55.

So, L.K.H. and Dodd, B. (1995) The acquisition of phonology by Cantonese-speaking children. *Journal of Child Language* 22(3), 473–95.

So, L.K.H. and Zhou, J. (1997) *Putonghua Segmental Phonology Test* (Research Version). Department of Speech and Hearing Sciences: University of Hong Kong.

So, L.K.H. and Zhou, J. (1998) Acquisition of Putonghua (Mandarin) phonology: Influence from the mother tongue. *Proceedings of the Asia Pacific Conference on Speech, Language and Hearing Disorders* (pp. 167–68).

So, L.K.H. and Zhou, J. (2000) *Putonghua Segmental Phonological Test*. Nanjing: Nanjing Normal University Press.

St. Louis, K. and Ruscello, D. (1981) *The Oral Speech Mechanism Screening Examination*. Baltimore: University Park Press.

Stackhouse, J. and Wells, B. (1997) *Children's Speech and Literacy Difficulties*. London: Whurr.

Stampe, D. (1969) The acquisition of phonetic representation. *Papers from the Fifth Regional Meeting of the Chicago Linguistic Society* (pp. 433–44). Chicago: Chicago Linguistic Society.

Stampe, D. (1979) *A Dissertation on Natural Phonology*. New York: Garland.

Stemberger, J.P. (1988) Between-word processes in child phonology. *Journal of Child Language* 5, 39–61.

Stepanof, E.R. (1990) Procesos phonologicos de niños Puertorriqueños de 3 y 4 años evidenciado en la prueba APP-Spanish. (Phonological processes evidenced on the APP-Spanish by 3- and 4-year-old Puerto Rican children). *Opphla* 8, 15–20.

Stoel-Gammon, C. (1985) Phonetic inventories, 15–24 months: A longitudinal study. *Journal of Speech and Hearing Research* 28, 505–12.

Stoel-Gammon, C. and Buder, E.H. (1999) Vowel length, post-vocalic voicing and VOT in the speech of two-year-olds. *Proceedings of the 14th International Congress of the Phonetic Sciences* (pp. 2485–88). University of California, Berkeley.

Stoel-Gammon, C. and Dunn, C. (1985) *Normal and Disordered Phonology in Children*. Austin: Pro-ed.

Stoel-Gammon, C. and Stone, J. (1991) Assessing phonology in young children. *Clinics in Communication Disorders* 2, 25–39.

Stokes, S.F. (2002) Levels of complexity in phonological disorders: Evidence from Cantonese. *Clinical Linguistics and Phonetics* 16, 35–57.

Stokes, S.F. and To, C.K.S. (2002) Feature development in Cantonese. *Clinical Linguistics and Phonetics* 16, 443–59.

Stokes, S.F. and Wong, I.M. (2002) Vowel and diphthong development in Cantonese-speaking children. *Clinical Linguistics and Phonetics* 16, 597–617.

Su, A.-T. (1985) The acquisition of Mandarin phonology by Taiwanese children. MA thesis, Fu Jen Catholic University.

Teizel, T. and Ozanne, A. (1999) Variability in single word production of typically developing toddlers. Paper presented at the 20th Child Phonology Conference, July. Bangor, M.E.

Templin, M.C. (1957) Certain language skills in children: Their developments and inter-relationships. *Institute of Child Welfare Monographs* (Vol. 26). Minneapolis: University of Minnesota Press.

Ternes, E. (1987) *Einführung in die Phonologie*. Darmstadt: Wissenschaftliche Buchgesellschaft.

Teutsch, A., and Fox, A.V. (2004) Vergleich der Effektivität von artikulatorischer vs. Phonologischer Therapie in der Behandlung kindlicher phonologischer Störungen (A comparison of intervention efficacy in childhood speech disorders: Articulation versus phonological intervention). *Sprache-Stimme-Gehör* 28, 178–185.

Thomas, C.H. (1967) Welsh intonation – a preliminary study. *Studia Celtica* 2, 8–28.

Topbaş, S. (1988) The frequency effect and the acquisition of /k, t, tʃ/ sounds in Turkish. MA thesis, The City University, London.

Topbaş, S. (1994) Assessment of speech and language disordered children by phonological approach and describing the phonological characteristics in the disordered children. Published doctoral dissertation, no. 1106. Eskisehir: Anadolu University Press.

Topbaş, S. (1996) Phonological analysis of speech disordered children: A suprasegmental study. Abstracts of VII International Congress for the Study of Child Language (IASCL) Boğaziçi University, Istanbul.

Topbaş, S. (1997) Turkish children's phonological acquisition: Implications for phonological disorders. *European Journal of Disorders of Communication* 2, 377–97.

Topbaş, S. (2004a) Does the phonology of Turkish-speaking children differ from children learning other languages? Paper presented at ICPLA 10, 26–29 February. University of Louisiana, Lafayette, LA.

Topbaş, S. (2004b) *Türkçe Sesletim-Sesbilgisi Testi* (SST) [Turkish articulation and phonology test (SST): Picture book]. Ankara: Milli Egitim Bakanlığı 4. Akşam Sanat Okulu Matbassı.

Topbaş, S. (2005) *Türkçe Sesletim-Sesbilgisi testi* (SST) [Turkish articulation and phonology Test (SST): Manual book]. Ankara: Milli Egitim Bakanlığı 4. Akşam Sanat Okulu Matbassı.

Topbaş, S. and Bleile, K. (2004) Early phoneme acquisition in Turkish and English. Paper presented at the 2nd National Congress in Speech and Language Disorders. 28–30 May, Anadolu University, Eskişehir, Turkey.

Topbaş, S. and Dinçer, B. (2002) Universal and language specific aspects of variability in phonological patterns. Paper presented at IASCL-SRCLD Conference, July 16–21, University of Wisconsin, Madison, WI.

Topbaş, S. and Konrot, A. (1997) Phonological acquisition of Turkish children: Implications for phonological disorders. *European Journal of Disorders of Communication* 32, 377–96.

Topbaş, S. and Konrot, A. (1998) Variability in phonological disorders: Can we search for systematicity? Evidence from Turkish-speaking children. In W. Ziegler and K. Deger (eds) *Clinical Phonetics and Linguistics* (pp. 79–87). London: Whurr Publishers.

Topbaş, S. and Kopkallı-Yavuz (1998) The onset of a linguistic system: Is there evidence from the acquisition of final devoicing in Turkish? *Proceedings of the GALA (Generative Approaches to Language Acquisition) Conference*, Edinburgh University Press.

Toronto, A. (1977) *Southwest Spanish Articulation Test*. Austin, TX: National Education Laboratory Publishers, Inc.

Treiman, R. (1989) The internal structure of the syllable. In G.N. Carlson and M.K. Tanenhaus (eds) *Linguistic Structure in Language Processing* (pp. 27–52). Dordrecht: Kluwer.

Tse, C.Y. (1991) The acquisition process of Cantonese phonology: A case study. Unpublished MPhil thesis, University of Hong Kong.

Tse, J. (1978) Tone acquisition in Cantonese: A longitudinal case study. *Journal of Child Language* 5, 191–204.

Tse, S.M. (1982) The acquisiton of Cantonese phonology. Unpublished PhD thesis, University of British Columbia.

Valdés, G. and Figueroa, R. (1994) *Bilingualism and Testing: A Special Case of Bias*. Norwood, NJ: Ablex Publishing Company.

Vasanta, D. (1986) Derivation of frequency importance functions for a feature recognition test material. Doctoral dissertation submitted to the University of Memphis, Memphis, TN, USA.

Vasanta, D. (1994) Phonological systems of Telugu deaf children: Procedures for analysis and remediation. Final technical report of the project (No. F-1/JS-MC) funded by the University Grants Commission, New Delhi, India.

Vasanta, D. (1997) Coarticulation in the temporal domain: Evidence from Telugu speaking prelingually deaf children. *Asia Pacific Journal of Speech, Language and Hearing* 2, 139–47.

Vasanta, D. (1998) Phonological vs. orthographic strategies in Telugu deaf children: Implications for reading and spelling instruction. In A. Weisel (ed.) *Proceedings of the 18th International Congress on the Education of the Deaf* (Vol. II) (pp. 158–67). Israel: Ramot Publications.

Vasanta, D. (2001) Phonology, orthography and reading: Insights from the spelling errors of Telugu deaf children. In B. Vijayanarayana, K. Nagamma Reddy and Aditi Mukherjee (eds) *Language Matters: Papers in Honour of Prof. Cekuri Ramarao* (pp. 245–71). Hyderabad: Booklinks Corporation.

Vasanta, D. (2003) Phonological awareness and orthographic knowledge in the processing of Telugu words by 4th and 6th Grade children. Paper presented at the Child Language Seminar held at the University of Newcastle, Newcastle Upon Tyne, UK.

Vasanta, D. (2004) Processing phonological information in a semi-syllabic script: Developmental data from Telugu. *Reading and Writing: An Interdisciplinary Journal* 17, 59–78.

Vasanta, D. and Dodd, B. (1991) *A Psycholinguistic Assessment Model for Disordered Phonology* (pp. 342–45). In Congress of Phonetic Sciences, Aix-en-Provence, Universite de Provence.

Velleman, S.L. (2002) Phonotactic therapy. *Seminars in Speech and Language* 23(1), 43–55.

Vennemann, T. (1988) *Preference Laws for Syllable Structure and the Explanation of Sound Change*. Berlin: Mouton.

Vihman, M. (1996) *Phonological Development: The Origins of Language in the Child*. Oxford: Blackwell.

Vihman, M., Ferguson, G. and Elbert, M. (1986) Phonological development from babbling to speech: Common tendencies and individual differences. *Applied Psycholinguistics* 7, 3–40.

Vivaldi, A. (1990) Phonological process use and dissolution in the acquisition of Puerto Rican Spanish. Unpublished doctoral dissertation, New York University, New York.

Vogel, I. (1975) One system or two: An analysis of a two-year old Romanian-English bilingual's phonology. *Papers and Reports on Child Language Development* 9, 43–62.

Walters, J.R. (1999) A study of the segmental and suprasegmental phonology of Rhondda Valleys. Unpublished doctoral thesis, University of Glamorgan.

Wang, W.S.-Y. (1973) The Chinese language. *The Scientific American* 228(2), 50–60.

Waterson, N. (1987) *Prosodic Phonology: The Theory and its Application to Language Acquisition and Speech Processing*. Newcastle upon Tyne: Grevatt & Grevatt.

Watson, I. (1991) Phonological processing in two languages. In E. Bialystok (ed.) *Language Processing in Bilingual Children* (pp. 25–48). Cambridge: Cambridge University Press.

Weindrich, D., Jennen-Steinmetz, C., Laucht, M., Esser, G. and Schmidt, M. (1998) At risk for language disorders? Correlates and course of language disorders in preschool children born at risk. *Acta Pediatrics* 87, 1288–94.

Weiner, F. (1979) *Phonological Process Analysis*. Baltimore, MD: University Park Press.

Weiner, F. (1981) Systematic sound preference as characteristic of phonological disability. *Journal of Speech and Hearing Disorders* 41, 281–86.

Weinreich, U. (1953) *Languages in Contact: Findings and Problems*. New York: The Linguistic Circle of New York.

Weitzman, R. (2004) Postings on info-childes@mail.talkbank.org.

Welden, A. (1980) Stress in Cairo Arabic. *Studies in the Linguistic Sciences* 2, 99–120.

Wellman, B., Case, I., Mengert, I. and Bradbury, D. (1931) Speech sounds of young children, University of Iowa Study. *Child Welfare* 5(2).

Wells, J.C. (1982) *Accents of English* (3 vol). Cambridge: Cambridge University Press.

Whitehurst, G.J. (1997) Language processes in context: Language learning in children reared in poverty. In L.B. Adamson and M.A. Romski (eds) *Communication and Language Acquisition: Discoveries from Atypical Development* (pp. 233–65). Baltimore: Paul Brookes.

Wiese, R. (1996) *The Phonology of German*. Oxford: Clarendon Press.

Williams, B. (1985) Pitch and duration in Welsh stress perception: The implications for intonation. *Journal of Phonetics* 13, 381–406.

Williams, A. and Kerswill, P. (1999) Dialect levelling: Continuity vs. change in Milton Keynes, Reading and Hull. In P. Foulkes and G.J. Docherty (eds) *Urban Voices* (pp. 141–62). London: Arnold.

Winitz, H. (1969) *Articulatory Acquisition and Behavior*. New York: Appleton-Century-Crofts.

Winter, K. (2001) Numbers of bilingual children in speech and language therapy: Theory and practice of measuring their representation. *International Journal of Bilingualism* 5(4), 465–95.

Wode, H. (1980) Phonology in L2 acquisition. In S. Felix (ed.) *Second Language Development: Trends and Issues*. Tubingen: Gunter Narr.

Wong, W.W.-Y. and Stokes, S.F. (2001) Cantonese consonantal development: A nonlinear account. *Journal of Child Language* 28(1), 191–212.

Woodyatt, G. and Dodd, B. (1995) A treatment case study of speech disorder: A child with multiple underlying deficits. In B. Dodd (ed.) *Differential Diagnosis and Treatment of Children with Speech Disorder*. London: Whurr.

Wu, C. and Yin, B. (1984) Putonghua shehui diaocha. (A survey of Putonghua). *Wenzi Gaige* 11, 37–38.

Xu, Fang and Ha, Ping-An (1992) Articulation disorders among speakers of Mandarin Chinese. *AJSLP* 1(4), 15–16.

Yasuda, A. (1970) Articulatory skills in three-year-old children. *Studia Phonologica* 5, 52–71.

Yavaş, M. (1996) Differences in voice onset time in early and later Spanish-English bilinguals. In J. Jensen and A. Roca (eds) *Spanish in Contact: Issues in Bilingualism*. Somerville, MA: Casadilla Press.

Yavaş, M. (1998) *Phonology Development and Disorder*. San Diego, London: Singular Publishing Group, Inc.

Yavaş, M. (2002) Voice onset time patterns in bilingual phonological development. In F. Windsor, M.L. Kelly and N. Hewlett (eds) *Investigations in Clinical Phonetics and Linguistics* (pp. 341–51). London: Lawrence Erlbaum Associates.

Yavaş, M. (2003) Role of sonority in developing phonologies. *Journal of Multilingual Communication Disorders* 1(2), 79–98.

Yavaş, M. and Topbaş, S. (2004) Liquid development in Turkish: Salience vs. frequency. *Journal of Multilingual Communication Disorders* 2, 110–23.

Yavaş, M. and Gogate, L.J. (1999) Phoneme awareness in children: A function of sonority. *Journal of Psycholinguistic Research* 28(3), 245–60.

Yavaş, M. and Goldstein, B. (1998) Speech sound differences and disorders in first and second language acquisition: Theoretical issues and clinical applications. *American Journal of Speech and Language Pathology* 7, 43–54.

Yavaş, M. and Lamprecht, R. (1988) Processes and intelligibility in disordered phonology. *Clinical Linguistics and Phonetics* 2, 329–45.

Yeni-Komshian, G.H., Caramazza, A. and Preston, M.S. (1977) A study of voicing in Lebanese Arabic. *Journal of Phonetics* 5, 35–48.

Zhu Hua (2000) Phonological development and disorder of Putonghua (Modern Standard Chinese)-speaking children. PhD thesis, University of Newcastle upon Tyne, UK.

Zhu Hua (2002) *Phonological Development in Specific Contexts: Studies of Chinese-speaking Children*. Clevedon: Multilingual Matters.

Zhu Hua and Dodd, B. (2000a) The phonological acquisition of Putonghua (Modern Standard Chinese). *Journal of Child Language* 27(1), 3–42.

Zhu Hua and Dodd, B. (2000b) Putonghua (Modern Standard Chinese)-speaking children with speech disorder. *Clinical Linguistics and Phonetics* 14(3), 165–91.

Zlatin, M. and Koenigsknecht, R. (1976) Development of the voicing contrast: A comparison of voice onset time values in stop perception and production. *Journal of Speech and Hearing Research* 19, 92–111.

Appendix

Websites for speech and language therapists' professional organisations in each country
The following list is adapted from RCSLT website.

Australia: Speech Pathology Australia
http://www.speechpathologyaustralia.org.au/

Canada: CASLPA
http://www.caslpa.ca/

China: The Amity Foundation
http://www.amityfoundation.org/
Website for a centre for hearing impaired children in China sponsored by a Christian organisation.

Czech Republic: Logopedické Centrum
http://home.tiscali.cz:8080/~cz417522/

Finland: Suomen logopedis-foniatrinen yhdistys
http://users.utu.fi/jyrtuoma/pkty/

France: ORL France
http://www.orl-france.org/francenet.htm

Germany: Deutscher Bundesverband für Logopädie e.V
http://www.dbl-ev.de/

Greece: Panhellenic Association of Logopedists
http://www.logopedists.gr/

Hong Kong: Association of Speech Therapists
http://www.speechtherapy.org.hk/
India: All India Institute of Speech and Hearing
http://www.mylibnet.org/aiish.html

Ireland: Irish Association of SLTs
http://www.iaslt.com/

Italy: Federazione Logopedisti Italiani
http://space.tin.it/salute/ddainott/

Korea: Korean Academy of Speech-Language Pathology
http://www.kasla.or.kr/

Malaysia: Association of Speech-Language & Hearing
http://www.geocities.com/mash1995/index.html

New Zealand: NZSTA
http://www.nzsta-speech.org.nz/

Palestine: Avenir Childhood Foundation
http://www.palnet.com/ ~ pacf/

Singapore: Speech-Language & Hearing Association
http://web.singnet.com.sg/ ~ speech/

South Africa: SASLHA
http://www.saslha.org.za/

Spain: AELFA
http://www.aelfa.org/

Sweden: SLOF
http://www.dik.se/

Taiwan: Speech-Language-Hearing Association
http://www.slh.org.tw/

UK: Royal College of Speech and Language Therapists
http://www.rcslt.org/

UK: The Association of Speech and Language Therapists in Independent Practice
http://www.asltip.co.uk/main.asp
The Association has two main functions: to provide information on independent speech and language therapists throughout the United Kingdom and to support therapists in independent practice.

UK: Bilingualism Database
http://www.edu.bham.ac.uk/bilingualism/database/ctlefl.htm
A vast resource on links surrounding bilingualism. Based in the University of Birmingham's School of Education.

USA: American Speech-Language-Hearing Association
http://www.asha.org

USA: American Speech-Language-Hearing Foundation
http://www.ashfoundation.org/

International Organisation

Communication Therapy International
http://www.ctint.co.uk/
CTI is an association set up to encourage the promotion of communication therapy in developing countries.

International: International Association of Logopedics and Phoniatrics
http://www.ialp.info/
The IALP (International Association of Logopedics and Phoniatrics) is a global organisation promoting the improvement of care for people with communication disorders.

International: Speech Communication Association
http://www.isca-speech.org/
Regularly-updated website with information on specific interest groups, publications, conferences, grants available and worldwide SLT recruitment.

Europe: CPLOL
http://www.cplol.org
Website for the European SLT association including 19 member countries and 21 professional/scientific organisations of SLTs.

Information on Asian countries:
http://members.tripod.com/Caroline_Bowen/Asia.htm
A list of contacts for those countries where speech and language therapy is under-developed.

Index

25 word consistency test, 21, 69
Affricates, 5, 57, 92, 95, 104, 110, 118, 123-4, 131, 137,139, 144, 163-9, 172, 175, 177, 180, 182, 185-7, 251-2, 255, 260,267, 275-6, 305, 313, 330, 333, 347, 351, 361
Affrication,32, 54, 93-8, 101-3, 119, 122-4, 129, 130, 175, 238, 255-6, 258, 293, 303-5, 323-5, 340, 422-3, 439-40, 442
Ambient language, 12, 31, 66, 78, 124, 193, 309, 310
Apical, 137, 139, 347, 394
Approximants, 53, 58, 83, 111, 138-9, 159-64, 77, 236, 261, 268, 347-8, 359-63, 377,402-3, 431, 444-5
Articulation disorder, 77, 79, 98, 114, 125, 133-4, 243, 447
Aspiration, 11, 93-6,101-2, 113, 122-4, 128-9, 137, 155, 180, 268, 272, 289, 293, 302, 306, 309, 323, 325, 331, 347, 348, 351, 393, 415, 419-20, 422-6, 433, 435, 438-40, 443, 447
Assimilation, 32, 33, 54, 63-4, 67, 93-4, 98, 100, 102, 104-5, 113, 119, 121-5, 129-30, 137, 141-4, 185, 210, 226, 229-30, 238-9, 253-4, 256, 258, 271, 286, 323, 338-9, 342, 382, 390, 402-3, 438, 440-2
Auditory, 140, 193, 202, 234, 247, 289, 397
Avoidance, 19, 168

Backing, 11, 32, 63-7, 70, 74-5, 93-6, 100-104, 122-23, 129, 131-2, 228, 238-40, 255-6, 258, 293-4, 304, 307, 313-4, 321, 323, 325, 331, 339, 419-26, 439, 442, 447
Biological model, 6, 435

Chronology of error patterns, 93 94, 178, 256, 260, 372
Cluster Simplification/reduction, 32, 36, 40, 41, 44, 54, 63-4, 67, 73-4, 113, 119, 121, 125, 129-31, 133, 162, 166, 169-71, 174, 210, 212, 214, 221-6, 230, 232, 238-9, 253, 256, 258, 260, 271-2, 283, 286, 293, 302, 304, 306, 311, 313-5, 317-25, 331, 343-4, 352, 368-70, 373, 381-2 390, 419-20, 438, 440, 442, 444-5
Code-switching, 136, 385, 388-89, 404-6, 410
Consistency, definition of, 20
  See also inconsistency
Consonant cluster
– acquisition, 62, 211
– description, 83, 184-6, 277, 445
– error pattern, 170
  See also cluster reduction
Consonant assimilation/harmony, 94, 98, 100, 102, 104, 162, 170, 293, 313, 352, 369, 373
Cross-linguistic effect/intralingual effect, 12, 311
Cross-linguistic similarity and difference, 5, 8, 65, 96, 161, 310-1
Customary production, age of, 17, 31, 158, 209, 214, 221, 23001

Deaffrication, 32-3, 40, 44, 54, 63, 122-3, 129, 240, 255-6, 258, 293, 303-4, 313, 323, 325, 339, 419-20, 422-3, 426, 439-40, 442
Deaspiration, 94-5, 101-2, 119, 122-4, 128-31, 293, 302, 323, 325, 419-20, 422, 423, 439-40, 442
De-emphasisation, 210, 214, 221-5, 228, 439
Depalatalisastion,23
Developmental verbal dyspraxia, 50, 51
Devoicing, 33, 54, 63-4, 67, 149, 163, 173, 210, 212, 214, 221-5, 227, 229-30, 239-40, 255-8, 266, 272, 304, 311, 347, 360, 382
Diphthong, 84, 94-5, 101, 103, 140, 142, 183, 188, 196, 236, 348-9, 351, 432, 441

Diphthong reduction, 94-5, 101, 103, 441
Distinctive features, 27, 93, 141, 180

Emergence, 26, 31, 87, 89, 92-3, 125, 242, 245-6, 248-9, 251, 302, 309, 417, 419, 421-2
Emphatic, 391-3, 408, 439
Epenthesis, 42, 143, 211, 226
Error patterns, definition & classification of, 20, 128, 243, 444

Favourite sound/articulation, 223, 229-30, 229, 368-9, 373
Feature, 164, 166, 168, 180, 196, 367, 389, 415, 425, 433-4, 439
Feature hierarchy, 5, 114
Final consonant deletion, 32, 36, 54, 63, 67, 122-3, 129-30, 162, 170, 210, 212, 214, 221-27, 230, 268, 271-2, 289, 293, 304, 313, 323, 331, 344, 368-9, 373, 381-2, 419-23, 426, 438, 440, 447
Flaps, 185, 278, 330
Fricatives, 5, 27, 44, 54, 65, 70, 75-6, 95, 104, 110, 113, 118, 123-4, 131, 139, 144, 1660-1, 164-5, 167-9, 172, 175, 180, 182-3, 185-7, 190, 211, 227-30, 235, 238-40, 251-2, 255, 257-60, 267-8, 270-1, 276, 278, 281, 283, 294, 300, 302
Fronting, 32-3, 36, 40-1, 44, 54, 63-4. 67. 73-4. 93-5, 98, 100, 102, 104, 113, 119, 122-4, 129-31, 149, 157, 163, 172, 210, 212, 214, 221-5, 228, 230, 238-9, 247, 249, 255-6, 258, 271, 286, 293-4, 302, 304, 307, 313, 323-5, 339, 341-2, 352, 360-1, 369, 373, 381-2, 419-23, 439-40, 42
Functional load, 4, 6-7, 19, 124-5, 134, 363, 391

Generative phonology, 66
Germination, 196, 434, 441
Gliding, 32-3, 40-1, 44, 54, 93-5, 98, 101-2, 104, 122-3, 129, 131, 149, 163. 172, 230, 239, 257-60, 272, 283, 293, 303-4, 306, 313, 315-18, 323-4, 331, 338-9, 344, 352, 361, 369, 373, 382, 390, 402, 419-20, 426, 439-42, 447
Glottal replacement, 63-5, 210, 228, 239, 361, 441

Hearing impairment, 7-8, 15, 18, 59, 96, 115-16, 193-4, 234, 287

Imitation, 19-20, 22, 29, 36, 41-2, 44, 69, 154, 214, 246, 288-9, 307, 357
Implicational feature hierarchy, 114-5, 165, 167, 187, 230, 280
Incidence, 47, 51, 136, 434
Inconsistency, 20-1, 47, 50, 64, 70-1, 73-4, 76-7, 80, 97-9, 132, 134, 366
Individual differences, 6, 30, 114, 232, 383, 391, 393
See also Variables
Initial consonant deletion, 11, 93, 96, 122-3, 129, 162, 171, 239-40, 272, 293, 303-4, 309, 311, 325, 331, 343-4, 419-20, 426, 439-40, 442, 447
Input, 408-11
Intelligibility, 45, 50, 197, 240, 272, 283, 306, 308
Interdentality, 63-5, 72-4, 77, 79, 441
Intonation, 149, 205, 350
Inventory, 126, 210, 223, 248

Jakobson, Roman, 4-5, 27, 65, 230

Labialisation, 139
Language interaction, 8, 11-2, 283, 292, 311, 363, 385, 404, 438, 444-5
Language interference, 11, 265-6, 311, 314, 321, 385, 390 395, 409-11, 413-4, 424-6, 434, 438
Language-specific, 5-7, 10-11, 65, 105-8, 124-5, 164, 238, 260, 306-7, 309-10, 355, 359, 368-70, 376, 434, 438-48
Lateralisation, 149, 163, 172, 257-60, 402, 441, 445
Law of irreversible solidarity, 435
Liquid gliding, 33, 44, 283, 361, 382, 439-40, 442, 447
Literacy, 46, 193, 328, 366
Locke, John, 4, 6, 96, 124, 232, 327

Markedness, 4-5, 242, 311, 438
Mastery, age of, 17, 31
Minimal pairs, 124, 137, 157, 182, 196-7, 199, 102, 235-7, 317, 350
Morphophonemic development, 166
Mutation, 19, 348-52, 356, 370, 379

Natural phonology, 14, 31, 66
Nonlinear, 66, 158

One or two systems, 9-10
Oral reading, 198-201
Orthography, 149-189, 191-3, 351

Palatalisation, 321
Perception, 7, 11, 32, 183, 186-7, 196, 394
Phoneme emergence, 16, 31, 242, 245, 248
Phoneme stabilisation, 16, 31, 248
Phonemic acquisition, 5, 7, 17, 20, 28, 31, 60-1, 64-6, 96, 113, 124, 166, 214, 238, 244, 286, 298, 344, 364, 417, 422
Phonemic awareness, 188, 203
Phonetic acquisition, 20, 31, 41-44, 61, 92, 107, 290, 299-301, 434-7
Phonetic disorders, definition of, 243
Phonological awareness, 45-6, 55, 191-2, 202
Phonological disorders, definition of, 233, 243
Phonological processes, definition of, see Error patterns
Phonological saliency, 7-8, 106-8, 434
Phonotactics, 143, 166, 169-70, 174-5, 349, 386, 433
Pitch, 7, 84, 110, 149, 205, 232, 237, 240, 350
Prosody, 110, 149, 195, 240, 350

Reduplication, 32, 54, 162, 170-1, 238, 253, 256, 293, 323, 338-9, 341, 344, 440-3
Regression, 17-8, 162, 166, 168, 170, 249, 292, 294
Relational analysis, 214
Religion and language, 329
Repertoire, definition of, see Inventory
Retroflex, 93, 95-6, 104, 181, 183, 185-6, 268, 333, 338, 340, 404, 419, 422, 425

Sequential bilingual, see Successive
Severity, 47, 49, 51, 68, 76, 126, 224, 227, 241
Shriberg, Lawrence, 46, 68, 155, 193, 195, 224, 240, 248
Sibilant deviation, 212, 214, 221-7, 230
Simultaneous bilingual, 9, 10, 272, 302, 374, 390
Socio-economic status, 38-9, 43, 48-51, 59, 213
Socio-phonetic features, 400, 435
Sonorant, 95, 165, 167, 187-8, 237, 267, 269, 349, 432
Sonority, 279, 280-2, 285, 434-4, 445
Sound preferences, see Favourite sound
Speech accuracy, 43-4, 260, 291-2, 294-5, 298, 302, 307-8, 445-8

Speech disorder
 – classification, 75, 78, 98, 125-6, 195, 234, 239, 243
 – underlying deficits, 46, 78, 356
Spelling, 57, 197-8, 201, 203, 403
Spontaneous speech, 300-1, 316, 138-9, 341, 416
Stabilisation, 16, 31, 88, 92-3, 160, 166, 248, 251-2
Stampe, David, 14, 31, 65-6
Stimulability, 35, 246
Stopping, 32-3, 36, 40-1, 44, 54, 63-4, 67, 70, 75, 93-5, 98, 100, 102, 104, 113, 119, 121, 123-4, 128-31, 156, 163, 172, 228-9, 238-9, 255-60, 271-2, 286, 293-4, 302-4, 307, 313, 323-5, 331, 339, 342, 344, 360, 381-2, 419-20, 244-3, 439-42
Stress, 20, 26, 124-5, 142-4, 149, 156, 184-5, 189, 205, 209, 237, 240, 270, 287, 350, 356, 379, 438
Stress-timed languages, 149
Substitution analysis, 212-4, 221
Successive bilingual, 9, 10, 11, 290, 309-11
Suprasegmental, see Prosody
Syllable position, 16, 19, 21-2, 132, 166, 348
Syllable shape/structure, 170, 184, 198, 205, 209, 211, 213, 224, 237-8, 278, 352, 355, 379, 386, 415, 438
Syllable-final consonant
 – age and order of acquisition, 118, 211, 417
 – error pattern, 32, 36, 54, 63, 67, 1034, 122-3, 129-30, 162, 170, 210, 212, 214, 221-7, 230, 239, 268, 271-2, 289, 293, 303-4, 313, 323, 331, 344, 368-9, 373, 381-2, 419-3, 426, 436, 440, 442, 447
Syllable-initial consonant
 – description, 53, 186, 188, 350-1, 370, 379
 – error pattern, 11, 93, 96, 105, 108, 119, 122-3, 129, 132, 162, 171, 188, 239-40, 272, 293, 302-4, 309, 311, 323, 325, 331, 343-4, 419-20, 426, 439-40, 447
Syllable-timed languages, 237, 270

Taps, 139, 403-4
Template, 186-7
Tone
 – description, 12, 84, 91, 106-7, 110, 113, 125, 149, 415

– age of acquisition, 86, 114-5, 119-20, 124, 417
– error patterns, 98, 113-4, 119-20, 133-4, 290, 293, 323, 325, 330
Tone sandhi, 86
Transcription reliability, 150, 156, 248
Trills, 139, 185, 348, 403
Triphthong reduction, 94-5, 101, 103

Underspecification, 311
Universals, 3, 5-6, 65-6, 113, 124, 125, 150, 154, 165, 168, 171, 176, 202, 230, 232, 241, 260, 266, 279-82, 320-1, 364, 366-7, 414
Uvular, 58, 206, 228-9, 330, 347, 360, 377, 392

Variability, 20-1, 51, 105, 153, 168-9, 239, 241, 243, 274, 359, 362-3, 365, 368, 376, 384, 385, 392-3, 397, 400, 410-1, 447
See also Inconsistency
Variables
– age, 22, 34-55, 249-50, 292
– gender, 18, 22, 27, 34-55, 98, 152, 249-50, 295, 382, 393
Variations, *see* Individual differences, Inconsistency,

Velar, 21, 32, 58, 67, 83, 93, 95, 104, 110-1, 119, 123, 131, 134, 137-9, 142, 164, 181, 206, 210, 212, 214, 221-5, 228, 230, 235, 251-2, 254-5, 261, 267, 270-1, 331, 347-8, 352, 360-3, 377, 381, 417, 419, 426, 431, 439, 441
Velarisation, 94-5, 98, 101-2, 239, 257, 258-60
Vihman, Marilyn, 3, 6-7, 30, 106, 155, 402
Vocalisation, 32, 156, 400, 402
Voice onset time (VOT), 389-99, 405-6, 409
Voiceless, 5, 57, 83, 137, 141, 144, 161, 165, 168, 175, 181, 183-6, 190, 206, 230, 232, 235-6, 240, 251, 266-72, 278, 300, 302, 347-8, 356, 360, 379, 389, 394-5, 398, 405, 415, 431
Voicing, 5, 11, 32, 40, 41, 44, 54, 63-4, 67, 113, 139, 141, 144, 182, 197, 196, 200-1, 210, 230, 247, 255-8, 272, 289, 302-5, 313, 323, 325, 331, 386, 394-9, 409

Weak stress, 20, 438
Weak syllable deletion, 20, 32, 36, 39, 44, 54, 63, 162, 170, 212, 271, 293, 323-4, 331, 382, 438